2006
YEAR BOOK OF
DERMATOLOGY
AND
DERMATOLOGIC
SURGERY™

The 2006 Year Book Series

Year Book of Allergy, Asthma, and Clinical Immunology™: Drs Rosenwasser, Boguniewicz, Milgrom, Routes, and Weber

Year Book of Anesthesiology and Pain Management™: Drs Chestnut, Abram, Black, Gravlee, Lee, Mathru, and Roizen

Year Book of Cardiology®: Drs Gersh, Cheitlin, Elliott, Graham, Sundt, and Waldo

Year Book of Critical Care Medicine®: Drs Dellinger, Parrillo, Balk, Bekes, Dorman, and Dries

Year Book of Dentistry®: Drs McIntyre, Belvedere, Buhite, Davis, Henderson, Johnson, Jureyda, Ohrbach, Olin, Scott, Spencer, and Zakariasen

Year Book of Dermatology and Dermatologic Surgery™: Drs Thiers and Lang

Year Book of Diagnostic Radiology®: Drs Osborn, Birdwell, Dalinka, Gardiner, Levy, Maynard, Oestreich, and Rosado de Christenson

Year Book of Emergency Medicine®: Drs Burdick, Hamilton, Handly, Quintana, and Werner

Year Book of Endocrinology®: Drs Mazzaferri, Bessesen, Clarke, Howard, Kennedy, Leahy, Meikle, Molitch, Rogol, and Schteingart

Year Book of Family Practice®: Drs Bowman, Apgar, Dexter, Miser, Neill, and Scherger

Year Book of Gastroenterology™: Drs Lichtenstein, Burke, Campbell, Dempsey, Drebin, Ginsberg, Katzka, Kochman, Morris, Rombeau, Shah, and Stein

Year Book of Hand Surgery and Upper Limb Surgery®: Drs Chang and Steinmann

Year Book of Medicine®: Drs Barkin, Frishman, Garrick, Loehrer, Phillips, Pillinger, and Snydman

Year Book of Neonatal and Perinatal Medicine®: Drs Fanaroff, Maisels, and Stevenson

Year Book of Neurology and Neurosurgery®: Drs Gibbs and Verma

Year Book of Nuclear Medicine®: Drs Coleman, Blaufox, Royal, Strauss, and Zubal

Year Book of Obstetrics, Gynecology, and Women's Health®: Dr Shulman

Year Book of Oncology®: Drs Loehrer, Arceci, Glatstein, Gordon, Hanna, Morrow, and Thigpen

Year Book of Ophthalmology®: Drs Rapuano, Cohen, Eagle, Flanders, Hammersmith, Myers, Nelson, Penne, Sergott, Shields, Tipperman, and Vander

Year Book of Orthopedics®: Drs Morrey, Beauchamp, Peterson, Swiontkowski, Trigg, and Yaszemski

Year Book of Otolaryngology-Head and Neck Surgery®: Drs Paparella, Gapany, and Keefe

2006

The Year Book of DERMATOLOGY AND DERMATOLOGIC SURGERY™

Editor-in-Chief
Bruce H. Thiers, MD
Professor and Chair, Department of Dermatology, Medical University of South Carolina, Charleston, South Carolina

Associate Editor
Pearon G. Lang, Jr, MD
Professor of Dermatology, Pathology, Otolaryngology, and Communicative Sciences, Medical University of South Carolina, Charleston, South Carolina

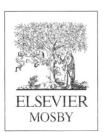

ELSEVIER
MOSBY

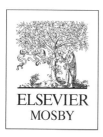

Vice President, Continuity: John A. Schrefer
Senior Manager, Continuity Production: Idelle L. Winer
Developmental Editor: Ali Gavenda
Senior Issue Manager: Pat Costigan
Illustrations and Permissions Coordinator: Linda S. Jones

2006 EDITION

Printed in the United States of America
Composition by Thomas Technology Solutions, Inc.
Printing/binding by Sheridan Books, Inc.

Editorial Office:
Elsevier
Suite 1800
1600 John F. Kennedy Blvd
Philadelphia, PA 19103-2899

International Standard Serial Number: 0093-3619
International Standard Book Number: 1-4160-3294-0
                                     978-1-4160-3294-6

Contributors

Margaret M. Boyle, BS
Research Associate, Dermatoepidemiology Unit, Brown University, Providence, Rhode Island

Joel Cook, MD
Associate Professor of Dermatology and Otolaryngology, Medical University of South Carolina, Charleston, South Carolina

Gillian M. P. Galbraith, MD
Professor of Biomedical Science, University of Las Vegas School of Dental Medicine, Las Vegas, Nevada

David Green, MD
Clinical Assistant Professor of Dermatology, Howard University Hospital, Washington, DC

John C. Maize, Sr, MD
Clinical Professor and Chairman Emeritus, Department of Dermatology, Medical University of South Carolina, Charleston, South Carolina

Sharon Raimer, MD
Professor of Dermatology and Pediatrics; Chair, Department of Dermatology, University of Texas Medical Branch, Galveston, Texas

Martin A. Weinstock, MD, PhD
Professor of Dermatology and Community Health, Brown University; Chief of Dermatology, VA Medical Center; Director, Pigmented Lesion Unit and Photomedicine, Rhode Island Hospital, Providence, Rhode Island

Table of Contents

Journals Represented

Journals represented in this YEAR BOOK are listed below.

Acta Dermato-Venereologica
Acta Paediatrica
Allergy
American Journal of Clinical Pathology
American Journal of Dermatopathology
American Journal of Epidemiology
American Journal of Medicine
American Journal of Psychiatry
American Journal of Surgical Pathology
American Surgeon
Annals of Allergy, Asthma, & Immunology
Annals of Internal Medicine
Annals of Rheumatic Diseases
Annals of Surgery
Annals of Surgical Oncology
Annals of Thoracic Surgery
Archives of Dermatology
Archives of Disease in Childhood
Archives of Physical Medicine and Rehabilitation
Archives of Surgery
Arthritis and Rheumatism
British Journal of Cancer
British Journal of Dermatology
British Journal of Plastic Surgery
British Medical Journal
Burns
Cancer
Cancer Epidemiology, Biomarkers and Prevention
Carcinogenesis
Chest
Circulation
Clinical Cancer Research
Clinical Infectious Diseases
Dermatologic Surgery
Dermatology
Diseases of the Colon and Rectum
European Journal of Cancer
European Journal of Plastic Surgery
Experimental Dermatology
Fertility and Sterility
Human Pathology
International Journal of Cancer
International Journal of Radiation, Oncology, Biology, and Physics
Journal of Clinical Investigation
Journal of Clinical Microbiology
Journal of Clinical Rheumatology
Journal of Cutaneous Pathology
Journal of Experimental Medicine
Journal of Immunology

Journal of Investigative Dermatology
Journal of Pediatric Surgery
Journal of Pharmacology and Experimental Therapeutics
Journal of Rheumatology
Journal of Ultrasound in Medicine
Journal of Vascular Surgery
Journal of the American Academy of Dermatology
Journal of the American College of Surgeons
Journal of the American Medical Association
Journal of the European Academy of Dermatology and Venereology
Journal of the National Cancer Institute
Lancet
Nature
Nephrology, Dialysis, Transplantation
Neurology
New England Journal of Medicine
Pediatric Dermatology
Pediatric Research
Plastic and Reconstructive Surgery
Proceedings of the National Academy of Sciences
Science
Thorax
Urology
World Journal of Surgery

STANDARD ABBREVIATIONS

The following terms are abbreviated in this edition: acquired immunodeficiency syndrome (AIDS), cardiopulmonary resuscitation (CPR), central nervous system (CNS), cerebrospinal fluid (CSF), computed tomography (CT), deoxyribonucleic acid (DNA), electrocardiography (ECG), health maintenance organization (HMO), human immunodeficiency virus (HIV), intensive care unit (ICU), intramuscular (IM), intravenous (IV), magnetic resonance (MR) imaging (MRI), ribonucleic acid (RNA), ultrasound (US), and ultraviolet (UV).

NOTE

The YEAR BOOK OF DERMATOLOGY AND DERMATOLOGIC SURGERY™ is a literature survey service providing abstracts of articles published in the professional literature. Every effort is made to assure the accuracy of the information presented in these pages. Neither the editors nor the publisher of the YEAR BOOK OF DERMATOLOGY AND DERMATOLOGIC SURGERY™ can be responsible for errors in the original materials. The editors' comments are their own opinions. Mention of specific products within this publication does not constitute endorsement.

To facilitate the use of the YEAR BOOK OF DERMATOLOGY AND DERMATOLOGIC SURGERY™ as a reference tool, all illustrations and tables included in this publication are now identified as they appear in the original article. This change is meant to help the reader recognize that any illustration or table appearing in the YEAR BOOK OF DERMATOLOGY AND DERMATOLOGIC SURGERY™ may be only one of many in the original article. For this reason, figure and table numbers will often appear to be out of sequence within the YEAR BOOK OF DERMATOLOGY AND DERMATOLOGIC SURGERY™.

COLOR PLATE I

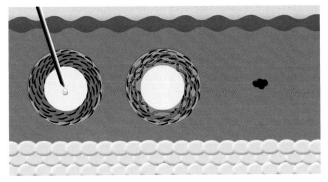

Green Fig 1

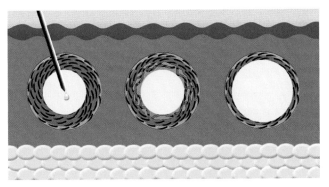

Green Fig 2

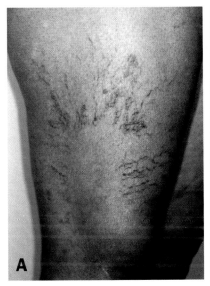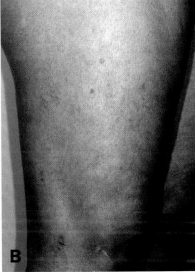

Green Fig 3, A-B

COLOR PLATE II

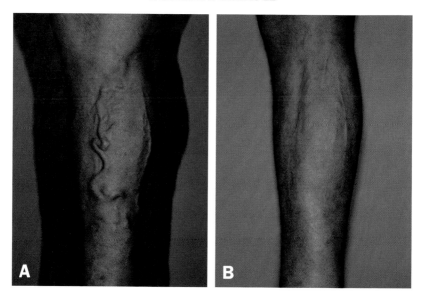

Green Fig 4, A-B

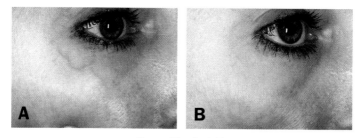

Green Fig 5, A-B

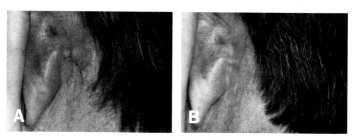

Green Fig 6, A-B

COLOR PLATE III

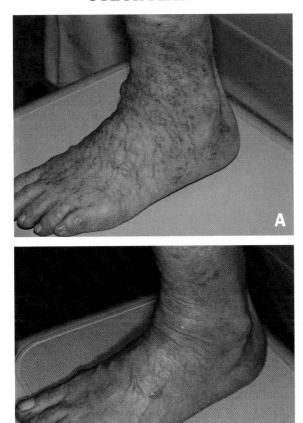

Green Fig 7, A-B

COLOR PLATE IV

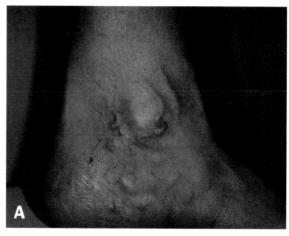

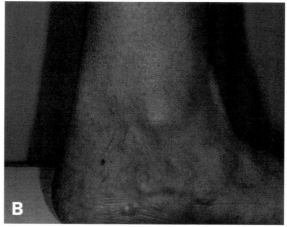

Green Fig 8, A-B

COLOR PLATE V

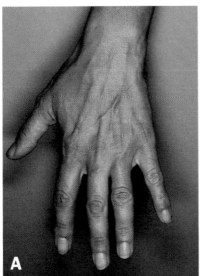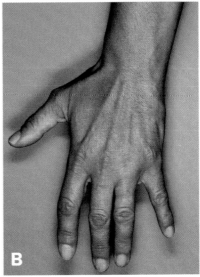

Green Fig 9, A-B

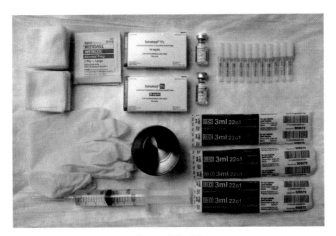

Green Fig 10

COLOR PLATE VI

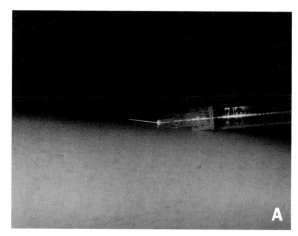

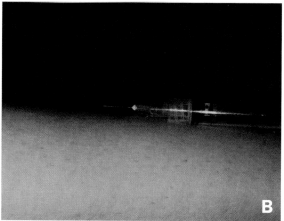

Green Fig 11, A-B

COLOR PLATE VII

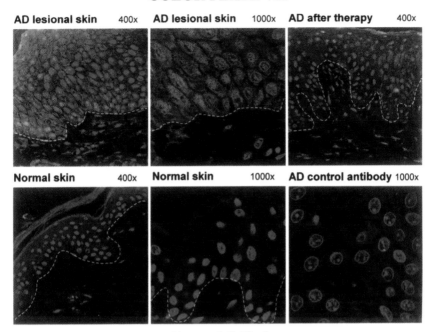

Abstract 1-8 Fig 1

COLOR PLATE VIII

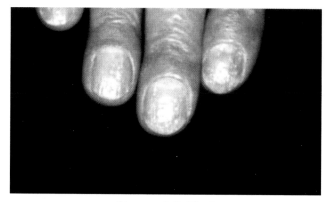

Abstract 2-9 Fig 8

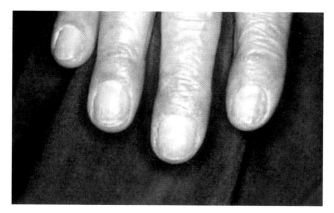

Abstract 2-9 Fig 9

COLOR PLATE IX

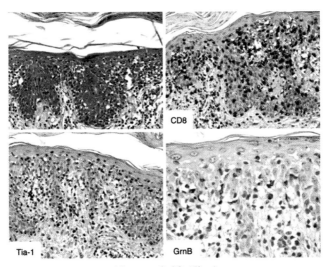

Abstract 2-28 Fig 1

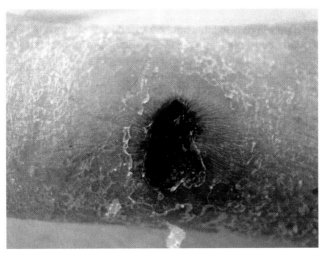

Abstract 3-26 Fig 3

COLOR PLATE X

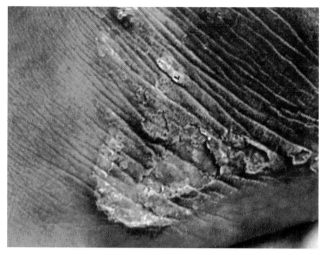

Abstract 4-13 Fig 1, B

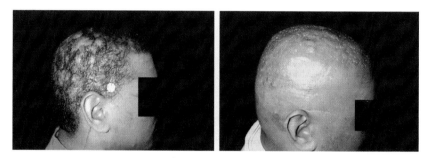

Abstract 7-20 Fig 1

COLOR PLATE XI

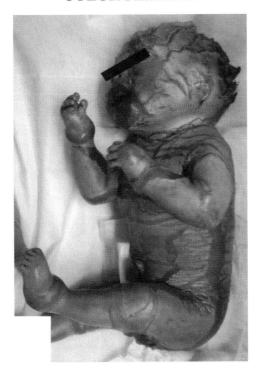

Abstract 11-1 Fig 1, A

COLOR PLATE XII

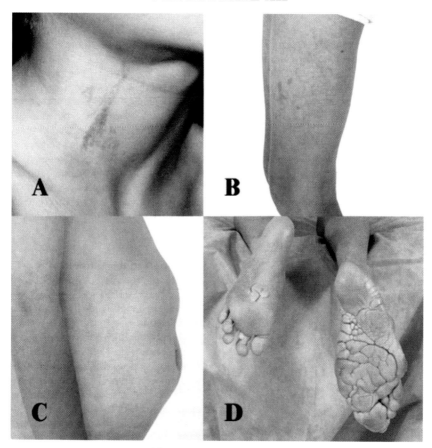

Abstract 11-3 Fig 1, A-D

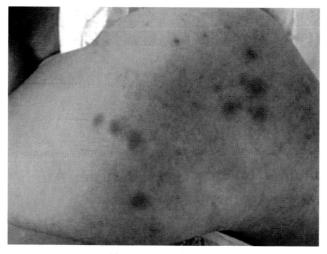

Abstract 15-16 Fig 1

COLOR PLATE XIII

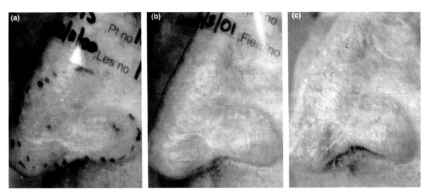

Abstract 16-24 Fig 4

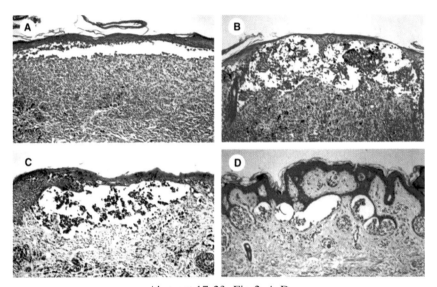

Abstract 17-23 Fig 2, A-D

COLOR PLATE XIV

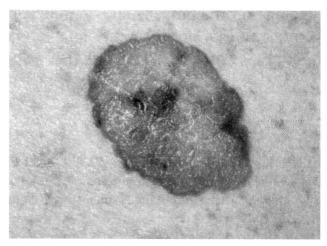

Abstract 17-28 Fig 1

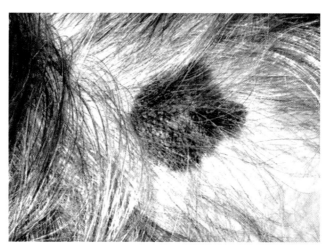

Abstract 17-28 Fig 2

COLOR PLATE XV

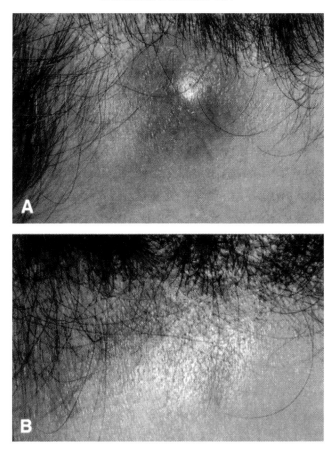

Abstract 18-10 Fig 1, A-B

COLOR PLATE XVI

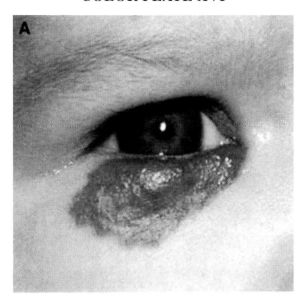

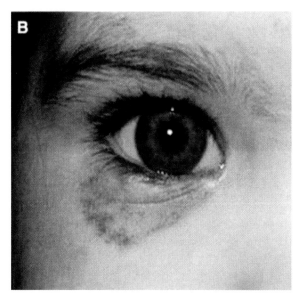

Abstract 19-15 Fig 1, A-B

Sclerotherapy: A Clinical Primer

DAVID GREEN, MD
Clinical Assistant Professor of Dermatology, Howard University Hospital, Washington, DC

Introduction

Introduced more than 150 years ago as a serendipitous concomitant of the development of the hypodermic needle, sclerotherapy remains the most effective procedure for the permanent eradication of pathologically enlarged as well as cosmetically undesirable but otherwise normal veins. Innovative devices have been introduced within the past 10 years that utilize electromagnetic energy sources to target vein wall constituents directly or indirectly and either transcutaneously or intravascularly, but these procedures are significantly less effective and reproducible than sclerotherapy for permanently eradicating unwanted veins.

This primer attempts to concisely review all pertinent aspects of sclerotherapy about which every physician should understand. It is even incumbent on those physicians who do not perform sclerotherapy to understand this procedure and its indications so as to be able to correctly and authoritatively advise patients who will invariably consult them about unwanted veins.

Venous System Anatomy of the Lower Extremity

The veins of the lower extremity are categorized into 2 axially directed systems based on their anatomic location relative to the deep fascia. These are the deep and superficial venous systems. The deep venous system comprises veins that course within and between the muscles of the limb, lying with the deep fascia. The deep venous system is the primary course through which most of the blood from the lower extremity is transported proximally. The superficial venous system consists of veins that course, primarily, within the cutaneous and subcutaneous tissue, outside of the deep fascia. Any visible vein of the lower extremity—whether a normal appearing and hemodynamically competent vein or an abnormally dilated and hemodynamically incompetent vein—no matter what its size, is a constituent of the superficial venous system. The 2 systems are directly connected at junctions where veins of the superficial venous system empty into those of the deep venous system. In addition, there is a third category of veins that are transversely directed and known as perforating or communicating veins. These veins are usually only several centimeters in length.

Venous System Hemodynamics and Implications of Vein Removal

The venous system has several functions, but it primarily serves as a conduit to passively return deoxygenated blood to the right side of the heart from where it is actively pumped to the lungs for oxygenation. This is accomplished through 1-way valves that are present in most veins larger than 1 mm in diameter. In axially directed veins of the superficial and deep venous systems of the extremities, these valves direct blood centripetally—toward the heart. In transversely directed veins (ie, perforating veins), these valves direct blood from the superficial to the deep venous system. When venous valves fail to function properly, they are unable to promote the 1-way flow of blood and are considered incompetent. Blood is then able to travel centrifugally— away from the heart—in axially directed veins and from the deep into the superficial veins through perforating veins. This explains why an erect posture causes an incompetent vein of the lower extremity to distend while leg elevation (above the level of the heart) empties the blood within the vein. Such veins become inefficient or ineffective channels for transporting blood to the heart.

Varicose and telangiectatic veins are not only anatomically enlarged but functionally (ie, hemodynamically) incompetent. Once a vein is rendered hemodynamically incompetent, it is no longer relied on to transport blood back to the heart and lungs. The removal of hemodynamically incompetent veins does not adversely affect venous return and is not associated with the development of new veins, competent or otherwise. By the time varicose and telangiectatic veins have appeared, competent pre-existing veins, which provide overlapping venous drainage, have compensated for their functional absence. This is an empirical fact: The presence of uncomplicated varicose or telangiectatic veins—that is, in the absence of incompetent venous junctions or incompetent perforating veins—are rarely ever associated with any adverse circulatory or cutaneous changes. It is the presence of incompetent veins, not their removal, that stimulates the detouring of blood flow through adjacent competent veins. The vascular system has no functional need, before or after varicose veins are removed, to produce new veins at that site. However, this does not imply that new varicose or telangiectatic veins will not develop. New varicosities are likely to appear at sites of pre-existing varicose veins if predisposing factors persist, such as the presence of incompetent perforating veins.

Often those who inquire about vein removal concomitantly express concern about the safety of removing their unwanted veins, believing that vein removal will adversely affect their circulation. However, they can be assured that they will suffer no adverse circulatory consequence from the successful removal of a varicose or telangiectatic vein.

Mechanism of Action of Sclerotherapy

Sclerotherapy is the procedure in which chemical energy is used to eradicate a vein. The chemical energy is delivered intravascularly in the form of a solution that is capable of denaturing those biologic molecules that comprise the vein wall. For permanent eradication of the vein, it is necessary to produce full mural denaturation, or at least enough mural injury requisite to preclude mural reconstitution. If this is attained, the mural layers will be resorbed, and the lumen that it surrounded will be obliterated (Fig 1; see color plate I). The vein will permanently disappear. The persistence of a vein after treatment is evidence that full mural denaturation was not achieved (Fig 2; see color plate I). This can usually be attributed to treatment technique and not because of any inherent limitation of sclerotherapy. Once a vein has been completely resorbed, there should not be any discernible remnant, clinically—either by visualization or palpation—or

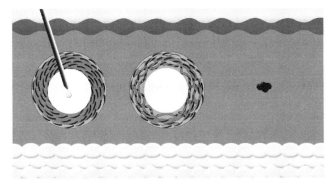

FIGURE 1.—Complete mural denaturation with resorption of mural layers and lumen obliteration.

ultrasonographically. For any given segment of a vein, a single treatment should result in full mural denaturation and its eventual disappearance.

As alluded to above, sclerotherapy targets the mural constitutents and not the blood in the vein lumen. Decades ago, however, physicians believed blood was their target and, as such, their goal was intraluminal thrombosis. For that reason, patients were often treated while standing to promote gravitational venous pooling. Under such a condition, the infused sclerosant would enter a vein distended with blood, ensuring maximal thrombosis. Unfortunately and much to their chagrin, these sclerotherapists eventually realized that many such treated varicose veins usually persisted or reappeared months to years later, when the thrombus was resorbed and the vein wall reconstituted.[1]

Although unnecessary and undesirable, thrombosis almost always develops within the lumen of every treated vein. This is because, once infusion of the sclerosant is terminated, some blood returns into the lumen, which at that time is still intact even though full mural denaturation may have been attained. The presence of subendothelial collagen and other coagulation cascade initiators causes the blood to coagulate (ie, thrombose). Thrombosis does not affect the extent of mural denaturation and does not usually affect

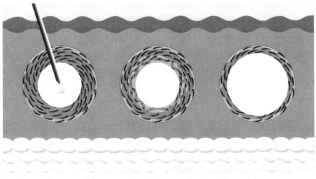

FIGURE 2.—Incomplete mural denaturation with reconstitution of mural layers and lumen persistence.

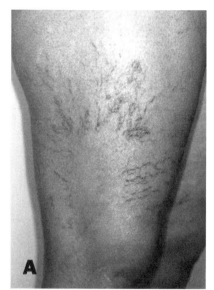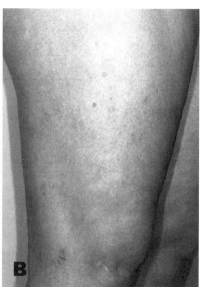

FIGURE 3.—Right thigh: **a**, Before; **b**, after.

the ultimate outcome of treatment. However, it prolongs the course of vein resorption and thus the duration for its eventual disappearance.

Indications and Contraindications for Sclerotherapy

Veins of any size, from small venous telangiectases (Fig 3; see color plate I) to large varicose veins (Fig 4; see color plate II), and at any site, from the face (Fig 5; see color plate II) and scalp (Fig 6; see color plate II) to the foot (Fig 7; see color plate III) and ankle (Fig 8; see color plate IV), can be permanently eradicated by sclerotherapy. However, this does not mean that every patient or varicose vein is a candidate for treatment. If there are incompetent venous junctions or incompetent perforating veins communicating with the varicose vein, interruption of these points of reflux (eg, surgical ligation) and division should be considered before sclerotherapy. That's because sclerotherapy is effective in eradicating a segment of an axial vein, but unlike ligation and division, it cannot reliably target a finite point (eg, saphenofemoral or saphenopopliteal junction, or a short segment of a perforating vein) without also infusing sclerosant into the deep venous system.

Sclerotherapy is usually directed at nonfunctional, pathologically enlarged veins, but it can effectively remove functionally normal although cosmetically undesirable veins. The most commonly requested sites for the latter are the dorsum of the hand (Fig 9; see color plate V) and the dorsum of the foot.

There are few contraindications to sclerotherapy. Anyone who previously experienced an allergic reaction to a sclerosant should not be treated with that agent. Women who are pregnant or lactating are not treated, although

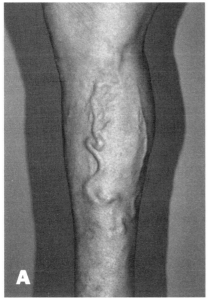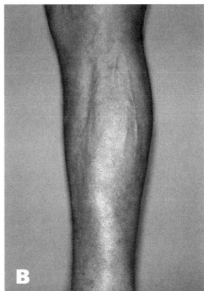

FIGURE 4.—Right leg: **a**, Before; **b**, after.

thousands of pregnant women have been treated in the past with sodium tetradecyl sulfate without any adverse effect.[2] There are no specific medical diseases that, when present, would contraindicate sclerotherapy. However, treatment is individualized and a patient's medical condition should always be considered as to the propriety of this treatment. Those with a history of deep vein thrombophlebitis, as well as those with collagen vascular, endocrinologic, hematologic, infectious (including human immunodeficiency disease), inflammatory, and neoplastic disorders, have been safely treated without adverse effect. Many of these patients are treated not simply for cosmetic appearance but to remove very superficial veins that have spontaneously eroded and bled through an atrophic overlying epidermis and dermis or in which such erosions seem imminent. This circumstance is primarily encountered on the feet, ankles, and distal legs. This same phenomenon of spontaneous erosion and bleeding through the overlying skin has been observed with angiokeratomas, although these are not treated by sclerotherapy. Pa-

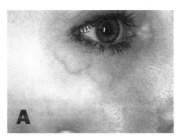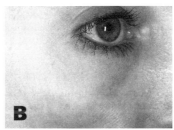

FIGURE 5.—Right lower eyelid: **a**, Before; **b**, after.

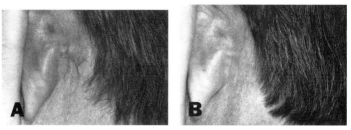

FIGURE 6.—Left posterior auricule and scalp: **a,** Before; **b,** after.

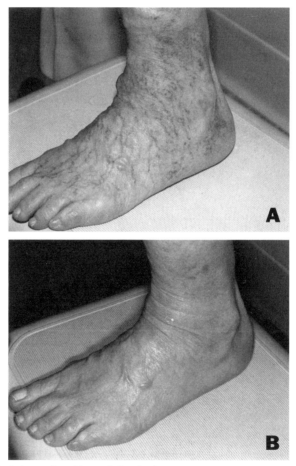

FIGURE 7.—Left anterolateral foot: **a,** Before; **b,** after.

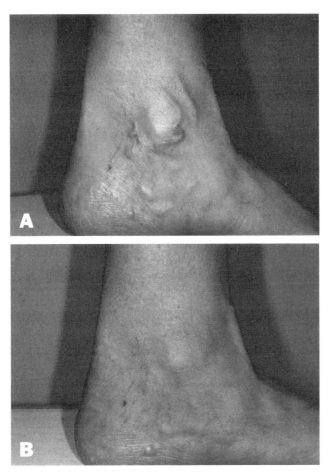

FIGURE 8.—Left medial foot: a, Before; b, after.

tients who have a personal or family history of thrombophlebitis before treatment should be evaluated for hypercoagulablility, including congenital and acquired conditions (eg, anti-phospholipid antibody syndrome).

Presclerotherapy Consultation

Before treatment is initiated, a consultation visit allows for examination of the unwanted veins and a thorough explanation of the procedure, the course of treatment, and potential adverse effects. During this visit, the patient's medical history is reviewed with special attention to past allergic reactions (especially to sclerosing agents); past episodes of lightheadedness, fainting, or other symptoms of vagus nerve hyperactivity; and whether she is pregnant or lactating. None of the sclerosing agents are known to be teratogenic and sodium tetradecyl sulfate has been used extensively in pregnant and lactating women; however, unless under extraordinary circumstances, pregnant and lactating women are not treated.[2] Based on the clinical exam-

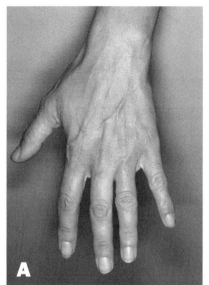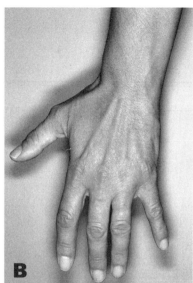

FIGURE 9.—Left dorsal hand: a, Before; b after.

ination, it may be appropriate to perform simple bidirectional Doppler or more sophisticated duplex ultrasound examination to confirm a clinical impression of venous junction or perforating vein incompetence. In the presence of uncomplicated venous telangiectasias and varicose veins, routine duplex ultrasound scanning is not necessary, especially if the findings will not alter the recommended course of treatment.

Presclerotherapy Preparation

Before treatment, the patient should have bathed to remove all lotions and oils. In men with a significant amount of hair, localized areas of skin are trimmed or shaved before sclerotherapy so that all of the veins can be visualized.

Neither medication that impacts the coagulation cascade nor platelet function affect the success of sclerotherapy; however, they can predispose to ecchymoses, especially in those with cutaneous atrophy as occurs in senescent skin and skin that is actinically damaged. This is because such skin has diminished connective tissue supporting the vasculature. If a high dose of aspirin, a nonsteroidal anti-inflammatory drug, or vitamin E is consumed in order to minimize ecchymoses, it is recommended that each be discontinued an appropriate time before treatment if there is no risk in so doing. However, those who arc taking coumadin or aspirin for treatment of or prophylaxis against hematological or cardiovascular disorders are always permitted to continue these medications without concerns about diminishing the effectiveness of treatment.

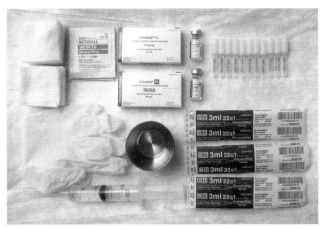

FIGURE 10.—Sclerotherapy supply tray.

Sclerotherapy Supplies

All of the supplies for sclerotherapy are disposable items as displayed in Fig 10 (see color plate V). These include:

- 3 mL syringes
- 27-gauge and 30-gauge needles, plastic not metal hubs
- gloves
- alcohol pads
- gauze
- sclerosant
- 0.9% saline as diluent
- cup for sclerosant

A 3-mL syringe is most practical because it accomodates a useful volume of solution and permits comfortable handling so that it is easy to control the rate of infusion. A syringe in which there is consistent and acceptable plunger resistance as it moves through the barrel is essential. For that reason, disposable plastic syringes provide much better control than glass syringes.

Needles should be smaller than the lumen of the vein to be cannulated. A 30-gauge needle (outer diameter of 0.3 mm) is adequate to treat all venous telangiectases. Those vessels that are too narrow to be cannulated with a 30-gauge needle are likely capillary telangiectasias and are not appropriately treated by sclerotherapy.[3] A 27-gauge needle (outer diameter of 0.46 mm) is appropriate for treating even the largest of varicose veins because it permits an infusion rate sufficient to produce full mural denaturation. Needles should have plastic hubs to visualize retrograde blood flow, which ensures the intraluminal localization of the needle tip. Needles are used only once to minimize discomfort as the needle pierces the skin—each time a needle passes through the skin, the point is somewhat dulled.

In the United States, the choice of sclerosants for varicose and telangiectatic veins of the lower extremity is limited to 2 surfactant sclerosants and hyperosmotic saline.

Sclerosing Solutions: Agents, Concentrations, Volumes, and Dilutions

All sclerosing agents, no matter what their chemical nature, share the functional capacity to denature biologic molecules, including those that provide the structural integrity to the vein wall.[4] This action is achieved by their ability to disrupt chemical bonds intramolecularly and intermolecularly. As such, all molecular constituents—including collagen, glycoaminoglycans, elastin, as well as cellular constituents within the mural layers and lining the tunica intima—are denatured. In decades past, a wider variety of chemicals had been used as sclerosing agents than are currently utilized. Presently, the most commonly used classes of chemicals are surfactants (ie, chemicals that possess both polar and nonpolar moieties) and hyperosmotic solutions (ie, any molecular species in a concentration that is hyperosmolar relative to that of tissue fluids). Although similar in purpose, these 2 classes of chemicals are quite dissimilar in their modes of actions and in their efficacy. By the nature of their interaction with biologic molecules, especially proteins, the surfactants that are currently used are significantly more effective as sclerosants (ie, denaturants) than any hyperosmotic solution. For that reason, hyperosmotic sclerosants are not recommended for treating varicose veins wider than 4 mm. However, both hyperosmotic and surfactant sclerosants yield excellent results in the eradication of smaller veins and venous telangiectases.

The only US Food and Drug Administration (FDA) approved sclerosant for ectatic vessels of the superficial venous system of the lower extremity is sodium tetradecyl sulfate.[5] Sodium morrhuate,[6] a rarely used sclerosant, has been marketed in the past without FDA sanctions, although it is not FDA approved. Like many drugs, its use predates the currently used vigorous standards required for FDA approval, so controlled clinical trials demonstrating safety and efficacy were never undertaken. The FDA has never intervened to halt the manufacturer from producing and distributing it. However, the FDA reserves the right to require safety and efficacy studies, as sanctioned by the 1938 FD&C Act and the 1962 FDA Act. Polidocanol, although commonly used worldwide, is not approved for use in the United States. Unlike sodium morrhuate, it is not marketed in the United States because the FDA and state authorities have, in rare circumstances, imposed sanctions and penalties for its use. There are no FDA approved hyperosmotic sclerosants. However, because hyperosmotic sodium chloride has been marketed as an abortifacient, its off-label use as a sclerosing agent is certainly legal. Other well-established sclerosing agents that are not FDA approved or sanctioned are illegal for use by physicians in the United States.

The use of sclerosing agents that have been aerated or "foamed" have recently been promoted.[7] There may be advantages and disadvantages to this technique. Aerated solutions do provide more effective and sustained blood displacement than nonaerated solutions, thus delaying the dilution of the sclerosing solution in the lumen and prolonging its effect on the mural layers of the vein. However, with large volumes of an aerated solution, there is the potential risk of air embolism. This process may increase the efficacy of some sclerosing agents, yet almost any segment of a vein can be denatured with currently available agents that have not been aerated.

Surfactant Sclerosing Agents

SODIUM TETRADECYL SULFATE

Sodium tetradecyl sulfate (sodium 1-isobutyl 4-ethyloctyl sulfate) is an anionic surfactant that was introduced in 1946. It is widely used throughout the world with a very low incidence of adverse effects and a high rate of success due to the fact that the mural layers are quite vulnerable to this agent. It is commercially available in the United States as Sotradecol (Bioniche Pharma USA, Bogart, Ga) and outside the United States as Tromboject (Omega Laboratories Ltd, Montreal) and STD (STD Pharmaceutical Products Ltd, Hereford, England) among other brands, in up to a 3% concentration. Most formulations contain 2% benzyl alcohol. Depending on the concentration injected, there may be minimal to mild discomfort, often described as cramping, for the duration of infusion or shortly thereafter. Sodium tetradecyl sulfate is effective over a range of concentrations from 0.1% to 3%. The denaturing potential of sodium tetradecyl sulfate is directly related to its concentration. The recommended maximum daily dose of sodium tetradecyl sulfate is 10 mL of a 1% solution or the equivalent thereof, eg, 5 mL of 2%, or 3.33% of 3%.[8] For the calculation to dilute sodium tetradecyl sulfate to achieve a lower final concentration, see Appendix 1.

SODIUM MORRHUATE

Sodium morrhuate is an anionic surfactant sclerosant that was introduced in the 1920s.[9] It consists of sodium salts of saturated and unsaturated fatty acids of cod liver oil. As such, it has a fishy odor. It is commercially available in the United States as Scleromate (Glenwood LLC, Englewood, NJ) in a 5% concentration. Depending on the concentration injected, there may be mild to moderate discomfort, often described as cramping, for the duration of infusion or shortly thereafter. Sodium morrhuate is effective over a range of concentrations from 0.1% to 5%. The denaturing potential of sodium morrhuate is directly related to its concentration. Its use has waned because of serious adverse effects that were reported in decades past. In particular, anaphylactic reactions had occurred due to presumed contamination with cod liver proteins. The purification process has improved since this drug was first formulated so that contaminant cod liver proteins have been eliminated, but this agent is rarely used and has no advantage compared with sodium tetradecyl sulfate.

POLIDOCANOL

Polidocanol (hydroxypolyethoxydodecane) is a nonionic surfactant that was first synthesized in 1936. Its continued worldwide use and very low incidence of adverse effects attests to its safety and efficacy. However, FDA approval has been elusive. It is marketed commercially outside the United States as Aethoxysklerol (Chemische Fabrik Kreussler & Co GmbH, Wiesbaden, Germany) and Sclerovein (Resinag AG, Zurich, Switzerland) among other brands, in up to a 5% concentration. Most commercially available formulations contain 5% ethyl alcohol and 0.5% chlorobutanol. Polidocanol is effective over a range of concentrations from 0.1% to 5%. Infusion is usually painless for concentrations below 1%. As with sodium tetradecyl sulfate, the denaturing potential of polidocanol is directly related to its concentration. The recommended maximum daily dose of 1% polidocanol is based on body weight as follows: 50 kg, 10 mL; 60 kg, 12 mL; 70 kg, 14 mL; 80 kg, 16 mL.[10] For the calculation to dilute polidocanol to achieve a lower final concentration, see Appendix 1.

Hyperosmotic Sclerosing Solutions

HYPEROSMOTIC SODIUM CHLORIDE

Hyperosmotic saline (ie, any concentration greater than 0.9%) has been used since the 1920s. In the United States, it is commercially available as a 23.4% solution. Because this is the concentration that is most readily available, it has by default become the concentration most often used. However, up to 30% has been used. Unlike the surfactant sclerosants, there is a narrow range of effective concentrations for hyperosmotic saline. Below 20%, full thickness mural denaturation for even small veins is not often achieved. In this circumstance, the veins will persist and subsequent treatments will be required. Lowering the concentration to 11.7% was demonstrated to be more tolerable than 23.4%, but the success rates were diminished.[11] Because it is not formulated with a preservative, there is no risk of an allergic reaction. It is readily available and inexpensive. Its primary disadvantages are the pain and muscle cramping that it engenders due to the high sodium concentration that is transiently induced in the environment of the nearby nerves and muscles, respectively.

HYPEROSMOTIC SODIUM CHLORIDE PLUS GLUCOSE

To reduce the pain and cramping associated with infusion of hyperosmotic saline, without reducing the osmolarity of the solution, the sodium concentration may be reduced and dextrose added. Sclerodex (Omega Laboratories Ltd, Montreal) consists of 10% NaCl + 25% dextrose. Although such a solution is associated with less pain and cramping than an isosmolar solution consisting only of sodium chloride, it is a less effective sclerosant than the latter because hyperosmotic dextrose is an even weaker denaturant of biologic molecules than is hyperosmotic sodium chloride. Sclerodex is formulated with 8% phenylethyl alcohol and 10% propylene glycol. This solution is not FDA approved and is not marketed in the United States.

For individuals with renal or cardiac disease, the total volume of sodium chloride infused cannot be ignored. For the calculation of the quantity of sodium that a patient will be subjected to with treatment, see Appendix 2.

Sclerotherapy Technique

Sclerotherapy is technique-sensitive procedure. With optimal technique, this procedure should approach a success rate of 100% for any vein after a single treatment. At the time of treatment, there should be minimal discomfort associated with the procedure, except when the sclerosant is hyperosmotic saline (as described above in "Sclerosing Solutions: Agents, Concentrations, Volumes, and Dilutions"). The following treatment techniques and recommendations will facilitate optimal outcomes after sclerotherapy.

POSITIONING

The treatment environment should be comfortable and relaxing for the patient. The patient should be recumbent during treatment—for comfort and to promote venous emptying. To this end, a motorized examination table facilitates positioning a patient to achieve these goals and it optimizes the physician's access to veins. The physician will perform more effectively if seated—rather than standing—during treatment.

VEIN VISUALIZATION: LIGHTING AND MAGNIFICATION

Immediately before injection, the skin is wiped with isopropyl alcohol. This removes any surface oil and debris and also improves the visualization of the veins. Veins are more easily visualized after wetting with alcohol, especially if the skin is dry. That's because the refractive index of epidermis increases if it is dry, thickened, or dyskeratotic and such skin surfaces' reflectivity is increased. Wetting the skin surface lowers its refractive index, facilitating light transmission through—rather than reflection, refraction, and scattering by—the skin. Adequate lighting is invaluable for optimal visualization of veins. If overhead room lighting is being relied on, it is much easier to visualize veins under fluorescent rather than incandescent light. Specifically, cool white fluorescent light (rated at 4100°K or cooler) highlights the blue green color of veins. The use of cross-polarized light—with a head-mounted light source and glasses each with appropriate polarized filters, or a free-standing floor lamp with the same optics—provides the most clarity to visualize veins. At least 2.5D magnification is recommended.

INTRAVASCULAR INJECTION

The cannula of the needle should be angled so that it can enter the vein parallel to its course in the skin (Fig 11; see color plate VI). The bevel of the needle should always be toward the skin surface. This ensures that if extravasation of sclerosant occurs, it will be superficial to the needle and readily visualized as a wheal or bleb and not deposited deeper where it may not be initially noticed. Once a vein is identified for injection, the skin and

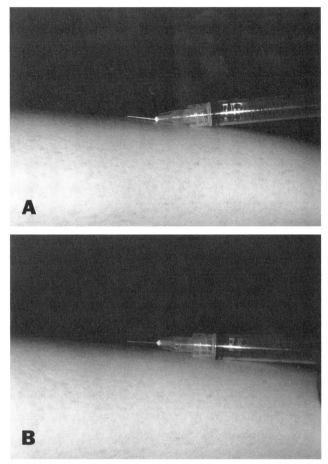

FIGURE 11.—Needle cannula: **a,** Bent, to allow easy access into vein; **b,** straight.

the vein are briskly pierced to minimize discomfort to the patient and trauma to the vein, respectively. After the vein has been cannulated and the intraluminal localization of the needle tip confirmed, infusion may begin. The intraluminal location of the needle tip is always confirmed by the passive retrograde flow of blood through the needle cannula and into the needle hub. For that reason, needles with plastic (not metal) hubs are preferred. The solution should be injected intravascularly—injection should be halted if the needle tip becomes extravascular or extravasation of blood appears. The infusion of solution intravascularly requires minimal pressure on the plunger of the syringe. If greater effort is required to move the plunger through the barrel of the syringe, it is likely that the solution is not being infused intraluminally and injection should be halted.

VOLUME OF SCLEROSANT INFUSION

The volume infused should be sufficient to produce irreversible mural denaturation for the entire length of the targeted veins. If there are tributaries, injection can slowly continue until all of the veins have been exposed to sclerosant. This is readily determined because as the colorless solution is infused into the lumen, it displaces the blood, which, as it recedes, makes the vein appear to disappear. Often, the entire 3 mL of sclerosant in the syringe is deposited during any one injection into a cluster of venous telangiectases and is the norm for varicose veins.

CONCENTRATION OF SCLEROSANT

The concentration of the injected sclerosant is determined by the mural thickness of the vein, which is directly correlated with the lumen diameter. In general, for any anatomic site, the greater the vein diameter, the greater the concentration of sclerosant that will be needed. Injection of too low a concentration will be inadequate to produce full mural denaturation. Injection of too high a concentration can produce extravascular tissue devitalization. See Appendix 3 for recommended ranges of sclerosants for different size veins.

RATE OF INJECTION

In addition to the concentration of sclerosant, the most important factor determining the extent of mural denaturation is the duration that the solution is in contact with the intraluminal surface. Therefore, the rate of infusion should, deliberately, be slow to maximize this contact time while minimizing the requisite volume.

EMPTY VEIN TECHNIQUE

Infusion of sclerosant is optimally into an empty vein. Because a vein conforms to the volume of blood within its lumen, an empty vein requires a low volume of sclerosant compared with a vein that is distended. More importantly, an empty vein is devoid of blood which, when present, can dilute the sclerosant, reducing the concentration that contacts the luminal surface. Therefore, leg elevation at or above the level of the heart ensures that minimal blood will remain intraluminally and minimal dilution of sclerosant can be expected.

INJECTION PRESSURE

During infusion, the injection pressure should be minimal. A high injection pressure can rupture the vein, causing extravasation of solution and blood. Also, if injection pressure is higher than necessary during treatment of venous telangiectases, retrograde flow is possible, forcing sclerosant into the more proximal capillaries or arterioles. Gentle pressure on the plunger of the syringe as it transits the barrel is all that should be necessary during infusion. If firm pressure is required, injection should be discontinued.

COMPRESSION AFTER SCLEROTHERAPY

Immediate and sustained compression after sclerotherapy serves one primary purpose—to minimize the volume of the thrombus that, almost invariably, develops within the lumen of the treated vein. A vein, to some extent, functions as a distensible tube, conforming to the volume of blood within its lumen. This volume will be determined by both intravascular and extravascular pressure, the latter of which will be increased by externally applied compression. Sustained compression, if sufficient, will prevent the vein from attaining its maximum distensible volume. This is important because, as the volume of coagulated blood within the vein's lumen is increased, the duration for its resorption will be prolonged. In addition, undesirable side effects that are related to residual blood within the vein's lumen will be favorably affected by compression. In particular, the degree of post-sclerotherapy hyperpigmentation and the incidence of symptomatic thrombosis (ie, thrombophlebitis) will be reduced compared with such treatment without compression.

Compression does not significantly affect the success of sclerotherapy in permanently eradicating a vein. This observation has been made in the past by investigators who found that the rates of treatment failure were independent of the duration of compression.[12] In addition, this finding is confirmed by the observation that the success rate for the eradication of nonextremity veins (eg, periocular veins)—for which post-sclerotherapy compression is not applied—reproducibly approaches 100%.[13] This is because compression does not enhance any chemical interaction between the sclerosant and the vein wall, nor does it prolong the contact time between them. By the time compression is applied—even within a minute after infusion of sclerosant—the full extent of mural denaturation is likely determined, as is the ultimate outcome of treatment (ie, eventual disappearance or persistence of the vein). The sclerosant exerts its denaturing effect on the mural layers of the vein for a brief duration, usually only seconds. In as short a period as 30 seconds after infusion of sclerosant, histopathological changes within the vein wall can be discerned.[2]

After sclerotherapy, sustained external compression to a superficial vein of the lower extremity must be maintained with circumferential compression, as provided by gradient compression hosiery and wrap-around bandages. Bandages, including cotton balls secured with tape, which are not circumferential, provide inadequate, if any, compression. Gradient compression hosiery provides the most practical approach to sustained compression because, in addition to being effective, it is well tolerated.

Gradient compression hosiery is so called because the compression that is maintained is progressively higher more distally, promoting venous and lymphatic system emptying. Unlike gradient compression hosiery, wrap-around bandaging provides an inconsistent force of external compression, which depends on the elasticity of the bandaging material and the tautness with which it is applied. Furthermore, there is significant variability in the tension different physicians attain with wrap-around bandaging, even though the tension exerted by any individual physician may be uniform.[14,15] In addition, most patients do not reapply wrap-around bandages to achieve an adequate amount of compression after it has been removed for bathing. When applied over a short segment, wrap-around bandaging behaves as a tourniquet and may produce distal swelling, especially of the foot and ankle.

FACTORS AFFECTING THE NECESSARY DEGREE OF COMPRESSION

The degree of compression necessary after sclerotherapy directly correlates with the maximal intravascular pressure that the vein sustains. Optimally, to prevent any blood return into the lumen of the denatured vein, external compression must exceed the maximal intravascular pressure to which the treated vein may be subjected. In some circumstances, such as when a varicose vein in the leg directly communicates with an incompetent perforating vein, this would require compression that would exceed arterial pressure. Clearly, such high compression would be contraindicated. For this reason, some coagulated blood accumulates within the vein lumen, in spite of correctly administered sclerotherapy followed by sustained circumferential compression. However, the volume of the thrombus should be smaller with sustained compression compared with no compression at all. After sclerotherapy of varicose veins, this author's patients are routinely fitted with class 2 (30 mm Hg to 40 mm Hg) gradient compression hosiery. If the treated varicose vein is routinely subjected to high pressures as a consequence of its direct communication with an incompetent venous junction or perforating vein, class 3 (40 mm Hg to 50 mm Hg) gradient compression hosiery is prescribed. Some will experience foot and ankle pain, cramping, numbness, or other symptoms of arterial insufficiency when compression hosiery is worn while the extremity is elevated, such as when in bed. Those who suffer from this reduction in arterial blood flow to the ankle and foot when elevated, however, usually tolerate the recommended level of external compression during the daytime when the lower extremity is in a dependent position.

FACTORS AFFECTING THE NECESSARY DURATION OF COMPRESSION

The duration of compression necessary after sclerotherapy directly correlates with mural thickness. The mural thickness of a vein is usually directly proportional to the diameter of the distended vein's lumen. Optimally, compression must be sustained for as long as a potentially viable lumen persists.[16] It can take weeks or even months after treatment before enough vein resorption has occurred to obliterate this channel precluding any blood from entering it. Compression should be maintained until that time.[17] If it is not maintained, then blood from patent connecting veins can flow into the lumen of the denatured vein if its hydrostatic or hydrodynamic pressure exceeds the denatured vein's intravascular pressure.[18] This causes the lumen of the denatured vein to become distended with blood.[19] Blood that enters this denatured vein interacts with exposed mural constituents producing thrombosis that prolongs the time for complete vein resorption.[20] Clinically, post-sclerotherapy delayed-onset thrombosis is frequently observed when compression has been, retrospectively, prematurely terminated. Compression after sclerotherapy does not promote adherence of the apposing walls of the denatured vein.[4] Unfortunately, there is no mural substance that bonds these walls when they are in apposition.

DURATION OF POST-SCLEROTHERAPY COMPRESSION

The following suggested durations for the continuous use of gradient compression hosiery are what this author has, empirically, found most useful. These suggestions represent the minimal time interval that the compression should be maintained. When the hosiery is removed, at the conclusion of these time periods, the vein will not yet be fully resorbed and may be still palpable as a firm cord. However, it is a duration beyond which post-sclerotherapy delayed-onset thrombosis is not usually observed. The continued use of compression hosiery beyond these minimal durations may aid in the resorption of the treated vein. Unless otherwise stated, these durations are for class 2 gradient compression hosiery.

Venous Telangiectases

In many circumstances, compression does not aid in the rate of removal of venous telangiectases—or in the reduction of side effects—after they are treated by sclerotherapy. However, in this author's experience, for those venous telangiectases that would benefit from compression (ie, especially those that protrude above the plane of the skin), compression should be maintained for at least 7 days but preferably 2 weeks; for some venous telangiectases, compression should be maintained for up to 4 weeks.

Varicose Reticular Veins

Varicose reticular veins that are treated should be subjected to compression for at least as long as venous telangiectases. Usually, 2 weeks are required but sometimes 4 weeks, or longer, are necessary. This duration will be dictated by the size of the veins, their location on the extremity, and the intraluminal venous pressures to which they are subjected. Those that protrude above the plane of the skin derive greater benefit from compression than those at the skin plane.

Varicose Veins

Unlike venous telangiectases and varicose reticular veins where the benefits of compression may not always be appreciated, there is, almost invariably, significant reduction in lumen diameter with compression of varicose veins. Because varicose veins comprise a wide range of sizes and are subjected to a wide range of intraluminal pressures, there is a wide variation in suggested compression intervals. Varicose veins may require sustained compression for at least 3 weeks but the need for 12 weeks of compression is sometimes mandated.

Post-Sclerotherapy Course

INFLAMMATION

Within minutes after injection, inflammation—including erythema, edema, and sometimes pruritus—may be observed at or around treated veins. Often, a linear wheal parallels the course of the solution through the treated vein. This urticarial reaction is due to nonspecific, nonimmunologic mast cell degranulation and does not represent an allergic reaction to the sclerosant. It has been observed with all sclerosants, including hyperosmotic saline, and usually resolves within 30 minutes. It is more commonly observed after treatment of venous telangiectases—which are intradermal, and in the vicinity of a greater number of mast cells—than varicose veins, which are subdermal. Beginning hours or beyond, more persistent swelling, not necessarily with erythema, may appear at or distal to treated veins. Primary swelling—that is, swelling that appears around the treated veins—may persist for a few days to weeks. Secondary swelling—that is, swelling that appears distal to treated veins and is a result of the gravitational effect on the primary swelling as well as compression of lymphatic vessels—may persist for a similar duration. For example, it is not uncommon to observe secondary swelling of the feet and ankles after the proximal legs have been treated. In general, primary swelling is more pronounced the more distal are the treated veins. That is, swelling is usually more apparent after veins of the ankle, foot, or hand are treated compared to more proximally treated areas. Tenderness around treated veins can usually be correlated with the degree of inflammation that develops. As inflammation wanes, so do symptoms.

ECCHYMOSIS

Ecchymosis may develop at or around treated sites. Its incidence may be increased in the presence of drugs in the serum that affect the coagulation cascade or platelet adhesiveness. Ecchymosis will be more evident on actinically damaged and atrophic, ie, senescent, skin due to its diminished structural support of vascular tissue by virtue of its reduced collagen content and integrity.

INTRAVASCULAR THROMBOSIS

Immediately after sclerotherapy, almost invariably, some blood returns into the vein's lumen even if appropriate compression has been applied. Once blood enters the treated channel, it quickly becomes thrombosed (ie, coagulated) due to the presence of exposed subendothelial collagen and other coagulation cascade initiators. The result is treatment-associated superficial vein thrombosis. Often, the skin and supporting tissue around this thrombosed vein become inflamed. The result is treatment-associated superficial vein thrombophlebitis. This may be observed after treatment of veins of all sizes—from the smallest telangiectasia to large varicose vein—and always resolves uneventfully after a few weeks to a few months, as the vein and blood are resorbed. However, if the inflammation is significant or the patient is symptomatic, it may be treated in a manner appropriate for superficial thrombophlebitis. Although treatment-associated superficial vein thrombophlebitis is common, deep vein thrombophlebitis is not a direct risk of treatment. Theoretical concerns about thrombi developing within or emboli emanating from deep veins is clinically unfounded. Any properly administered sclerosant that has been infused into a superficial vein and has entered the deep venous system will be diluted to an extent as to render it impotent, as far as producing mural denaturation or intravascular coagulation.

HYPERPIGMENTATION

Within weeks after treatment, linear hyperpigmentation appears overlying the course of the treated vein. This pigmentation usually represents hemosiderin, a metabolic by-product of hemoglobin, that has remained in the vein's lumen.[21] As such, it should not be considered a complication of treatment but rather a concomitant of treatment. It is part of the resorption process—not much different than the green (ie, biliverdin) or yellow (ie, bilirubin) pigmentation that appears in the course of resorption of an ecchymotic patch. Less commonly, the pigmentation represents postinflammatory incontinence of melanin from the overlying epidermis. Rarely, linear pigmentation may be due to minocycline moieties along the course of the treated vein if this antibiotic is ingested at the time of—or subsequent to—treatment.[22]

DURATION FOR VEIN DISAPPEARANCE

Treated veins require weeks to months for their disappearance. During this time, the vein may feel firm and tender along its course. The duration for resorption depends upon a number of variables, including the vein size and the volume of blood that has re-entered its lumen after sclerotherapy. Compression attempts to minimize the volume of blood in the vein and thus the duration for resorption.

POST-SCLEROTHERAPY ACTIVITY

Immediately after treatment—of veins of all diameters and lengths—the patient may participate in all activities, without restriction, whether or not gradient compression hosiery has been prescribed. This includes strenuous activities, including running and aerobics. For those who are required to wear compression hosiery, after the first 12 hours, it can be removed, for a short time, to bathe. Thereafter, it can be removed whenever bathing is desired. Otherwise, it should be kept on at all times, including at bedtime, if tolerated (as described above in "Factors Affecting the Necessary Degree of Compression"). Shaving is permitted but, to avoid nicking the skin, care should be exercised directly over treated veins, where swelling may cause this skin to be above the plane of the adjacent, noninvolved skin.

Lotion and bath oil may be applied to the skin after treatment. In fact, their application is recommended, especially in those who are required to wear gradient compression hosiery, which has the effect of absorbing moisture—and the sebum that retains it—from the skin, especially during the winter months in temperate climates.

In those for whom compression hosiery is not required, or for those who have worn compression hosiery for the prescribed duration, immersion in water (eg, swimming pool, hot tub) is permitted as is massage.

Although the pharmocokinentics of sclerosing agents, including sodium tetradecyl sulfate, have not been extensively studied, for over 20 years this author has treated patients at an interval of 24 hours—with the maximum recommended quantity of sclerosing agent—without any adverse effects observed.

Adverse Effects

HYPERSENSITIVITY REACTION

Although rarely reported, an immediate hypersensitivity reaction to a sclerosing agent or its preservative could appear. Such a reaction would be treated as would any other type of immediate hypersensitivity. For a mild urticarial reaction, an antihistamine should be administered. For symptomatic urticaria, subcutaneous epinephrine could be considered. If any signs or symptoms of anaphylaxis develop, then subcutaneous epinephrine should be given. The usual initial dose is 0.5 mL of epinephrine 1:1000.

VASOVAGAL REACTION

Some patients manifest a vasovagal reaction (ie, lightheadedness, nausea, perspiration) with a sudden drop in blood pressure, associated with treatment. When such a reaction occurs, it is usually in someone who has experienced a similar episode in the past, unrelated to sclerotherapy. For those susceptible to this reaction, it may be observed prior to the actual injection of the sclerosant. If the decrease in blood pressure is significant and sudden, a transient loss of consciousness (ie, fainting) due to inadequate cerebral perfusion, can be observed. Although unlikely when a patient is recumbent—the position in which treatment is performed—it is nonetheless possible, especially in those with an especially active vagus nerve response (ie, vagotonia). The treatment requires measures to promote cerebral perfusion. To that end, the patient should be placed in a supine position with the lower extremities elevated above the level of the heart. Most often, these episodes resolve within a few minutes. For a more severe response, the intravenous administration of atropine rapidly reverses this reaction. The usual dose of atropine is 0.5 mg. If no response is observed within a minute, a second dose of 0.5 mg should be administered. If a patient requires sclerotherapy but is likely to develop this reaction, it is usually prevented by pretreatment with, the longer acting anticholinergic agent, glycopyrrolate. The usually dose is 0.2 mg intravenously administered within 30 minutes before treatment. Intravenous access is most reliably achieved with a catheter, which should be readily accessible for just such a circumstance. The most appropriate size is 22 gauge with a 1-inch needle.

HYPERTRICHOSIS

Hypertrichosis is a rare side effect that can develop overlying the course of the treated vein. When observed, it usually appeared weeks to months after the vein had been treated. Although it has been observed overlying a treated cluster of venous telangiectases, this rare reaction more often overlies the course of a large varicose vein. Spontaneous regression has always been observed, usually after 12 months to a few years—long after the treated vein has disappeared. To expedite the process, once the vein has been resorbed, an epilating laser can be used.

TELANGIECTATIC CAPILLARY MATTING

The appearance of capillary telangiectasias—thread-like, red vessels that are less than 0.2 mm in diameter—at and around sclerotherapy-treated veins is reported with an incidence up to 18%.[23] When these capillaries are densely clustered, they are described as a telangiectatic capillary matte.[24] Some people are predisposed to their development: It is especially common in those who manifest benign vascular mottling of the lower extremities and in those have previously developed telangiectatic capillaries after sclerotherapy. It is more likely to develop—whether one is predisposed or not—if a higher than necessary concentration of sclerosant is used or if injection pressure is high enough to permit retrograde flow of sclerosant. However, capillary telangiectases can develop when sclerotherapy is properly performed even in those with no predisposing factors. If it has developed, it often regresses spontaneously but can take 12 months or longer to do so. If regression has not occurred, if they are large enough, treatment by photothermal ablation with a vascular laser may be attempted. However, usually, the individual capillaries that comprise the telangiectatic capillary matte are too small to respond to such photothermal treatment. The capillary telangiectases within a matte do not respond to sclerotherapy and, if attempted, the matte may enlarge.

CUTANEOUS DEVITALIZATION

Although uncommon, cutaneous devitalization and subsequent scarring can develop after sclerotherapy. The pathophysiology of such devitalization could be excessive inflammation that unexpectedly develops at a treatment site but may also be attributed to retrograde flow of sclerosant from the treated vein into more proximal capillaries and arterioles at the time of infusion. Although necrosis is usually attributed to inadvertent extravasation of sclerosant, this is an unlikely cause. Rarely is extravasated sclerosant—which would appear as a wheal or bleb—apparent at the time of treatment, prior to the development of cutaneous devitalization. However, blanching of the skin—a manifestation of interruption of blood flow into the area of the skin being served by the afferent circulation—is a well-recognized precursor of cutaneous devitalization. Wound care is directed at preventing dessication. This can be achieved with an occlusive ointment or, if possible, a hydrogel polymer sheet that ensures hydration and promotes wound healing (eg, Vigilon [Bard Medical Division, C. R. Bard, Inc, Covington, Ga] and 2nd Skin [Spenco Med Corp, Waco, Texas]). Inflammation, which is an impediment to healing, is common in the absence of infection and is usually ameliorated with an oral antibiotic. Infection within these wounds is rare but, if cultured, there will always be a bacterial presence. This represents contamination and not the presence of a primary pathogen. Cleansing the skin with soap and water is essential. Compression, almost always, promotes healing, and it should be maintained until the ulcer is healed. Although it can require months for healing, spontaneous resolution almost always occurs.

References

1. Fentem PH, Goddard M, Gooden BA, et al: Control of distension of varicose veins achieved by leg bandages, as used after injection sclerotherapy. *Br Med J* 2:725-727, 1976.
2. Fegan G: Varicose Veins: Compression Sclerotherapy. William Heinemann Medical Books Limited, London, 1967, p 63.
3. Green D. Treatment of lower extremity telangiectases: Sclerotherapy and photo-thermal coagulation. *Cosmetic Dermatol* 12:21-25, 1999.
4. Green, D: Mechanism of action of sclerotherapy. *Semin Dermatol* 12:88-97, 1993.
5. Approved Drug Products With Therapeutic Equivalence Evaluations, Sotradecol ANDA 40-0541 [Nov 12, 2004] Bioniche Pharma USA, Inc, 25 Ed, US Department of Health and Human Services, Food and Drug Administration 2005.
6. Palidsades Pharmaceuticals, Inc: Sodium morrhuate product information. Physicians Desk Reference. 51st ed, Montvale, NJ, Medical Economics: 1998 pp 1184-1185.
7. Bergan J, Pascarella L, Mekenas L: Venous disorders: treatment with sclerosant foam. *J Cardiovasc Surg (Torino)* 47:9-18, 2006.
8. Product Information Sotradecol® Bioniche Pharma USA Inc Bogart, Ga.
9. Higgins TT, Kittel PB: The use of sodium morrhuate in treatment of varicose veins by injection. *Lancet* 1:68-69, 1930.
10. Product Information Aethoxysklerol® Chemische Fabrik Kreussler & Co GmbH, Wiesbaden, Germany
11. Sadick NS: Sclerotherapy of varicose and telangiectatic leg veins: Minimal sclerosant concentration of hyperosmotic saline and its relationship to vessel diameter. *J Dermatol Surg Oncol* 20:65-70, 1991.
12. Raj TB, Makin GS: A random controlled trial of two forms of compression bandaging in outpatient sclerotherapy of varicose veins. *J Surg Res* 31:440-445, 1981.
13. Green D: Removal of periocular veins by sclerotherapy. *Ophthalmology* 108:442-448, 2001.
14. Fentem PH, Goddard M, Gooden BA, et al: Control of distension of varicose veins achieved by leg bandages, as used after injection sclerotherapy. *Br Med J* 2:725-727, 1976.
15. Raj TB, Goddard M, Makin GS: How long do compression bandages maintain their pressure during ambulatory treatment of varicose veins? *Brit J Surg* 67:122-124, 1980.
16. Green D: Sclerotherapy for the permanent eradication of varicose veins: Theoretical and practical considerations. *J Amer Acad Dermatol* 38:461-475, 1998.
17. Fegan WG: Continuous uninterrupted compression technique of injecting varicose veins. *Proc R Soc Med* 53:837-840, 1960.
18. Fegan WG: Continuous compression technique for injecting varicose veins. *Lancet* 2:109-112, 1963.
19. Weissberg D: Treatment of varicose veins by compression sclerotherapy. *Surg Gynecol Obstet* 151:353-356, 1980.

20. Fegan WG: Injection with compression as a treatment for varicose veins. *Proc R Soc Med* 58:874-876, 1965.
21. Goldman MP, Kaplan RP, Duffy DM: Postsclerotherapy hyperpigmentation: A histologic evaluation. *J Dermatol Surg Oncol* 13:547-550, 1987.
22. Green D: Post-sclerotherapy pigmentation aggravated by minocycline—Three cases and a review of post-sclerotherapy pigmentation. *J Cosmet Dermatol* 4:173-182, 2003.
23. Weiss RA, Weiss MA: Resolution of pain associated with varicose and telangiectatic leg veins after compression sclerotherapy. *J Dermatol Surg Oncol* 16:333-336, 1990.
24. Duffy DM: Small vessel sclerotherapy: An overview. *Adv Dermatol* 3:221-242, 1988. Year Book Medical Publishers, Inc.

Appendix 1
Calculation of Dilution Volumes for Sclerosants

Commercially available sodium tetradecyl sulfate is available in concentrations of 0.5%, 1%, and 3%, and polidocanol is available in concentrations of 1%, 2%, 3%, and 5%. Usually, it is necessary to dilute the commercially available solution to a concentration appropriate for the veins that are being treated. The following equation is used to calculate the diluent volume, using 0.9% saline solution, to achieve any concentration of sclerosant. This can be used for any sclerosing agent, including sodium tetradecyl sulfate and polidocanol:

$$C_f = [C_i][V_s \div (V_s + V_d)]$$

C_f = final concentration (in percent) of sclerosant

C_i = initial concentration (in percent) of sclerosant

V_s = initial volume in ml of undiluted sclerosant

V_d = diluent volume in ml of 0.9% saline solution

The following chart provides final concentrations of sodium tetradecyl sulfate based upon an initial volume of 1 mL of a 3% solution using 0.9% sterile saline as a diluent. These dilutions would be the same for a 3% solution of any sclerosant, including polidocanol. To prepare a smaller final volume than in the table below, the initial volume of the undiluted 3% sodium tetradecyl sulfate would be reduced and the added volume of 0.9% saline would be reduced proportionally. Likewise, to prepare a larger final volume, the initial volume of 3% sodium tetradecyl sulfate would be increased and the added volume of 0.9% saline would be increased proportionally. For example, to obtain 6ml of a 1% solution of sodium tetradecyl sulfate, start with 2 mL of 3% sodium tetradecyl sulfate and add 4 mL of 0.9% normal saline.

For a Final Concentration	Added Volume of 0.9% Saline	Initial Volume of 3% Sodium Tetradecyl Sulfate	Final Volume of Desired Concentration
0.10%	29.00 mL	1 mL	30.00 mL
0.20%	14.00 mL	1 mL	15.00 mL
0.30%	9.00 mL	1 mL	10.00 mL
0.40%	6.50 mL	1 mL	7.50 mL
0.50%	5.00 mL	1 mL	6.00 mL
0.75%	3.00 mL	1 mL	4.00 mL
1.00%	2.00 mL	1 mL	3.00 mL
1.50%	1.00 mL	1 mL	2.00 mL
2.00%	0.50 mL	1 mL	1.50 mL

The above volumes were determined by the following equation, using 1 mL of a 3% solution of sodium tetradecyl sulfate:

$$C_f = [3\%][1 \div (1 + V_d)]$$

C_f = desired final concentration (in percent) of sodium tetradecyl sulfate

3 = initial concentration (in percent) of sodium tetradecyl sulfate

1 = initial volume in mL of 3% sodium tetradecyl sulfate

V_d = diluent volume in mL of 0.9% saline solution

Example 1: Determination of the volume of 0.9% saline (V_d) that must be added to 1 mL of 3% to prepare a 0.2% solution of sodium tetradecyl sulfate:

1) $C_f = [C_i][V_s \div (V_s + V_d)]$
2) $0.2 = [3][1 \div (1 + V_d)]$
3) $0.2 \div 3 = 1 \div (1 + V_d)$
4) $0.2 + 0.2V_d = 3$
5) $0.2V_d = 2.8$
6) $V_d = 14$ mL

Therefore, it is necessary to add 14 mL of 0.9% normal saline to 1 mL of 3% sodium tetradecyl sulfate to have a final concentration of 0.2%.

Example 2: Determination of the volume of 0.9% saline (V_d) that must be added to 1 mL of 3% to prepare a 1% solution of sodium tetradecyl sulfate:

1) $C_f = [C_i][V_s \div (V_s + V_d)]$
2) $1 = [3][1 \div (1 + V_d)]$
3) $1 \div 3 = 1 \div (1 + V_d)$
4) $1 + 1V_d = 3$
5) $1V_d = 2$
6) $V_d = 2$ mL

Therefore, it is necessary to add 2 mL of 0.9% normal saline to 1 mL of 3% sodium tetradecyl sulfate to have a final concentration of 1%.

Appendix 2
Calculation of Sodium Load Provided by Hyperosmotic Saline

The sodium load that someone will be subjected to with treatment, for any concentration of hyperosmotic saline, will depend on the volume infused. This can be calculated for a 23.4% sodium chloride solution (which contains 91.3 mg/mL Na^+ and 142.7 mg/mL of Cl^-) as follows:

Milligrams of Na^+ = number of milliliters of solution infused $\times$ 91.3 mg/mL

For example, if 10 mL of 23.4% sodium chloride solution are infused, the sodium load is 913 mg as follows: 10 mL $\times$ 91.3 mg/mL = 913 mg Na^+

Similarly, if 20 mL of 23.4% sodium chloride are infused, the sodium load is 1826 mg as follows: 20 mL of 23.4% NaCl = 1826 mg Na^+

Appendix 3
Sclerosant Concentrations

The following are the usual range of concentrations for treating venous telangiectases to varicose veins with the most commonly used sclerosants. There are variables that affect the outcome of treatment in addition to sclerosant concentration, including the volume infused and duration of contact. Slow infusion prolongs the time the sclerosant directly interacts with the mural layers and may allow a lower concentration and a lower volume to achieve the same effect. The last column has a wide range of concentrations, because there is a wide range in diameters of varicose veins. The higher end of the concentration range is reserved only for the largest of varicose veins that are greater than 10 mm.

Vein Diameter ⟍ Sclerosant	<1 mm	1 mm-5 mm	>5 mm
Sodium Tetradecyl Sulfate	0.15%-0.2%	0.2%-0.4%	0.4%-3%
Polidocanol	0.25%-0.4%	0.4%-0.7%	0.7%-5%
Hyperosmotic Saline	23.4%	23.4%	N/A

Statistics of Interest to the Dermatologist

MARTIN A. WEINSTOCK, MD, PHD, AND MARGARET M. BOYLE, BS
Brown University Dermatoepidemiology Unit, Providence, Rhode Island

TABLE 1.—New Cases of Selected Reportable Infectious Diseases in the United States

	1940	1950	1960	1970	1980	1990	2000	2005*
AIDS	—	—	—	—	—	41,595	40,758	30,568†
Anthrax	76	49	23	2	1	0	1	—
Congenital Rubella	—	—	—	77	50	11	9	—
Congenital Syphilis	—	—	—	—	—	3865	529	273
Diphtheria	15,536	5796	918	435	3	4	1	—
Gonorrhea	175,841	286,746	258,933	600,072	1,004,029	690,169	358,995	314,370
Hansen's Disease	—	44	54	129	223	198	91	89
Lyme Disease	—	—	—	—	—	—	17,730	21,304
Measles	291,162	319,124	441,703	47,351	13,506	27,786	86	62‖
Plague	1	3	2	13	18	2	6	7
Rocky Mountain Spotted Fever	457	464	204	380	1163	651	495	1843
Syphilis (primary and secondary)†	—	23,939	16,145	21,982	27,204	50,223	5979	8020
Toxic Shock Syndrome‡	—	—	—	—	—	322	135	96
Tuberculosis‡	102,984§	121,742§	55,494	37,137	27,749	25,701	16,377	11,547
US population (millions)	132	151	179	203	227	249	281	296

Note: Dash indicates that data not available.
*For 52 weeks ending December 31, 2005.
†Last update December 3, 2005.
‡Reporting criteria changed in 1975.
§Data include newly reported active and inactive cases.
‖Of 62 cases reported, 51 were indigenous, and 11 were imported from another country.
(Data from Centers for Disease Control and Prevention: Summary of Notifiable Diseases, United States, 2005. Morb Mortal Wkly Rep 54[51&52] :1320-1330, 2006; Centers for Disease Control and Prevention: Summary of Notifiable Diseases, United States, 2000. Morb Mortal Wkly Rep 49[51&52] :1167-1174, 2001; Centers for Disease Control and Prevention: Annual Summary 1994: Reported morbidity and mortality. Morb Mortal Wkly Rep 43[53] :70-71, 1994; Centers for Disease Control and Prevention: Annual Summary 1984: Reported morbidity and mortality. Morb Mortal Wkly Rep 33 :124-129, 1986.)

TABLE 2.—Estimates of HIV/AIDS, 2005

REGION	Adults and Children Living With HIV	Adults and Children Newly Affected With HIV	Adult Prevalence (%)	Adult and Child Deaths Due to AIDS
Sub-Saharan Africa	23.8-28.9 million	2.8-3.9 million	6.6-8.0	2.1-2.7 million
North Africa and Middle East	230,000-1.4 million	35,000-200,000	0.1-0.7	25,000-150,000
South and Southeast Asia	4.5-11 million	480,000-2.4 million	0.4-1.0	290,000-740,000
East Asia	440,000-1.4 million	42,000-390,000	0.05-0.2	20,000-68,000
Oceania	25,000-48,000	2,100-13,000	0.2-0.7	1,700-8,200
Latin America	1.4-2.4 million	130,000-360,000	0.5-0.8	52,000-86,000
Caribbean	200,000-510,000	17,000-71,000	1.1-2.7	16,000-40,000
Eastern Europe and Central Asia	990,000-2.3 million	140,000-610,000	0.6-1.3	39,000-91,000
Western and Central Europe	570,000-890,000	15,000-39,000	0.2-0.4	<15,000
North America	650,000-1.8 million	15,000-120,000	0.4-1.1	9,000-30,000
Total	40.3 million 36.7-45.3 million	4.9 million 4.3-6.6 million	1.10% 1.0-1.3	3.1 million 2.8-3.6 million

(Data from AIDS Epidemic Update, Joint United Nations Programme on HIV/AIDS (UNAIDS) World Health Organization (WHO), December 2005.)

TABLE 3.—AIDS Cases by Age Group and Exposure Category, and
Cumulative Totals Through 2004, United States

	2004		Cumulative Total*	
	No.	(%)	No.	(%)
Adult/adolescent exposure category				
Male-to-male sexual contact	15,607	(35%)	402,722	(44%)
Injecting drug use	6919	(16%)	219,053	(24%)
Male-to-male sexual contact And injection drug use	1696	(4%)	60,038	(7%)
Hemophilia/coagulation disorder	92	(0%)	5427	(1%)
Heterosexual contact	8651	(19%)	117,887	(13%)
Receipt of blood transfusion, blood components, or tissue†	196	(0%)	9274	(1%)
Other/risk factor not reported or identified	11,454	(26%)	94,504	(10%)
Adult/adolescent SUBTOTAL	44,615	(100%)	908,905	(100%)
Pediatric (<13 years old) exposure category				
Hemophilia/coagulation disorder	0	(0%)	230	(2%)
Mother with/at risk for HIV infection	104	(85%)	8576	(91%)
Receipt of blood transfusion, blood components, or tissue†	0	(0%)	388	(4%)
Other/risk not reported or identified	18	(15%)	187	(2%)
Pediatric SUBTOTAL	122	(100%)	9381	(100%)
TOTAL	44,737	(100%)	918,286	(100%)

Note: Total includes 2 person of unknown sex.
*Includes persons with a diagnosis of AIDS, reported from the beginning of the epidemic through 2004.
†Forty-seven adults/adolescents and 3 children developed AIDS after receiving blood screened negative for HIV antibodies. Fourteen additional adults developed AIDS after receiving tissue, organs, or artificial insemination from HIV-infected donors. Four of the 14 received tissue or organs from a donor who was negative for HIV antibody at the time of donation.
(Data from Centers for Disease Control and Prevention: *HIV/AIDS Surveillance Rep* 16:32, 2004.)

TABLE 4.—Selected Causes of Death, United States, 1993 and 2003

Cause of Death	Number of Deaths	
	1993	2003
Malignant melanoma	6712	7818
Infections of the skin	778	1587
Motor vehicle traffic accidents	40,899	43,340
Accident involving animal being ridden	66	101
Accidental drowning and submersion	3807	3306
Lightning	57	47
Homicide and legal intervention	26,009	18,155
All cancer	529,904	556,902
All causes	2,288,553	2,448,288

(Data from National Center for Health Statistics, Division of Vital Statistics, personal communication, March 2006.)

TABLE 5.—Annual Change in Cancer Incidence in the United States

Top 20 Highest Incidence Sites	Average Annual Percent Change	
	1991-2003	1973-1990
Prostate	−1.9	3.5
Breast	0.1	1.9
Lung and bronchus	−0.8	1.8
Colon/rectum	−1.0	0.2
Corpus and uterus, NOS	−0.1	−2.3
Urinary bladder	0.1	0.7
Non-Hodgkin lymphoma	0.4	3.6
Melanoma of the skin	2.5	4.1
Leukemia	−0.5	0.1
Kidney and renal pelvis	1.7	2.2
Oral cavity and pharynx	−1.4	−0.4
Pancreas	0.0	−0.2
Cervix uteri	−2.8	−2.6
Stomach	−1.7	−1.6
Thyroid	4.7	0.8
Brain and ONS	−0.4	1.5
Myeloma	−0.4	1.1
Testis	0.8	2.5
Liver and intrahepatic bile duct	3.0	2.3
Esophagus	0.3	0.8
All sites	−0.5	+1.2

Note: SEER 9 registries and NCHS public use data file for the total United States. Rates are per 100,000 and age-adjusted to the 2000 US standard population.
  Rates are for invasive cancers only.
  (Data from Ries LAG, Harkins D, Krapcho M, et al (eds): *SEER Cancer Statistics Review: 1975-2003*, National Cancer Institute, Bethesda, Md, http://seer.cancergov/csr/1975_2003/, based on November 2005 SEER data submission, posted to the SEER Web site, 2006; Surveillance, Epidemiology, and End Results (SEER) Program SEER Stat Database: Incidence—SEER 9 Registries, November 2005 Sub (1973-2003), National Cancer Institute, DCCPS, Surveillance Research Program, Cancer Statistics Branch, released April 2006 based on the November 2005 submission.)

TABLE 6.—Melanoma Incidence and Mortality Rates, United States

Year	Incidence*	Mortality†
1975	7.9	2.1
1976	8.1	2.2
1977	8.9	2.3
1978	8.9	2.3
1979	9.5	2.4
1980	10.5	2.3
1981	11.1	2.4
1982	11.2	2.5
1983	11.1	2.5
1984	11.4	2.5
1985	12.8	2.6
1986	13.3	2.6
1987	13.7	2.6
1988	12.9	2.6
1989	13.7	2.7
1990	13.8	2.8
1991	14.6	2.7
1992	14.8	2.7
1993	14.6	2.7
1994	15.6	2.7
1995	16.4	2.7
1996	17.2	2.8
1997	17.6	2.7
1998	17.8	2.8
1999	18.1	2.6
2000	18.7	2.7
2001	19.4	2.7
2002	18.6	2.6
2003	18.7	2.7

2006 estimate: 62,190 newly diagnosed cases and 7910 deaths

*Surveillance, Epidemiology and End-Results (SEER) Program, (9 registries of the National Cancer Institute).

†National Center for Health Statistics, United States population. Rates per 100,000 per year, and age-adjusted to the 2000 US standard population. All races.

(Data from American Cancer Society, Inc, Surveillance Research. *Cancer Facts & Figures 2006 4:2006;* Surveillance, Epidemiology, and End-Results (SEER) Program, SEER Stat Database: Incidence SEER 9 Registries Public Use, November 2005 sub. (1973-2003); Linked to County Attributes—Total US, 1969-2003 Counties, National Cancer Institute DCCPS, Surveillance Research Program, Cancer Statistics Branch, released April 2006, based on the November 2005 submission; Surveillance, Epidemiology, and End-Results (SEER) Program, SEER Stat Database: Mortality-All COD, Public-Use with State, Total US (1969-2003), National Cancer Institute CDDPS, Surveillance Research Program, Cancer Statistics Branch, released April 2006, based on the November 2005 submission. Underlying mortality data provided by the National Center for Health Statistics.)

TABLE 7.—Melanoma Five-Year Relative Survival

Year	Whites (%)	Blacks (%)
Year at Diagnosis		
1960-1963	60	—
1970-1973	68	—
1974-1976	81	67
1977-1979	83	50
1980-1982	83	56
1983-1985	85	74
1986-1988	88	67
1989-1991	89	78
1992-1994	89	59
1995-1997	91	76
1998-2002	91	*
Stage at Diagnosis (1996-2002)		
Local	99	95
Regional	65	38
Distant	15	27

Notes: Dash indicates insufficient data. Relative survival is the observed survival divided by the survival expected in a demographically similar subgroup of the general population. Survival estimates among blacks are imprecise due to small numbers of cases observed.

*The statistic could not be calculated.

†The relative cumulative rate increased from a prior interval and has been adjusted.

(Data from Surveillance, Epidemiology, and End Results (SEER) Program, SEER Stat Database: Incidence—SEER Registries, (1973-2003 varying)—Linked To County Attributes-Total US, 1969-2003 Counties, National Cancer Institute, DCCPS, Surveillance Research Program, Cancer Statistics Branch, released April 2006, based on the November 2005 submission, and personal communication, SEER Program, May 2006.)

TABLE 8.—Contact Dermatitis in Belgium: Proportion of Positive Patch Tests to Standard Chemicals in 290 Patients With at Least 1 Positive Reaction (Among 522 Patients Tested in 2005)

Chemical	%
Nickel sulphate	33.4
Paraphenylenediamine	15.5
Fragrance mix	12.4
Cobalt chloride	8.6
Balsam of Peru	8.3
Colophonium	7.6
Potassium dichromate	6.5
Wood alcohols	4.5
Methyldibromo glutaronitrile	4.1
Thiuram mix	3.8
Paratertiarybutylphenol-formaldehyde resin	3.4
Benzocaine	3.1
Mcthyl(chloro)isothiazolinone	3.1
Formaldehyde	2.8
Epoxy resin	2.1
Tixocortol pivalate	2.1
Clioquinol	1.7
Budesonide	1.4
Mercapto mix	1.4
Paraben mix	1.4
Sesquiterpene lactone mix	1.4
Mercaptobenzothiazole	1.0
Neomycin sulphate	1.0
Isopropyl-phenylparaphenylenediamine	0.7
Quaternium-15	0.7
Primin	0.3

(Data from Goossens A, University Hospital, Katholieke Universiteit Leuven, Belgium, personal communication, January 2006.)

TABLE 9.—Dermatology Trainees in the United States

Year Residency to Be Completed	Male Residents	Female Residents	Unknown	Total
MD Programs				
2006	141	210	1	352
2007	136	213	1	350
2008	129	235	0	364
DO Programs				
2006	8	9	3	20
2007	14	10	5	29
2008	16	8	0	24

(Data from American Academy of Dermatology, personal communication, January 2006.)

TABLE 10.—Diplomates Certified by The American Board of Dermatology
From 1933 to 2005

Decade Totals (Inclusive Dates)	Average Number Certified per Year
1933-1940	69
1941-1950	74
1951-1960	76
1961-1970	112
1971-1980	247
1981-1990	271
1991-2000	295
2001-2005	320
Individual Year Totals	Actual Number Certified
1999	286
2000	283
2001	305
2002	309
2003	307
2004	329
2005	352
TOTAL 1933 through 2005	12,909

(Data from The American Board of Dermatology, Inc, personal communication, January 2006.)

TABLE 11.—Physicians Certified in Dermatologic Subspecialties

Physicians Certified for Special Qualification in Dermatopathology, 1974-2005

Year	Dermatologists	Pathologists	Total
		Average Number Certified	
1974-1975	108	44	302
1976-1980	54	49	515
1981-1985	37	34	351
1986-1990	11	14	125
1991-1995	20	20	196
1996-2000	14	32	227
		Actual Number Certified	
2001	10	34	44
2002	14	55	69
2003	14	48	62
2004	16	45	61
2005	23	47	70
TOTAL Certified 1974-2005	970	1055	2025

Dermatologists Certified for Special Qualification in
Clinical and Laboratory Dermatological Immunology, 1985-2005

Year	Number Certified
1985	52
1987	16
1989	22
1991	15
1993	5
1997	5
2001	6
TOTAL 1985-2005	121

Dermatologists Certified for Special Qualification in
Pediatric Dermatology, 2004

2004	90

Notes: No special qualification examination for Dermatopathology was administered in 1992, 1994, and 1996. No special qualification examination in Clinical and Laboratory Dermatological Immunology was administered in 1986, 1988, 1990, 1992, 1994, 1995, 1996, 1998, 1999, 2000, 2002, 2003 or 2004, or 2005. Special qualification in Pediatric Dermatology began in 2004. No special qualification examination in Pediatric Dermatology was administered in 2005.

(Data from American Board of Dermatology and American Board of Pathology, personal communication, January 2006.)

TABLE 12.—Visits to Non-Federal Office-Based Physicians in the United States, 2003

Diagnosis	Dermatologist		Type of Physician Other		All Physicians	
	Number of Visits (1000's)	Percent	Number of Visits (1000's)	Percent	Number of Visits (1000's)	Percent
Acne vulgaris	3772	12.7	*	*	4402	0.5
Eczematous dermatitis	2452	8.2	5676	0.7	8128	0.9
Warts	1400	4.7	1567	0.2	2967	0.3
Skin cancer	2103	7.1	1459	0.2	3562	0.4
Psoriasis	1100	3.7	*	*	1268	0.1
Fungal infections	*	*	2104	0.2	2555	0.3
Hair disorders	772	2.6	*	*	1690	0.2
Actinic keratosis	2653	8.9	*	*	3031	0.3
Benign neoplasm of the skin	2791	9.4	*	*	3935	0.4
All disorders	29,801	100.0	876,222	100.0	906,023	100.0

Note: Figures may not add to totals because of rounding.
*Figure suppressed due to small sample size.
(Data from National Ambulatory Medical Care Survey 2003. National Center for Health Statistics, Centers for Disease Control and Prevention, personal communication, January 2006.)

TABLE 13.—Health Insurance Coverage of the United States Population, 2004

	Children 1-17 Years (%)	Adults 18-64 Years (%)	Adults 65 Years and Over (%)
Individually Purchased Insurance	8	6	25
Employment-based Coverage	58	64	36
Public Insurance, all types	30	13	95
Medicaid	27	8	9
No Health Insurance	11	21	1

Note: Some individuals have both public and private insurance, so the numbers will not add to 100%.
(Data from the Employee Benefit Research Institute, estimates from the *Current Population Survey, March Supplement, 2005.* Washington, DC, personal communication, April 2006.)

TABLE 14.—Nonelderly Population With Selected Sources of Health Insurance, by Family Income, 2004

Yearly Family Income Level	Employment-Based Coverage (%)	Individually Purchased (%)	Public (%)	Uninsured (%)	Total (%)
under $5000	13	11	39	41	100
$5000-$9999	12	11	53	28	100
$10,000-$14,999	18	10	43	34	100
$15,000-$19,999	29	9	33	34	100
$20,000-$29,999	42	8	27	29	100
$30,000-$39,999	58	7	19	22	100
$40,000-$49,999	69	7	14	16	100
$50,000 and over	82	5	7	9	100
TOTAL	62	7	18	18	100

Note: Details may not add to totals because individuals may receive coverage from more than one source.
(Data from Fronstin P, "Sources of Coverage and Characteristics of the Uninsured: Analysis of the March 2005 Current Population Survey." *EBRI Issue Brief*, No. 287 [Washington, DC, Employee Benefit Research Institute], November 2005.)

TABLE 15.—Health Maintenance Organization (HMO)
Market Penetration in the United States,
January 1, 2005

HMO Penetration in Region	
Pacific	46%
Northeast	34%
Mid-Atlantic	27%
East North Central	23%
Mountain	23%
South Atlantic	23%
West North Central	19%
West South Central	13%
East South Central	10%

HMO Penetration Top Ten Most Highly Penetrated Metropolitan Statistical Areas	
Sacramento—Arden-Arcade—Roseville, California	67%
San Jose-Sunnyvale-Santa Clara, California	66%
Oakland-Fremont-Hayward, California	66%
San Francisco-San Mateo-Redwood City, California	58%
Los Angeles-Long Beach-Glendale, California	55%
Riverside-San Bernardino-Ontario, California	52%
Philadelphia, Pennsylvania	50%
San Diego-Carlsbad-San Marcos, California	50%
Buffalo-Cheektowaga-Tonawanda, New York	48%
Santa Ana-Anaheim-Irvine, California	43%

(Data from 2005 HealthLeaders-Interstudy Publications, *Managed Care Census,* Nashville, Tennessee, personal communication, April 2006.)

TABLE 16.—National Health Expenditure Amounts: Selected Calendar Years
(Billions of Dollars)

Spending Category	1980	1990	2000	2006*	2007*
Total national health expenditures	246	696	1310	2078	2233
Health services and supplies	234	670	1262	1998	2147
Personal health care	215	609	1138	1781	1911
Hospital care	102	254	417	624	663
Professional services	67	217	425	667	717
Physician and clinical services	47	158	289	454	487
Other professional services	4	18	39	60	64
Dental services	13	32	61	90	96
Other personal health care	3	10	37	64	70
Nursing home and home health	20	65	126	182	194
Home health care	2	13	32	55	60
Nursing home care	18	53	94	127	134
Retail outlet sale of medical products	26	73	171	309	338
Prescript on drugs	12	40	122	249	276
Other medical products	14	33	49	59	62
Durable medical equipment	4	11	18	22	23
Other non-durable medical products	10	23	31	37	39
Government administration and net cost of private health insurance	12	40	81	147	160
Government public health activities	7	20	44	69	75
Investment	12	26	48	80	86
Research†	6	13	29	51	55
Construction	7	14	19	29	31

Note: Numbers may not add to totals because of rounding.
*Projected values. The health spending projections were based on the 2003 version of the National Health Expenditures (NHE) released in January 2005.
†Research and development expenditures of drug companies and other manufacturers and providers of medical equipment and supplies are excluded from research expenditures but are included in the expenditure class in which the product falls, in that they are covered by the payment received for that product.
(Data from Centers for Medicare and Medicaid Services, Office of the Actuary, January 2006.)

TABLE 17.—Spending on Consumer Advertising of
Prescription Products, United States

Year	(Dollars in Millions)
2005	4132
2004	4084
2003	3082
2002	2514
2001	2479
2000	2150*
1999	1590
1998	1173
1997	844
1996	595
1995	313
1994	242
1993	165
1992	156
1991	56
1990	48
1989	12

*Estimated.
(Data from TNS Media Intelligence Copyright 2006, Magazine Publishers of America, Inc, personal communication, February 2006.)

TABLE 18.—Results of the American Academy of Dermatology Skin Cancer
Screening Program, 1985-2005

Year	Number Screened	Suspected Diagnosis		
		Basal Cell Carcinoma	Squamous Cell Carcinoma	Malignant Melanoma
1985	32,000	1056	163	97
1986	41,486	3049	398	262
1987	41,649	2798	302	257
1988	67,124	4457	474	435
1989	78,486	6266	761	593
1990	98,060	7959	1069	872
1991	102,485	8110	1193	1062
1992	98,440	8403	1280	1054
1993	97,553	7067	1068	2465*
1994	86,895	6908	1235	1010
1995	88,934	7503	1317	1353
1996	94,363	8713	1656	1399
1997	99,554	8730	1685	1469
1998	89,536	6687	1308	1078
1999	89,916	5790	1136	635
2000	65,854	5074	1053	653
2001	70,562	5192	1102	642
2002	64,492	4733	1009	692
2003	70,692	4481	1032	489
2004	71,243	4891	1165	760
2005	82,532	5659	1411	794
TOTAL	1,631,856	123,526	21,817	18,071

*Number of cases included melanoma, "rule out melanoma," and lentigo maligna.
(Data from American Academy of Dermatology: *2005 Skin Cancer Screening Program Statistical Summary Report*, March 2006.)

TABLE 19.—Leading Dermatology Journals

Journal	Total Citations in 2004	Number of Articles Published in 2004
Journal of Investigative Dermatology	16,817	311
Journal of the American Academy of Dermatology	13,508	350
British Journal of Dermatology	12,007	317
Archives of Dermatology	10,476	181
Dermatology	3592	154
Contact Dermatitis	3448	81
Acta Dermato-Venereologica	3011	67
International Journal of Dermatology	2802	220
Dermatologic Surgery	2538	203
Clinical and Experimental Dermatology	2112	152
Archives of Dermatological Research	1968	65
Burns	1751	156
American Journal of Dermatopathology	1750	79
Cutis	1670	120
Journal of Cutaneous Pathology	1598	103
Melanoma Research	1397	87
Pediatric Dermatology	1336	101
Mycoses	1301	100
Journal of Dermatology	1255	159
Experimental Dermatology	1155	102
Annals de Dermatologie et de Venereologie	1112	118
Dermatology Clinics	1100	51
Journal of Dermatological Science	1062	52
Wound Repair and Regeneration	1035	78
European Journal of Dermatology	991	86

(Data from *Journal Citation Reports Web Version 2004:JCR*, Science ed. Philadelphia, The Thomson Corporation, January 2006.)

CLINICAL DERMATOLOGY

CLINICAL DERMATOLOGY

1 Urticarial and Eczematous Disorders

Risk of First-Time Hospitalization for Angioedema Among Users of ACE Inhibitors and Angiotensin Receptor Antagonists

Johnsen SP, Jacobsen J, Monster TBM, et al (Aarhus Univ, Denmark; Inst of Cancer Epidemiology, Copenhagen; Internatl Epidemiology Inst, Rockville, Md; et al)

Am J Med 118:1428-1429, 2005   1–1

Background.—Angioedema develops in 0.1% to 0.2% of patients who receive angiotensin-converting enzyme (ACE) inhibitors and can be life-threatening. In angioedema, self-limited local swelling occurs in the deeper cutaneous and mucosal layers of various body areas. This is believed to result from increased concentrations of bradykinin, which is inactivated by ACE. Angiotensin receptor antagonists have no effect on bradykinin catabolism, so they have been viewed as carrying no increased risk of angioedema. However, some reports link angiotensin receptor antagonist therapy with angioedema. The relative risk of first-time hospitalization for angioedema for users of ACE inhibitors and angiotensin receptor antagonists was investigated.

Methods.—The study population was gathered from hospital discharge registries in 3 counties in Denmark. All patients had been hospitalized for the first time with nonhereditary angioedema. Ten control subjects matched for age, gender, and place of residence were chosen from the general population for each patient. The participants were divided into groups of ever users, current users, former users, and never users of ACE inhibitors, angiotensin receptor antagonists, and other drugs reportedly linked to angioedema.

Results.—Six hundred forty-one patients with angioedema and 6364 controls participated. The use of ACE inhibitors was associated with a high relative risk for angioedema, with an adjusted odds ratio (OR) of 10.2. New users had the highest risk (OR, 34.4); former users and patients with 2 to 4 or 5 or more prescriptions also had an increased risk. Patients currently using angiotensin receptor antagonists had no increased risk of angioedema, with an OR of 0.5.

Conclusions.—The use of ACE inhibitors was associated with an increased risk of angioedema that persisted long after use began. In contrast, the use of angiotensin receptor antagonists appeared to have no increased risk of angioedema. Further analysis is needed to completely rule out an increased risk of angioedema for new users of angiotensin receptor antagonists.

▶ The data presented by Johnsen et al provide a reminder that ACE inhibitors induce angioedema and that the risk persists even after long-term use.[1] However, the use of angiotensin receptor antagonists does not appear to be associated with an increased risk of angioedema.

B. H. Thiers, MD

Reference

1. Vleeming W, van Amsterdam JGC, Stricker BHC, et al: ACE inhibitor-induced angioedema. Incidence, prevention and management. *Drug Saf* 18:171-188, 1998.

Once-Daily Fexofenadine Treatment for Chronic Idiopathic Urticaria: A Multicenter, Randomized, Double-blind, Placebo-controlled Study
Kaplan AP, Spector SL, Meeves S, et al (Med Univ of South Carolina, Charleston; Cedars-Sinai Med Ctr, Los Angeles; Sanofi-Aventis Pharma, Bridgewater, NJ)
Ann Allergy Asthma Immunol 94:662-669, 2005   1–2

Background.—Chronic idiopathic urticaria (CIU) can have a profound effect on patients' health and quality of life.

Objective.—To evaluate the efficacy and safety of once-daily dosing of fexofenadine hydrochloride, 180 mg, on CIU.

Methods.—This randomized, double-blind, parallel-group, placebo-controlled study consisted of a placebo run-in period followed by a 4-week treatment period. Patients 12 years and older with active CIU were randomized 2:1 to receive once-daily fexofenadine, 180 mg, or placebo. The primary end points were change from baseline in mean daily number of wheals (MNW score) and mean daily severity of pruritus during treatment. Secondary efficacy measures included modified total symptom scores and MNW and pruritus severity scores evaluated weekly and instantaneously at trough drug levels.

Results.—Patients administered fexofenadine (n = 163) experienced significantly greater improvements in MNW and pruritus severity scores compared with the placebo group (n = 92) ($P < .001$ for both). Similarly, throughout treatment and at each individual week, the mean reductions in modified total symptom scores were significantly greater in the fexofenadine group ($P \leq .005$ for all comparisons vs placebo). The mean reductions in instantaneous MNW and pruritus severity scores were greater in patients in the fexofenadine group than in those who received placebo (MNW score: $P = .015$; pruritus severity score: $P < .001$). There were no significant differences in the frequency of treatment-emergent adverse events between the 2 treatment groups.

Conclusions.—A once-daily dose of fexofenadine hydrochloride, 180 mg, offered effective, well-tolerated relief for the management of CIU.

► I have found fexofenadine (Allegra) to be effective in the treatment of chronic urticaria, although rarely as monotherapy. More often, I tell patients to use it in the morning (because of its nonsedating properties) with the addition of doxepin or cetirizine at bedtime.

B. H. Thiers, MD

Evidence of a Role of Tumor Necrosis Factor α in Refractory Asthma
Berry MA, Hargadon B, Shelley M, et al (Univ Hosp of Leicester Natl Health Service Trust, England)
N Engl J Med 354:697-708, 2006   1–3

Background.—The development of tumor necrosis factor α (TNF-α) antagonists has made it feasible to investigate the role of this cytokine in refractory asthma.

Methods.—We measured markers of TNF-α activity on peripheral-blood monocytes in 10 patients with refractory asthma, 10 patients with mild-to-moderate asthma, and 10 control subjects. We also investigated the effects of treatment with the soluble TNF-α receptor etanercept (25 mg twice weekly) in the patients with refractory asthma in a placebo-controlled, double-blind, crossover pilot study.

Results.—As compared with patients with mild-to-moderate asthma and controls, patients with refractory asthma had increased expression of membrane-bound TNF-α, TNF-α receptor 1, and TNF-α–converting enzyme by peripheral-blood monocytes. In the clinical trial, as compared with placebo, 10 weeks of treatment with etanercept was associated with a significant increase in the concentration of methacholine required to provoke a 20 percent decrease in the forced expiratory volume in one second (FEV_1) (mean difference in doubling concentration changes between etanercept and placebo, 3.5; 95 percent confidence interval, 0.07 to 7.0; $P=0.05$), an improvement in the asthma-related quality-of-life score (by 0.85 point; 95 percent confidence interval, 0.16 to 1.54 on a 7-point scale; $P=0.02$), and a 0.32-liter increase in post-bronchodilator FEV_1 (95 percent confidence interval, 0.08 to 0.55; $P=0.01$).

Conclusions.—Patients with refractory asthma have evidence of upregulation of the TNF-α axis. (ClinicalTrials.gov number, NCT00276029.)

Tumour Necrosis Factor (TNFα) as a Novel Therapeutic Target in Symptomatic Corticosteroid Dependent Asthma

Howarth PH, Babu KS, Arshad HS, et al (Southampton Gen Hosp, England; St Mary's Hosp, Portsmouth, England; Wyeth Labs, Berkshire, England)
Thorax 60:1012-1018, 2005   1–4

Background.—Tumour necrosis factor α (TNFα) is a major therapeutic target in a range of chronic inflammatory disorders characterised by a Th1 type immune response in which TNFα is generated in excess. By contrast, asthma is regarded as a Th2 type disorder, especially when associated with atopy. However, as asthma becomes more severe and chronic, it adopts additional characteristics including corticosteroid refractoriness and involvement of neutrophils suggestive of an altered inflammatory profile towards a Th1 type response, incriminating cytokines such as TNFα.

Methods.—TNFα levels in bronchoalveolar lavage (BAL) fluid of 26 healthy controls, 42 subjects with mild asthma and 20 with severe asthma were measured by immunoassay, and TNFα gene expression was determined in endobronchial biopsy specimens from 14 patients with mild asthma and 14 with severe asthma. The cellular localisation of TNFα was assessed by immunohistochemistry. An open label uncontrolled clinical study was then undertaken in 17 subjects with severe asthma to evaluate the effect of 12 weeks of treatment with the soluble TNFα receptor-IgG$_1$Fc fusion protein, etanercept.

Results.—TNFα levels in BAL fluid, TNFα gene expression and TNFα immunoreative cells were increased in subjects with severe corticosteroid dependent asthma. Etanercept treatment was associated with improvement in asthma symptoms, lung function, and bronchial hyperresponsiveness.

Conclusions.—These findings may be of clinical significance in identifying TNFα as a new therapeutic target in subjects with severe asthma. The effects of anti-TNF treatment now require confirmation in placebo controlled studies.

▶ Unfortunately, no data exist to suggest that TNFα-targeted drugs are effective in related skin diseases such as atopic dermatitis or urticaria.

B. H. Thiers, MD

CD4⁺IL-13⁺ Cells in Peripheral Blood Well Correlates With the Severity of Atopic Dermatitis in Children

La Grutta S, Richiusa P, Pizzolanti G, et al (Children Hosp—ARNAS, Palermo, Italy; Università di Palermo, Italy; Università di Messina, Italy; et al)
Allergy 60:391-395, 2005   1–5

Background.—In atopic dermatitis (AD) a Th1/Th2 imbalance has been reported, and interleukin (IL)-13 seems to play a pivotal role in the inflammatory network. We tried to assess the correlation between the immunological marker D4⁺IL-13⁺ and the clinical phase of extrinsic AD in children.

Methods.—Twenty children with AD were studied. Assessed parameters were: clinical severity (SCORAD index), total serum immunoglobulin E (IgE), blood eosinophil count, and percentage of CD4$^+$ IFNγ$^+$, CD4$^+$ IL-4$^+$, CD4$^+$ IL-13$^+$ T cells. Determinations were carried out in the acute phase and after clinical remission were achieved. Ten nonatopic-matched children served as controls.

Results.—At baseline, AD was mild in 25%, moderate in 50% and severe in 25% of children. In the acute phase a significant relationship between the eosinophil count and the SCORAD index was found ($P = 0.0001$). Blood CD4$^+$ IL-4$^+$ were significantly higher in the AD group (median 17.0, range: 13.7–21.4) than in controls (12.6, 6.4–17.2, $P < 0.0001$). CD4$^+$ IL-13$^+$ cells in the AD group well correlated ($P = 0.0007$) with SCORAD index. At remission, a significant correlation between SCORAD index and eosinophil count was found ($P < 0.03$) and the percentage of CD4$^+$ IL-13$^+$ cells globally decreased (P 0.0001), while no difference was found among SCORAD classes.

Conclusion.—This study confirms the Th2 profile predominance in the peripheral blood of children with AD, and evidences close relationship between the number of CD4$^+$ IL-13$^+$ T cells and the disease's severity.

▶ Previous studies have provided strong evidence that atopic dermatitis is associated with increased production of Th2 cytokines, including IL-4 and IL-13, and that this correlates with disease severity. IL-13 mRNA expression has also been shown to be increased in acute AD lesional skin compared with the chronic disease. In the current study, 20 children with AD and evidence of hypersensitivity and 10 healthy nonatopic children were examined for their circulating T-lymphocyte profiles and cytokine expression. The results clearly showed that while there were no differences in percentages of CD4$^+$ IL-13$^+$ T cells (Th1) between patients and controls, there were highly significant increases in circulating CD4$^+$ IL-13$^+$ and IL-13$^+$ cells (Th2) in patients with acute AD. Furthermore, there was a dramatic correlation between the percentage of CD4$^+$ IL-13$^+$ cells and severity of the disease. The authors argue, justifiably, that these cells provide an excellent biomarker of AD, although they caution that CD4$^+$ IL-13$^+$ cell counts do not predict disease remission.

G. M. P. Galbraith, MD

CCL1-CCR8 Interactions: An Axis Mediating the Recruitment of T Cells and Langerhans-Type Dendritic Cells to Sites of Atopic Skin Inflammation

Gombert M, Dieu-Nosjean M-C, Winterberg F, et al (Heinrich-Heine Universitäat Düsseldorf, Germany; Centre de Recherches Biomédicales des Cordeliers, Paris; Helsinki Univ; et al)

J Immunol 174:5082-5091, 2005   1–6

Introduction.—Atopic dermatitis represents a chronically relapsing skin disease with a steadily increasing prevalence of 10–20% in children. Skin-infiltrating T cells, dendritic cells (DC), and mast cells are thought to play a crucial role in its pathogenesis. We report that the expression of the CC chemokine CCL1 (*I-309*) is significantly and selectively up-regulated in atopic dermatitis in comparison to psoriasis, cutaneous lupus erythematosus, or normal skin. CCL1 serum levels of atopic dermatitis patients are significantly higher than levels in healthy individuals. DC, mast cells, and dermal endothelial cells are abundant sources of CCL1 during atopic skin inflammation and allergen challenge, and *Staphylococcus aureus*-derived products induce its production. In vitro, binding and cross-linking of IgE on mast cells resulted in a significant up-regulation of this inflammatory chemokine. Its specific receptor, CCR8, is expressed on a small subset of circulating T cells and is abundantly expressed on interstitial DC, Langerhans cells generated in vitro, and their monocytic precursors. Although DC maintain their CCR8[+] status during maturation, brief activation of circulating T cells recruits CCR8 from intracytoplasmic stores to the cell surface. Moreover, the inflammatory and atopy-associated chemokine CCL1 synergizes with the homeostatic chemokine CXCL12 (*SDF-1α*) resulting in the recruitment of T cell and Langerhans cell-like DC. Taken together, these findings suggest that the axis CCL1-CCR8 links adaptive and innate immune functions that play a role in the initiation and amplification of atopic skin inflammation.

CCL18 Is Expressed in Atopic Dermatitis and Mediates Skin Homing of Human Memory T Cells

Günther C, Bello-Fernandez C, Kopp T, et al (Novartis Insts for Biomedical Research, Vienna; Vienna Internatl Research Cooperation Ctr; Vienna Med Univ)
J Immunol 174:1723-1728, 2005 1–7

Introduction.—CCL18 is a human chemokine secreted by monocytes and dendritic cells. The receptor for CCL18 is not yet known and the functions of this chemokine on immune cells are not fully elucidated. In this study, we describe that CCL18 is present in skin biopsies of atopic dermatitis (AD) patients but not in normal or psoriatic skin. CCL18 was specifically expressed by APCs in the dermis and by Langerhans and inflammatory dendritic epidermal cells in the epidermis. In addition, the serum levels of CCL18 and the percentages of CCL18-producing monocyte/macrophages and dendritic cells were significantly increased in AD patients compared with healthy controls. Furthermore, we demonstrate that CCL18 binds to CLA [+] T cells in peripheral blood of AD patients and healthy individuals and induces migration of AD-derived memory T cells in vitro and in human skin-transplanted SCID mice. These findings highlight a unique role of CCL18 in AD and reveal a novel function of this chemokine mediating skin homing of a subpopulation of human memory T cells.

▶ These 2 studies (Abstracts 1–6 and 1–7) investigated the expression of human chemokines and their role in T-lymphocyte recruitment in AD. Gombert et al (Abstract 1–6) reported that chemokine CCL1 mRNA expression was significantly increased in lesions of AD compared with normal skin, and that the CCL1 protein was readily detectable in the basal layer of the epidermis, epidermal endothelial cells, and dendritic cells of AD lesions but undetectable in normal or nonlesional skin. Furthermore, CCR8, which is the receptor for CCL1, was expressed by a significantly increased number of leukocytes infiltrating AD lesional skin compared with control subjects. Further studies showed that CCL1 protein production was increased by AD Langerhans cells activated by bacterial products such as lipopolysaccharide, and that challenge of AD patients with specific allergen resulted in increased CCL1 mRNA and protein expression in lesional skin. Serum levels of CCL1 were also found to be significantly increased in AD patients compared with control subjects.

In the second investigation (Abstract 1–7), Günther et al examined the expression of a less well characterized chemokine, CCL18, in patients with AD. They clearly demonstrated that this chemokine was detectable in association primarily with Langerhans cells in AD lesional skin and was undetectable in normal or psoriatic skin. Furthermore, CCL18 was found to be expressed by a strikingly increased percentage of circulating monocytic cells from patients with AD, and serum levels of the protein were also significantly increased in AD patients when compared with control subjects. The receptor for this chemokine has yet to be identified; however, these investigators showed that CCL18 bound to peripheral blood memory T lymphocytes in patients with AD and that this binding was significantly greater than in cells of healthy individuals. Experiments using in vitro T-cell migration assays and a SCID mouse model showed that memory T cells derived from patients with AD migrated in response to CCL18.

These 2 studies illustrate the complexity of the mechanisms underlying the pathogenesis of AD and the roles played by various immunoactive factors in this disease. Currently, it merely seems safe to say that multifactorial elements are at play.

G. M. P. Galbraith, MD

Increased Expression and a Potential Anti-inflammatory Role of TRAIL in Atopic Dermatitis
Vassina E, Leverkus M, Yousefi S, et al (Univ of Bern, Switzerland; Otto-von-Guericke Univ Magdeburg, Germany)
J Invest Dermatol 125:746-752, 2005   1–8

Introduction.—The tumor necrosis factor-related apoptosis-inducing ligand (TRAIL) induces apoptosis of many transformed but also of non-transformed cells. In addition, TRAIL receptor activation has been reported to activate non-apoptotic signaling pathways. Here, we report an increased expression of TRAIL in peripheral blood T cells and monocytes from patients with atopic dermatitis (AD) compared with control individuals. High TRAIL expression was also observed in skin-infiltrating T cells of AD patients. Topical tacrolimus treatment reduced the total number of T cells in the skin, but the relative proportion of TRAIL-positive cells within both

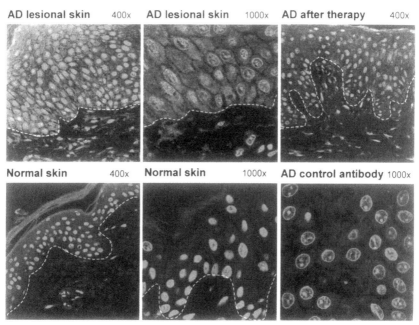

FIGURE 3.—Representative immunofluorescence stainings of interleukin-1 receptor antagonist (IL-1Ra) in the skin. Staining with an anti-IL-1Ra Ab reveals strong positive cells throughout the epidermis of lesional AD skin. Nuclei were counterstained with propidium iodide. After treatment, few keratinocytes in the suprabasal layers stained weakly positive. Weak staining was also observed in normal skin. The white dashed line indicates the border between the epidermis and the dermis. The original magnification is indicated in each panel. (Courtesy of Vassina E, Leverkus M, Yousefi S, et al: Increased expression and a potential anti-inflammatory role of TRAIL in atopic dermatitis. *J Invest Dermatol* 125:746-752, 2005. Reprinted by permission of Blackwell Publishing.)

CD4+ and CD8+ cell populations did not change. TRAIL was demonstrated to induce the expression of interleukin-1 receptor antagonist (IL-1Ra) in keratinocytes in a caspase-independent manner *in vitro*. Moreover, increased expression of IL-1Ra was observed in keratinocytes of AD lesional skin. These data suggest that TRAIL-expressing inflammatory skin cells may contribute to the epidermal activation of the IL-1Ra gene in AD (Fig 3; see color plate VII).

▶ TRAIL has received much attention as a biologic modulator. It appears to play an important role in tumor immunology and has immunoregulatory activities, including antiinflammatory effects. In this interesting study, the authors examined the expression of TRAIL in cells of 10 patients with moderate to severe AD and 9 healthy control individuals. The results showed significantly increased membrane expression in circulating leukocytes in AD, including monocytes and both CD4+ and CD8+ T cells, as well as in infiltrating T cells in lesional skin. The investigators were also interested in any possible correlation between TRAIL expression in AD and production of IL-1Ra, an intrinsic regulator of inflammation. Their studies clearly demonstrated an increased expression of IL-1Ra by epidermal keratinocytes in lesional skin of patients with AD.

Further studies of a keratinocyte cell line showed that TRAIL stimulation of these cells resulted in a 2- to 3-fold increase in IL-1Ra mRNA expression, with an up to 10-fold increase in the protein production. This effect was abrogated by pretreatment with a TRAIL-R2-Fc construct that inhibits TRAIL. Together, these data provide a novel insight into possible intrinsic inflammation control mechanisms in AD.

G. M. P. Galbraith, MD

Risk Factors for Atopic Dermatitis in New Zealand Children at 3.5 Years of Age
Purvis D, Thompson JMD, Clark PM, et al (Univ of Auckland, New Zealand)
Br J Dermatol 152:742-749, 2005   1–9

Background.—The prevalence of atopic dermatitis (AD) is increasing in Western societies. The hygiene hypothesis proposes that this is due to reduced exposure to environmental allergens and infections during early life.

Objectives.—To examine factors associated with a diagnosis of AD at 3.5 years of age, especially those factors implicated by the hygiene hypothesis.

Methods.—The Auckland Birthweight Collaborative study is a case-control study of risk factors for small for gestational age babies. Cases were born at term with birthweight $\leq$ 10th centile; controls were appropriate for gestational age, with birthweight > 10th centile. The infants were assessed at birth, 1 year and 3.5 years of age. Data were collected by parental interview and examination of the child. AD was defined as the presence of an itchy rash in the past 12 months with three or more of the following: history of flexural involvement; history of generally dry skin; history of atopic disease in parents or siblings; and visible flexural dermatitis as per photographic protocol. Statistical analyses took into account the disproportionate sampling of the study population.

Results.—Analysis was restricted to European subjects. Eight hundred and seventy-one children were enrolled at birth, 744 (85.4%) participated at 1 year, and 550 (63.2%) at 3.5 years. AD was diagnosed in 87 (15.8%) children seen at 3.5 years. The prevalence of AD did not differ by birthweight. AD at 3.5 years was associated with raised serum IgE > 200 kU L^{-1}, and wheezing, asthma, rash or eczema at 1 year. In multivariate analysis, adjusted for parental atopy and breastfeeding, AD at 3.5 years was associated with atopic disease in the parents: maternal atopy only, adjusted odds ratio (OR) 3.83, 95% confidence interval (CI) 1.20-12.23; paternal atopy only, adjusted OR 3.59, 95% CI 1.09-11.75; both parents atopic, adjusted OR 6.12, 95% CI 2.02-18.50. There was a higher risk of AD with longer duration of breastfeeding: < 6 months, adjusted OR 6.13, 95% CI 1.45-25.86; $\geq$ 6 months, adjusted OR 9.70, 95% CI 2.47-38.15 compared with never breastfed. These findings remained significant after adjusting for environmental factors and a personal history of atopy. AD at 3.5 years was associated with owning a cat at 3.5 years (adjusted OR 0.45, 95% CI 0.21-0.97) but not with owning a dog at 3.5 years, pets at 1 year, nor with older siblings.

Furthermore, AD at 3.5 years was not associated with gender, socioeconomic status, maternal smoking, parity, damp, mould, immunizations, body mass index or antibiotic use in first year of life.

Conclusions.—A personal and a parental history of atopic disease are risk factors for AD at 3.5 years. Duration of breastfeeding was associated with an increased risk of AD. No association was found with those factors implicated by the hygiene hypothesis. This study suggests that breastfeeding should not be recommended for the prevention of AD.

▶ Studies designed to assess factors that influence the development of AD in children continue to show conflicting results. In this investigation of 871 children of European ancestry born in New Zealand, 63% of whom were followed up for 3.5 years, parental history of atopic disease appears to be a major risk factor. A longer duration of breastfeeding was associated with an increased risk of AD. The authors point out that studies that find breastfeeding protective generally have looked at atopy during the first few years of life, whereas those finding no protective effect tend to look at the incidence of AD and other atopic disease in later childhood. It may be that if breastfeeding is protective, its effect is short lived and does not prevent expression of atopy in older children.

S. Raimer, MD

Atopic Dermatitis and the 'Hygiene Hypothesis': Too Clean to Be True?
Flohr C, Pascoe D, Williams HC (Univ of Nottingham, England; Univ of North Carolina, Chapel Hill)
Br J Dermatol 152:202-216, 2005   1–10

Background.—The so-called 'hygiene hypothesis' postulates an inverse relationship between atopic dermatitis (AD) and an environment that leads to increased pathogen exposure.

Objectives.—We sought to systematically identify, summarize and critically appraise: (i) the epidemiological evidence to suggest that environmental exposures that lead to an increase in microbial burden reduce the risk of AD; (ii) whether any specific infections have been shown to reduce AD risk; (iii) whether there is a link between immunizations, use of antibiotics and AD risk; and (iv) to comment on the new therapeutic approaches in AD that have evolved out of the 'hygiene hypothesis'.

Methods.—We searched Medline from 1966 until August 2004 to identify relevant studies for inclusion. Differences in study design and populations did not allow formal meta-analysis. Studies were therefore described qualitatively.

Results.—We identified 64 studies that were relevant to our review, 27 (42%) of which were of prospective design. There was prospective evidence to support an inverse relationship between AD and endotoxins, early day care and animal exposure. Two well-designed cohort studies have found a positive association between infections in early life and AD, and measles vaccination and AD. Antibiotic use was consistently associated with an increase in AD risk even into the antenatal period, although a few studies did not reach conventional statistical significance. A few small randomized controlled trials have suggested that probiotics can reduce AD severity and that probiotics may also be able to prevent AD to some degree.

Conclusions.—Although population-based studies have suggested a consistent inverse relationship between AD and increasing family size, this does not seem to be explained by a straightforward increased exposure to a single environmental pathogen. The effect seen with early day care, endotoxin and animal exposure may be due to a nonpathogenic microbial stimulus of a chronic or recurrent nature. This would also explain the risk increase associated with antibiotic use. Caution should prevail in the prescribing of antibiotics early in life, especially in children with a family history of AD. Larger well-designed pragmatic trials on probiotics and the prevention and treatment of AD are now needed to inform whether such interventions should be used in routine clinical practice.

▶ A number of articles reviewed in recent issues of the YEAR BOOK OF DERMATOLOGY AND DERMATOLOGIC SURGERY have examined the possible protective effect of microbial stimulation early in life on the eventual development of AD. The possible preventive effect of probiotics has also been discussed, although this approach may not be totally risk free.[1,2] As stated by Flohr et al, the validity of the "hygiene hypothesis" remains uncertain.

B. H. Thiers, MD

References

1. Matricardi PM, for the EAACI Task Force 7: Position paper: Microbial products in allergy prevention and therapy. *Allergy* 68:461-471, 2003.
2. Murch SH: Toll of allergy reduced by probiotics. *Lancet* 357:1057-1059, 2001.

Worm Infestation and the Negative Association With Eczema (Atopic/Nonatopic) and Allergic Sensitization

Schäfer T, Meyer T, Ring J, et al (Med Univ Lübeck, Germany; Univ Munich)
Allergy 60:1014-1020, 2005   1–11

Background.—Worm infestations may play a role in preventing allergies. There is a lack of epidemiological information from Western countries on the association between worm infestation and eczema.

Objective.—To investigate the association between worm infestation and eczema in a proper temporal sequence and under consideration of allergic sensitization.

Methods.—Two surveys were performed in East German school children. Questionnaire data included the history of eczema and worm infestation and their time of onset. Specific IgE antibodies to five common aeroallergens were measured and used to define nonatopic and atopic eczema. Logistic regression analyses were performed to control for relevant confounders (age, sex, parental school education and history of allergies). In order to confirm the findings a corresponding conditional regression analysis was applied on cases and controls matched by age and sex.

Results.—A total of 4169 children participated (response 75 and 76%) who were, on average, 9.2 years old (47% girls). Overall 17.0% reported a prior worm infestation (Ascaris 44%, Oxyuris 33%) and 18.1% had a history of eczema. Eczema occurred significantly less frequent in children who had a worm infestation (prior to the onset of eczema) compared with children without such a history (8.1% *vs* 16.5%, OR_{adj}: 0.45, 95% CI: 0.33-0.60). The finding was confirmed by the corresponding matched case-control analysis (OR_{adj}: 0.57, 95% CI: 0.41-0.79). Atopic eczema was affected more by a prior worm infestation (OR_{adj}: 0.31, 95% CI: 0.18-0.56) than the nonatopic eczema (OR_{adj}: 0.58, 95% CI: 0.40-0.84). A total of 29.1% exhibited specific IgE antibodies to at least one aeroallergen. Sensitized children gave significantly less frequent a history of worm infestation (14.2% *vs* 18.3%, OR_{adj}: 0.74, 95% CI: 0.60-0.92). Stratified analysis revealed that this effect most pronounced for a sensitization to house dust mite.

Conclusions.—A worm infestation is associated with a reduced frequency of subsequent eczema, especially the atopic type. Furthermore allergic sensitization, especially to house dust mite, and worm infestation are negatively associated. The data support the concept that a lack of immune-stimulation by parasitic infections contributes to the development of allergies.

▶ This is yet another small piece of evidence supporting the "hygiene hypothesis," which has been discussed in many articles previously reviewed in the YEAR BOOK OF DERMATOLOGY AND DERMATOLOGIC SURGERY. The "hygiene hypothesis" states that reduced immune stimulation by infections (as a consequence of improved sanitation, antibiotic use, and lifestyle factors) has contributed to the increasing prevalence of atopic dermatitis. In this large population-based study, Schäfer et al show that worm infestation is negatively associated with subsequent eczema, especially in atopic individuals.

B. H. Thiers, MD

Probiotics in the Treatment of Atopic Eczema/Dermatitis Syndrome in Infants: A Double-blind Placebo-controlled Trial
Viljanen M, Savilahti E, Haahtela T, et al (Univ of Helsinki; Valio Research and Development, Helsinki; STAT-Consulting, Tampere, Finland)
Allergy 60:494-500, 2005   1–12

Background.—Probiotic bacteria are suggested to reduce symptoms of the atopic eczema/dermatitis syndrome (AEDS) in food-allergic infants. We aimed to investigate whether probiotic bacteria have any beneficial effect on AEDS.

Methods.—Follow-up of severity of AEDS by the Severity Scoring of Atopic Dermatitis (SCORAD) index in 230 infants with suspected cow's milk allergy (CMA) receiving, in a randomized double-blinded manner, concomitant with elimination diet and skin treatment, *Lactobacillus* GG (LGG), a mixture of four probiotic strains, or placebo for 4 weeks. Four weeks after the treatment, CMA was diagnosed with a double-blind placebo-controlled (DBPC) milk challenge in 120 infants.

Results.—In the whole group, mean SCORAD (at baseline 32.5) decreased by 65%, but with no differences between treatment groups immediately or 4 weeks after the treatment. No treatment differences were observed in infants with CMA either. In IgE-sensitized infants, however, the LGG group showed a greater reduction in SCORAD than did the placebo group, -26.1 vs -19.8 ($P = 0.036$), from baseline to 4 weeks after the treatment. Exclusion of infants who had received antibiotics during the study reinforced the findings in the IgE-sensitized subgroup.

Conclusion.—Treatment with LGG may alleviate AEDS symptoms in IgE-sensitized infants but not in non-IgE-sensitized infants.

▶ In this study, 230 infants with atopic dermatitis were placed on a cow's milk elimination diet and also treated topically. They then were randomly assigned to receive LGG, a combination of 4 probiotic strains of bacteria (including LGG), or placebo for 4 weeks. Only IgE-sensitized infants, which the authors defined as any infant with positive skin prick test results or significant antigen-specific IgE concentrations to any antigen tested, showed more improvement than those receiving placebo. In this study, a benefit occurred in infants treated with LGG alone, but a benefit was not seen in the group in which LGG was combined with other probiotic strains; the maximum improvement in the LGG group was not noted until 4 weeks after the treatment period. The observed improvement may have resulted from increased serum IL-10 concentrations. In a previous study,[1] an increase in the IL-10 concentration was shown to occur 4 weeks after LGG treatment but not immediately. Further studies are needed to explore strain-specific effects of various probiotic bacteria on atopic dermatitis.

S. Raimer, MD

Reference

1. Pessi T, Sütas Y, Hurme M, et al: Interleukin-10 generation in atopic children following oral *Lactobacillus rhamnosus* GG. *Clin Exp Allergy* 30:1804-1808, 2000.

Effects of Probiotics on Atopic Dermatitis: A Randomised Controlled Trial
Weston S, Halbert A, Richmond P, et al (Univ of Western Australia, Perth; Princess Margaret Hosp for Children, Perth, Australia)
Arch Dis Child 90:892-897, 2005   1–13

Background.—The aim of the study was to investigate the effects of probiotics on moderate or severe atopic dermatitis (AD) in young children.

Methods.—Fifty six children aged 6-18 months with moderate or severe AD were recruited into a randomised double blind placebo controlled trial in Perth, Western Australia; 53 children completed the study. The children were given a probiotic (1 × 10⁹ *Lactobacillus fermentum* VRI-033 PCC; Probiomics) or an equivalent volume of placebo, twice daily for 8 weeks. A final assessment at 16 weeks was performed.

Results.—The main outcome measures were severity and extent of AD at the end of the study, as measured by the Severity Scoring of Atopic Dermatitis (SCORAD) index. The reduction in the SCORAD index over time was significant in the probiotic group (p = 0.03) but not the placebo group. Significantly more children receiving probiotics (n = 24, 92%) had a SCORAD index that was better than baseline at week 16 compared with the placebo group (n = 17, 63%) (p = 0.01). At the completion of the study more children in the probiotic group had mild AD (n = 14, 54%) compared to the placebo group (n = 8, 30%).

Conclusion.—Supplementation with probiotic *L fermentum* VRI-003 PCC is beneficial in improving the extent and severity of AD in young children with moderate or severe disease.

▶ In this relatively small study of 53 children aged 6 to 18 months with moderate to severe AD, administration of a probiotic (*L fermentum* VRI-033 PCC) resulted in significant improvement in the treated group versus the control group. This improvement persisted 2 months after treatment was completed. No adverse effects were reported. It is likely that some strains of bacteria considered to be probiotics will prove to be more effective than others, but perhaps it is time for the administration of probiotics to be more routine in the treatment of AD.

S. Raimer, MD

Deficiency of Dermcidin-Derived Antimicrobial Peptides in Sweat of Patients With Atopic Dermatitis Correlates With an Impaired Innate Defense of Human Skin In Vivo
Rieg S, Steffen H, Seeber S, et al (Eberhard Karls Univ, Tubingen, Germany; Friedrich Alexander Univ, Erlangen-Nurnberg, Germany)
J Immunol 174:8003-8010, 2005   1–14

Introduction.—Antimicrobial peptides are an integral part of the epithelial innate defense system. Dermcidin (DCD) is a recently discovered antimicrobial peptide with a broad spectrum of activity. It is constitutively expressed in human eccrine sweat glands and secreted into sweat. Patients with atopic dermatitis (AD) have recurrent bacterial or viral skin infections and pronounced colonization with *Staphylococcus aureus*. We hypothesized that patients with AD have a reduced amount of DCD peptides in sweat contributing to the compromised constitutive innate skin defense. Therefore, we performed semiquantitative and quantitative analyses of DCD peptides in sweat of AD patients and healthy subjects using surface-enhanced laser desorption ionization time-of-flight mass spectrometry and ELISA. The data indicate that the amount of several DCD-derived peptides in sweat of patients with AD is significantly reduced. Furthermore, compared with atopic patients without previous infectious complications, AD patients with a history of bacterial and viral skin infections were found to have significantly less DCD-1 and DCD-1L in their sweat. To analyze whether the reduced amount of DCD in sweat of AD patients correlates with a decreased innate defense, we determined the antimicrobial activity of sweat in vivo. We showed that in healthy subjects, sweating leads to a reduction of viable bacteria on the skin surface, but this does not occur in patients with AD. These data indicate that reduced expression of DCD in sweat of patients with AD may contribute to the high susceptibility of these patients to skin infections and altered skin colonization.

▶ The authors found that the sweat of patients with AD contained less DCD-derived peptides compared with those of the sweat of healthy individuals. The decreased DCD expression correlated with clinical infectious complications. They therefore concluded that DCD deficiency might contribute to the altered skin colonization noted in AD patients and to their propensity to recurrent bacterial and viral skin infections.

B. H. Thiers, MD

Topical Corticosteroids for Atopic Eczema: Clinical and Cost Effectiveness of Once-Daily vs. More Frequent Use
Green C, Colquitt JL, Kirby J, et al (Univ of Southamptom, England)
Br J Dermatol 152:130-141, 2005   1–15

Background.—Topical corticosteroids remain the mainstay of treatment for atopic eczema, yet there is uncertainty over the frequency of their use in terms of clinical and cost effectiveness.

Objectives.—To assess the clinical and cost effectiveness of once-daily vs. more frequent use of same-potency topical corticosteroids in atopic eczema.

Methods.—A systematic review of the clinical and cost-effectiveness literature was undertaken, together with a cost-minimization analysis.

Results.—The review identified a sparse literature, comprising one previous systematic review and 10 randomized controlled trials (RCTs). No published cost-effectiveness studies were identified. RCTs were focused on potent topical corticosteroids (eight RCTs), with no trials (RCTs/controlled clinical trials) identified on mild potency products. There was broad heterogeneity in trial methods, and therefore we considered outcomes according to: (i) at least a good response or 50% improvement, and (ii) eczema rated as cleared or controlled. Studies found little difference between once-daily and more frequent use of topical corticosteroids. The literature on moderately potent and potent corticosteroids offered no basis for favouring once-daily or more frequent use, although some significant differences favouring twice-daily treatment were identified. One RCT on very potent products favoured three times daily use on the basis of clinical response, but reported no difference in the numbers with at least a good response. Given the similar outcomes seen in clinical effectiveness a cost-minimization approach was adopted to consider cost effectiveness, in order to identify the least-cost option. However, cost-minimization analysis proved complex due to wide variations in product price, with the relative cost of product comparisons by frequency proving the most important factor in determining the least-cost alternative.

Conclusions.—This review has not identified any clear differences in outcomes between once-daily and more frequent application of topical corticosteroids. We would encourage prescribing clinicians to consider the once-daily use of topical corticosteroids when making treatment decisions for patients with atopic eczema. However, we find that the literature on clinical effectiveness is limited and a broader understanding of compliance and phobia associated with topical steroids is needed to inform on this issue.

▶ Many older, less-potent topical corticosteroids came to market with package inserts recommending application 3 or even 4 times each day. The newer, more-potent preparations are usually applied once or twice daily. I have always been quite skeptical that application of any corticosteroid more than twice daily confers additional benefit.

Once a product is approved for sale, the manufacturer generally is locked into recommending a specific prescribing frequency based on the structure of the requisite clinical trials and the instructions in the Food and Drug Administration–approved package insert. There is little incentive (and perhaps a disincentive) to set aside additional funds to document that a product can be used less often with similar efficacy.

B. H. Thiers, MD

Pharmacokinetics of Topical Calcineurin Inhibitors in Adult Atopic Dermatitis: A Randomized, Investigator-Blind Comparison

Draelos Z, Nayak A, Pariser D, et al (Dermatology Consulting Services, High Point, NC; Sneeze, Wheeze, and Itch Associates LLC, Normal, Ill; Eastern Virginia Med School, Norfolk; et al)
J Am Acad Dermatol 53:602-609, 2005   1–16

Objective.—We sought to compare pharmacokinetics of pimecrolimus cream 1% and tacrolimus ointment 0.1% in adults with extensive, moderate to severe atopic dermatitis. Secondary end points included efficacy and safety.

Methods.—Patients received twice-daily treatment for 13 days. Blood concentrations of pimecrolimus and tacrolimus were measured at days 1, 5, and 13. Treatment success was defined as an Investigators' Global Assessment score of 0 (clear) or 1 (almost clear).

Results.—Tacrolimus was detectable in 36% of blood samples and pimecrolimus was detectable in 12%. In patients with measurable blood drug concentrations, systemic exposure to tacrolimus (mean area under the curve$_{0-10h} < 9.7$ ng·h/mL; $n = 7$) was higher than to pimecrolimus (mean area under the curve$_{0\text{-}10h}$ < 2.5 ng·h/mL; n = 2). Whole-body treatment success (day 13) was achieved in 1 of 18 (5.6%) and 2 of 19 (10.5%) patients treated with pimecrolimus and tacrolimus, respectively, and face/neck treatment success in 5 of 18 (27.8%) and 5 of 19 (26.3%) patients, respectively. Patients included in the study were adult patients with severe atopic dermatitis. The results and conclusions drawn from this study population may not be applicable for the majority of patients with atopic dermatitis who have mild to moderate disease.

Conclusion.—Pimecrolimus appears to be associated with lower systemic drug exposure than tacrolimus.

Low Systemic Absorption and Good Tolerability of Pimecrolimus, Administered as 1% Cream (Elidel®) in Infants With Atopic Dermatitis—A Multicenter, 3-Week, Open-Label Study

Staab D, Pariser D, Gottlieb AB, et al (Charité Campus Virchow, Berlin; Eastern Virginia Med School, Norfolk; UMDNJ-Robert Wood Johnson Med School, New Brunswick, NJ; et al)

Pediatr Dermatol 22:465-471, 2005   1–17

Introduction.—Pimecrolimus cream 1%, a nonsteroid inhibitor of inflammatory cytokines, offers an alternative to corticosteroids in the treatment of atopic dermatitis. Here we evaluate pimecrolimus blood concentrations and tolerability to pimecrolimus cream 1% in 22 infants below 2 years of age with atopic dermatitis (10–92% body surface area affected at baseline). Efficacy was assessed as a secondary objective. Pimecrolimus cream 1% was applied twice daily for 3 weeks. Blood concentrations were low, typically (96% of total 100 concentrations measured) below 2 ng/mL, the majority (71%) remaining below 0.5 ng/mL. The highest concentration observed was 2.26 ng/mL. At steady state, there was no indication of accumulation. Pimecrolimus was well tolerated locally and systemically, with no serious adverse events recorded. Most adverse events recorded (35 in 17/22 patients) were typical of the young pediatric population studied, of mild to moderate severity, and not considered to be study-medication related, with the exception of four local adverse effects limited to the site of cream application. No clinically relevant change was observed in physical examination, vital signs, or laboratory safety parameters. A rapid onset of therapeutic effect was observed within the first four days of treatment. Pimecrolimus cream 1% is well tolerated in infants 3 to 23 months of age treated for 3 weeks, and results in minimal systemic exposure.

▶ Staab et al studied 22 infants aged 3 to 23 months who were treated twice daily for 3 weeks with 1% pimecrolimus cream. Serum concentrations of drug measured on days 1, 10, and 22 remained low in all infants. One infant developed a staphylococcal infection classified as severe. Pimecrolimus is a valuable medication for treating the face of infants with eczema, where extended use of topical corticosteroids is undesirable. There is no evidence at the present time that limited use of pimecrolimus is unsafe in infants.

S. Raimer, MD

Efficacy and Tolerability of Topical Pimecrolimus and Tacrolimus in the Treatment of Atopic Dermatitis: Meta-analysis of Randomised Controlled Trials

Ashcroft DM, Dimmock P, Garside R, et al (Univ of Manchester, England)
BMJ 330:516-522, 2005   1–18

Objective.—To determine the efficacy and tolerability of topical pimecrolimus and tacrolimus compared with other treatments for atopic dermatitis.

Design.—Systematic review and meta-analysis.

Data Sources.—Electronic searches of the Cochrane Library, Medline, and Embase.

Study Selection.—Randomised controlled trials of topical pimecrolimus or tacrolimus reporting efficacy outcomes or tolerability.

Data Extraction.—Efficacy: investigators' global assessment of response; patients' global assessment of response; proportions of patients with flares of atopic dermatitis; and improvements in quality of life. Tolerability: overall rates of withdrawal; withdrawal due to adverse events; and proportions of patients with burning of the skin and skin infections.

Data Synthesis.—4186 of 6897 participants in 25 randomised controlled trials received pimecrolimus or tacrolimus. Both drugs were significantly more effective than a vehicle control. Tacrolimus 0.1% was as effective as potent topical corticosteroids at three weeks and more effective than combined treatment with hydrocortisone butyrate 0.1% (potent used on trunk) plus hydrocortisone acetate 1% (weak used on face) at 12 weeks (number needed to treat (NNT) = 6). Tacrolimus 0.1% was also more effective than hydrocortisone acetate 1% (NNT = 4). In comparison, tacrolimus 0.03% was more effective than hydrocortisone acetate 1% (NNT = 5) but less effective than hydrocortisone butyrate 0.1% (NNT = −8). Direct comparisons of tacrolimus 0.03% and tacrolimus 0.1% consistently favoured the higher strength formulation, but efficacy differed significantly between the two strengths only after 12 weeks' treatment (rate ratio 0.80, 95% confidence interval 0.65 to 0.99). Pimecrolimus was far less effective than betamethasone valerate 0.1% (NNT = −3 at three weeks). Pimecrolimus and tacrolimus caused significantly more skin burning than topical corticosteroids. Rates of skin infections in any of the comparisons did not differ.

Conclusions.—Both topical pimecrolimus and topical tacrolimus are more effective than placebo treatments for atopic dermatitis, but in the absence of studies that show long term safety gains, any advantage over topical corticosteroids is unclear. Topical tacrolimus is similar to potent topical corticosteroids and may have a place for long term use in patients with resistant atopic dermatitis on sites where side effects from topical corticosteroids might develop quickly. In the absence of key comparisons with mild corticosteroids, the clinical need for topical pimecrolimus is unclear. The usefulness of either treatment in patients who have failed to respond adequately to topical corticosteroids is also unclear.

Tacrolimus Ointment Is More Effective Than Pimecrolimus Cream With a Similar Safety Profile in the Treatment of Atopic Dermatitis: Results From 3 Randomized, Comparative Studies

Paller AS, Lebwohl M, Fleischer AB Jr, et al (Northwestern Univ, Chicago; Mount Sinai School of Medicine, Winston-Salem, NC; Yale Univ, New Haven, Conn; et al)
J Am Acad Dermatol 52:810-822, 2005   1–19

Objective.—To compare the efficacy and safety of tacrolimus ointment and pimecrolimus cream in adult and pediatric patients with mild to very severe atopic dermatitis (AD).

Methods.—One thousand and sixty-five patients were randomized to treatment in 3 multicenter, randomized, investigator-blinded, 6-week studies.

Results.—Based on the Eczema Area Severity Index (EASI), tacrolimus ointment was more effective than pimecrolimus cream at the end of the study in adults (54.1% vs. 34.9%, respectively; $P < .0001$), in children with moderate/severe disease (67.2% vs. 56.4%, respectively; $P = .04$), in the combined analysis (52.8% vs. 39.1%, respectively; $P < .0001$), and at week 1 in children with mild disease (39.2% vs. 31.2%, respectively; $P = .04$). Tacrolimus was also more effective than pimecrolimus based on the Investigator Global AD Assessment (IGADA), improvement in percentage of total body surface area affected, and improvement in itch scores ($P \leq .05$), with a faster onset of action. There was no significant difference in the incidence of adverse events (AEs), including application site reactions in the 2 studies involving 650 children. Adults treated with tacrolimus experienced a greater number of local application site reactions on day 1; both groups reported a similar incidence of application site reactions thereafter. More pimecrolimus-treated patients than tacrolimus-treated patients withdrew from the studies because of a lack of efficacy ($P \leq .03$) or adverse events ($P = .002$; pediatric mild).

Conclusion.—Tacrolimus ointment is more effective and has a faster onset of action than pimecrolimus cream in adults and children with AD; their safety profiles are similar.

▶ Both of these studies (Abstracts 1–18 and 1–19) indicate that tacrolimus is more effective than pimecrolimus for the treatment of AD, particularly for patients with moderate or severe disease. The meta-analysis done by Ashcroft et al (Abstract 1–18) questions any advantage of topical calcineurin inhibitors over topical corticosteroids. Although in many situations, topical corticosteroids should be considered first-line therapy, the topical calcineurin inhibitors would seem to offer a clear advantage for treating persistent facial or intertriginous lesions, locations where atrophy from topical corticosteroids and/or increased absorption are of concern, or when long-term generalized treatment with topical corticosteroids suggest the potential for systemic adrenal suppression.

S. Raimer, MD

Review of the Potential Photo-Cocarcinogenicity of Topical Calcineurin Inhibitors: Position Statement of the European Dermatology Forum
Ring J, Barker J, Behrendt H, et al (Technische Universität München, Germany; St Thomas' Hosp, London; Inselspital Bern, Switzerland; et al)
J Eur Acad Dermatol Venereol 19:663-671, 2005   1–20

Introduction.—Topical Calcineurin Inhibitors (TCIs) used for the treatment of atopic eczema modify the immune regulatory function of the skin and may have the potential to enhance immunosuppressive ultraviolet (UV) effects. Current recommendations on UV protection in eczema patients treated with PCIs are inconsistent and have given rise to uncertainty and anxiety in patients. Therefore, the European Dermatology Forum (EDF) developed a position statement which reviews critically the available data with regard to the problem, especially analysing and commenting the limitations of rodent models for the human situation. There is no conclusive evidence from rodent trials to indicate that long-term application of TCIs is photococarcinogenic. There is a need for further studies to investigate the validity of mouse models as well as long-term cohort studies in patients using TCIs. Available data suggest that long-term application of TCIs is safe, that there is no evidence of increased skin cancer risk and that it is ethical to treat patients with TCIs when indicated.

▶ Systemic administration of certain TCIs has been associated with an increased risk of skin cancer. The question that remains is whether the same effect can be observed with topical application of related drugs. More specifically, are we putting our patients with a chronic inflammatory skin disease, such as atopic dermatitis, at risk by asking them to apply a drug that potentially enhances cutaneous carcinogenesis to sun-exposed areas of their skin over an extended period? Previous studies using a murine model have shown amazingly disparate results.[1,2] The bottom line is the only model of relevance is the human model, and it is unlikely that we will have the answer to this question for many years to come.

B. H. Thiers, MD

References

1. Jiang H, Yamamoto S, Nishikawa K, et al: Anti-tumor-promoting action of FK506, a potent immunosuppressive agent. *Carcinogenesis* 14:67-71, 1993.
2. Niwa Y, Terashima T, Sumi H: Topical application of the immunosuppressant tacrolimus accelerates carcinogenesis in mouse skin. *Br J Dermatol* 149:960-967, 2004.

Efficacy and Acceptability of a New Topical Skin Lotion of Sodium Cromoglicate (Altoderm) in Atopic Dermatitis in Children Aged 2-12 Years: A Double-blind, Randomized, Placebo-controlled Trial

Stainer R, Matthews S, Arshad SH, et al (St Mary's Hosp, Isle of Wight, England; Synexus Limited, Liverpool, England; Royal Hampshire County Hosp, England; et al)

Br J Dermatol 152:334-341, 2005

1–21

Background.—Atopic dermatitis (AD) is a common inflammatory allergic disease of children. The primary anti-inflammatory therapy is topical steroids. An effective treatment without the topical and systemic adverse effects of corticosteroids would be useful. Topical formulations of sodium cromoglicate have been researched in the past, but without consistent results. We report a trial of a new aqueous skin lotion of sodium cromoglicate (Altoderm) in children with AD.

Objectives.—To compare the efficacy, safety and acceptability of Altoderm lotion with a placebo control in the treatment of AD in children.

Methods.—A double-blind, controlled study in which children aged 2-12 years with AD were randomized to 12 weeks of treatment with a lotion containing 4% sodium cromoglicate (Altoderm) or the lotion base. To be included subjects had to have a SCORAD score of ≥ 25 and ≤ 60 at both of two clinic visits 14 days apart. Subjects continued using existing treatment, which included emollients and topical steroids. The primary outcome was the change in the SCORAD score. The two groups were compared for the change in the SCORAD score from the second baseline visit to the visit after 12 weeks of treatment using an analysis of variance. Secondary outcome measures included parents' assessment of symptoms, usage of topical steroids recorded on daily diary cards, and final opinions of treatment by parent and clinician. Parents were asked about adverse effects at each clinic visit and the responses recorded.

Results.—Fifty-eight children were randomized to Altoderm and 56 to placebo and all were included in the intention-to-treat analysis. The mean ± SD SCORAD scores at baseline were 41.0 ± 9.0 (Altoderm) and 40.4 ± 8.73 (placebo). These scores were reduced after 12 weeks by 13.2 (36%) with Altoderm and by 7.6 (20%) with placebo. The difference of 5.6 (95% confidence interval 1.0-10.3) is statistically significant ($P = 0.018$). Diary card symptoms improved with both treatments but the improvement was greater in the Altoderm-treated patients. Topical steroid usage was reduced in both groups and was larger in the Altoderm-treated patients. The differences were statistically significant for the mean of all symptoms, the overall skin condition and use of topical steroids. Those for itching and sleep loss were not. Treatment-related adverse events were reported in 11 subjects (Altoderm seven, placebo four). Most of these referred to irritation, redness and burning at the site of application. There were four reports of erythema and pruritus (Altoderm three, placebo one), and three reports of application site burning (Altoderm two, placebo one). None was reported as severe or very severe.

Conclusions.—These results show a clinically useful benefit of this sodium cromoglicate lotion in children with moderately severe AD.

▶ Sodium cromoglicate was developed originally as an inhaled powder for the treatment of asthma. It has now been used for more than 30 years with no long-term adverse effects reported. Unfortunately, it is a highly polar lipophobic drug that is poorly absorbed through the skin. To date, trials of various topical formulations of the drug have produced inconsistent results. This relatively small trial of an aqueous-based skin lotion of sodium cromoglicate showed a small but statistically significant improvement in SCORAD scores of children with AD using this formulation versus those using the base alone. Because of its long-term safety record, this agent, if effective, may have some use in the treatment of active disease but might be most beneficial as long-term maintenance therapy for children with AD.

S. Raimer, MD

Atopy and Contact Hypersensitivity: A Reassessment of the Relationship Using Objective Measures
Spiewak R (VU Univ Med Ctr, Amsterdam)
Ann Allergy Asthma Immunol 95:61-65, 2005   1–22

Background.—There is a big contradiction in the medical literature regarding the relationship between atopy and contact hypersensitivity. Some researchers believe that atopy would prevent, whereas others believe that it would promote, the development of contact allergy. Possible causes of this confusion range from different study populations to different definitions of atopy.

Objective.—To evaluate the relationship between atopy and contact hypersensitivity in a well-defined general population sample using objectively measurable markers.

Methods.—I studied 135 randomly selected students from 5 vocational schools: 73 women and 62 men aged 18 to 19 years. The following atopy markers were tested: positive skin prick test results, positive Phadiatop test results, and total IgE levels greater than 120 kU/L. Contact hypersensitivity was detected by using patch tests. Statistical analyses included the Fisher exact test, the Mann-Whitney U test, and calculation of odds ratios.

Results.—At least 1 positive skin prick test result was found in 23.7% (95% confidence interval [CI], 16.5%-30.9%) of study participants, positive Phadiatop test results were found in 20.0% (95% CI, 13.3%-26.7%), and total IgE levels greater than 120 kU/L were found in 23.7% (95% CI, 16.5%-30.9%). Positive patch test reactions were found in 28.1% (95% CI, 20.6%-35.7%) of participants, most frequently to thimerosal (18.5%; 95% CI, 12.0%-25.1%) and nickel (9.6%; 95% CI, 4.6%-14.6%). For persons with atopy markers, odds ratios for contact hypersensitivity ranged from 1.0 to 3.2, the highest being for nickel hypersensitivity among those with total

IgE levels greater than 120 kU/L. None of these relationships were statistically significant.

Conclusion.—Atopy and contact hypersensitivity are independent phenomena.

▶ This topic has been addressed by multiple authors with contradictory results. One reason for the desparate findings might be remarkable differences in the definition of atopy. Two previous studies[1,2] on the relationship between atopy and contact hypersensitivity performed in samples from the general population have suggested that there is no association between the 2 conditions.

B. H. Thiers, MD

References

1. Mortz CG, Lauritsen JM, Bindslev-Jensen C, et al: Contact allergy and allergic contact dermatitis in adolescents: Prevalence measures and associations: The Odense Adolescence Cohort Study on Atopic Diseases and Dermatitis (TOACS). *Acta Derm Venereol* 82:352-358, 2002.
2. Nielsen NH, Menne T: The relationship between IgE-mediated and cell-mediated hypersensitivities in an unselected Danish population: The Glostrup Allergy Study, Denmark. *Br J Dermatol* 134:669-672, 1996.

Contact Sensitization in 1094 Children Undergoing Patch Testing Over a 7-Year Period

Seidenari S, Giusti F, Pepe P, et al (Univ of Modena and Reggio Emilia, Italy)
Pediatr Dermatol 22:1-5, 2005   1–23

Introduction.—Contact sensitization in children is frequent. However, because exposure to sensitizing agents varies rapidly, it is of utmost importance to perform a periodic evaluation of patch test results. Our purpose was to compare our data on contact sensitization in children during the past 7 years to our previous 1988–1994 findings, in order to identify emerging allergens and update our pediatric series. From 1995 to 2001, 1094 consecutive children were examined. Of these, 997 patients were patch tested with our pediatric series, which includes 30 allergens, whereas 97 underwent patch testing with 46 allergens. A total of 570 children proved allergic (52.1%). The highest sensitization rate was observed in children under 3 years of age. No differences between atopic dermatitis patients and nonatopic ones were observed in the sensitization rate. Neomycin, nickel, wool alcohols, thimerosal, and ammoniated mercury gave most of the positive responses. With respect to 1988–1995 data, allergy to substances such as neomycin, nickel, wool alcohols, thimerosal, ammoniated mercury, propolis, potassium dichromate, and thiuram mix proved more frequent. In conclusion, as sensitization rates to different allergens show great variations over time, periodic evaluations of patch test results in children is necessary in order to update the test trays.

▶ The most common antigens to which a large series of children undergoing patch testing in Italy were shown to be sensitive are demonstrated in this study. As discussed by the authors, sensitization rates to different antigens can change over time. It is important to reevaluate patch test results periodically and to update patch test trays appropriately.

S. Raimer, MD

Fifteen-Year Follow-up of Hand Eczema: Predictive Factors
Meding B, Wrangsjö K, Järvholm B (Natl Inst for Working Life, Stockholm; Karolinska Institutet, Stockholm; Umeå Univ, Sweden)
J Invest Dermatol 124:893-897, 2005   1–24

Introduction.—The aim of this study was to identify factors of importance for the long-term prognosis of hand eczema in the general population. In a 15-y follow-up, 868 (78%) individuals with hand eczema, diagnosed and clinically examined in a previous population-based study, answered a postal questionnaire with questions concerning persistence of the disease. In a logistic regression model, the extent of eczema involvement at the initial examination was the strongest negative factor for the prognosis, followed by history of childhood eczema and age below 20 y at onset of hand eczema. These factors significantly influenced both the total time with hand eczema during the 15 y follow-up and occurrence of hand eczema the previous year. The predictive factor for hand eczema 15 y later was doubled for an individual with all three risk factors compared with one without them, 72% *vs* 35%. Contact allergy to any of the standard allergens also related significantly to current hand eczema. In conclusion, the main determinant for a poor long-term prognosis was widespread hand dermatitis at the initial examination. Other important factors were low age at onset of hand eczema, history of childhood eczema, and contact allergy.

▶ Meding et al provide useful prognostic information for patients with hand dermatitis. A history of childhood eczema, widespread hand dermatitis, younger than 20 years at onset of dermatitis and, to a lesser degree, contact allergy to standard allergens—all are negative prognostic influences.

B. H. Thiers, MD

Is the Risk of Lung Cancer Reduced Among Eczema Patients?

Castaing M, Youngson J, Zaridze D, et al (Internatl Agency for Research on Cancer, Lyon, France; Univ of Liverpool, England; Cancer Research Ctr, Moscow; et al)

Am J Epidemiol 162:542-547, 2005   1–25

Introduction.—Persons with a history of eczema have been shown to have a reduced risk of lung cancer, but the evidence has been inconclusive because of the small size of previous studies and their limited ability to control for confounding by smoking. The objective of this study was to determine the role of eczema in relation to lung cancer while overcoming the limitations of previous investigations. Study subjects included 2,854 cases and 3,116 population and hospital controls recruited during 1998-2001 from 16 areas in the Czech Republic, Hungary, Poland, Romania, Russia, Slovakia, and the United Kingdom. Odds ratios were calculated for self-reported history of eczema via multivariate logistic regression modeling. The odds ratio for a history of eczema was 0.61 (95% confidence interval: 0.48, 0.76) after control for age, sex, study center, and cumulative tobacco smoking. There was no heterogeneity in the results by sex or age at onset of eczema. Subjects reporting use of medication for eczema had a lower odds ratio than subjects not reporting such use. This study provides further evidence for an inverse association between history of eczema and lung cancer risk, which is unlikely to be due to chance, bias, or confounding.

▶ The data support the hypothesis that the altered immune function associated with atopic and allergic conditions (and eczema in particular) decreases the risk of lung cancer. The relatively large negative association that was noted in this study might be of significant clinical importance and certainly requires confirmation by other investigators.

B. H. Thiers, MD

2 Psoriasis and Lichenoid Disorders

Identification of Differentially Expressed Genes in Psoriasis Using Expression Profiling Approaches

Itoh K, Kawasaki S, Kawamoto S, et al (Natl Inst of Genetics, Mishima, Shizuoka, Japan; Kyoto Prefectural Univ of Medicine, Hirokoji-Kawaramachi, Kamigyo-ku, Japan; Nara Inst of Science and Technology, Ikoma, Nara, Japan; et al)

Exp Dermatol 14:667-674, 2005   2–1

Introduction.—To identify differentially expressed genes which play causal roles in pathogenesis and maintenance for psoriasis, we used BodyMapping and introduced amplified fragment length polymorphism approaches. From the BodyMap database, we selected 2007 genes which specifically expressed in epithelial tissues. Among 2007 genes, we surveyed genes which differentially expressed in involved or uninvolved psoriatic lesional skin samples compared with atopic dermatitis, mycosis fungoides, and normal skin samples. As a result of surveying 2007 genes, 241 genes were differentially expressed only in involved psoriatic skin but not in the other samples. Hierarchical cluster analysis of gene expression profiles showed that 13 independent psoriatic-involved skin samples clustered tightly together, reflecting highly similar expression profiles. Using the same 2007 gene set, we examined gene expression levels in five serial lesions from distal uninvolved psoriatic skin to involved psoriatic plaque. We identified seven genes such as alpha-1-microglobulin/bikunin precursor, calnexin, claudin 1, leucine zipper down-regulated in cancer 1, tyrosinase-related protein 1, Yes-associated protein 1, and unc-13-like protein (*Coleonyx elegans*) which show high-expression levels only in uninvolved psoriatic lesions. These seven genes, which were reported to be related to apoptosis or antiproliferation, might have causal roles in pathophysiology in psoriasis.

▶ The sheer apparent size and complexity of this study will be daunting to the uninitiated (which includes most of us). These authors examined gene expression in psoriasis, as have many previous investigators. However, they surveyed 2007 (!) genes, selected from the BodyMap database, which are known to be expressed in epithelium. Of these, 241 genes were found to be expressed at significant levels in psoriatic lesional skin. Seventeen were found to show major differences in expression between psoriatic skin and tissues from normal subjects or those with other dermatologic diseases. Furthermore, most of these had been previously reported to be either upregulated or down-regulated in psoriasis. However, this process also identified 14 genes that were shown to be uniquely upregulated in nonlesional skin of psoriatic patients. Seven of these appear to play a role in control of cell proliferation. The authors suggest that these 7 genes may bear further scrutiny for their potential role in the pathogenesis of psoriasis.

G. M. P. Galbraith, MD

Stat3 Links Activated Keratinocytes and Immunocytes Required for Development of Psoriasis in a Novel Transgenic Mouse Model

Sano S, Chan KS, Carbajal S, et al (Univ of Texas, Smithville; Louisiana State Univ, Shreveport; Osaka Univ, Japan; et al)
Nature Med 11:43-49, 2005   2–2

Introduction.—Here we report that epidermal keratinocytes in psoriatic lesions are characterized by activated Stat3. Transgenic mice with keratinocytes expressing a constitutively active Stat3 (K5.Stat3C mice) develop a skin phenotype either spontaneously, or in response to wounding, that closely resembles psoriasis. Keratinocytes from K5.Stat3C mice show upregulation of several molecules linked to the pathogenesis of psoriasis. In addition, the development of psoriatic lesions in K5.Stat3C mice requires cooperation between Stat3 activation in keratinocytes and activated T cells. Finally, abrogation of Stat3 function by a decoy oligonucleotide inhibits the onset and reverses established psoriatic lesions in K5.Stat3C mice. Thus, targeting Stat3 may be potentially therapeutic in the treatment of psoriasis.

▶ Stat3 (signal *t*ransducers and *a*ctivators of *t*ranscription) is a transcription factor that appears to have a critical role in various biological activities, including cell proliferation, survival, and migration. Sano et al found that Stat3 was activated in keratinocytes in the majority of human psoriatic lesions examined. This activation did not appear to be simply a consequence of epidermal hyperplasia because keratinocytes from other nonpsoriatic inflammatory skin disorders that display epidermal hyperplasia did not show nuclear localization of Stat3. Thus, they concluded that activation of Stat3 appears to be specific for psoriasis among nonmalignant dermatoses. Moreover, studies of K5.Stat3C mice demonstrated that constitutive activation of Stat3 in keratinocytes is associated with the development of skin lesions that mimic human psoriasis, both clinically and histologically, and is a process that appears to require a (misguided) T-cell response. Thus, Stat3 may serve as a link between the epidermis and the immune system, and this transcription factor may represent a new therapeutic target in psoriasis.[1]

B. H. Thiers, MD

Reference

1. Pittelkow M: Psoriasis: More than skin deep. *Nat Med* 11:17-18, 2005.

▶ These investigators examined the putative role of Stat3 in the pathogenesis of psoriasis. Stat proteins are a crucial component of signal transduction in many cell systems. In this study, lesional skin biopsies were obtained from 21 patients with psoriasis. Control biopsies were derived from 14 patients with nonpsoriatic inflammatory skin diseases and 3 healthy individuals. Immunohistochemical examination of these biopsies revealed the presence of activated Stat3 in the psoriatic epidermal keratinocyte nuclei, whereas staining in control samples was faint and limited to the cell cytoplasm. The authors then used a transgenic mouse model to further examine the potential role of Stat3 in psoriasis. These mice constitutively expressed activated Stat3 and developed psoriaticlike lesions at 2 weeks of age. Epidermal injury by full skin thickness wounding, tail-stripping, and application of tetradecanoylphorbol-13-actetate (TPA) induced severe lesions that were markedly similar to human psoriatic plaques; this was not seen in control mice. Stat3 staining of the murine lesions was very similar to that observed in the human psoriatic biopsies. Importantly, inhibition of Stat3 in the transgenic mice was shown to both prevent and reverse the psoriatic lesions induced by TPA. The authors conclude that Stat3 activation may be required for the development of psoriasis and suggest the need for further studies to elucidate the mechanism underlying activation of this signal transducer in human psoriasis.

G. M. P. Galbraith, MD

Psoriasis-like Skin Disease and Arthritis Caused by Inducible Epidermal Deletion of Jun Proteins
Zenz R, Eferl R, Kenner L, et al (Research Inst of Molecular Pathology, Vienna; Deutsches Krebsforschungszentrum, Heidelberg, Germany; Med Univ of Vienna)
Nature 437:369-375, 2005   2–3

Introduction.—Psoriasis is a frequent, inflammatory disease of skin and joints with considerable morbidity. Here we report that in psoriatic lesions, epidermal keratinocytes have decreased expression of JunB, a gene localized in the psoriasis susceptibility region *PSORS6*. Likewise, inducible epidermal deletion of *JunB* and its functional companion c-*Jun* in adult mice leads (within two weeks) to a phenotype resembling the histological and molecular hallmarks of psoriasis, including arthritic lesions. In contrast to the skin phenotype, the development of arthritic lesions requires T and B cells and signalling through tumour necrosis factor receptor 1 (TNFR1). Prior to the disease onset, two chemotactic proteins (S100A8 and S100A9) previously mapped to the psoriasis susceptibility region *PSORS4*, are strongly induced in mutant keratinocytes in vivo and in vitro. We propose that the abrogation of JunB/activator protein 1 (AP-1) in keratinocytes triggers chemokine/

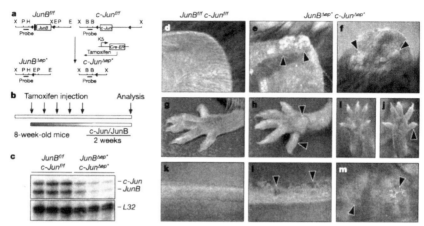

FIGURE 2.—Inducible deletion of *JunB* and *c-Jun* in the epidermis of adult mice. Mice carrying floxed alleles for the *JunB* and/or *c-Jun* locus were used to delete 1 or both genes in the epidermis by inducible Cre-recombinase activity. d–m, Macroscopic views of ear (**d–f**), paw (**g–j**), tail, (**k,l**) and back skin (**m**) from adult mice 2 weeks after inducible deletion of *JunB* and *c-Jun* in the epidermis. Scale-like skin irritations (marked by *arrows*) were observed on the front and back side of the ear (**e,f**), paw (**h,j**), tail, (**l**) and shaved back skin (**m**) of adult mutant mice. (Courtesy of Zenz R, Eferl R, Kenner L, et al: Psoriasis-like skin disease and arthritis caused by inducible epidermal deletion of Jun proteins. *Nature* 437:369-375, 2005. Reprinted by Nature Publishing.)

cytokine expression, which recruits neutrophils and macrophages to the epidermis thereby contributing to the phenotypic changes observed in psoriasis. Thus, these data support the hypothesis that epidermal alterations are sufficient to initiate both skin lesions and arthritis in psoriasis (Fig 2).

▶ Zenz et al describe a mouse model of psoriasis in which changes in the epidermis can lead to typical psoriatic skin lesions and an inflammatory joint disease analogous to psoriatic arthritis. This model should prove suitable for future preclinical studies aimed at better understanding the pathogenesis of this disease and developing interventions to effect a cure. Interestingly, ciprofloxacin seemed to delay the onset of the skin disease, and arthritis did not develop in some antibiotic-treated mice, which lends support to the hypothesis that certain forms of the disease, especially the juvenile form, can be triggered by resident bacteria or bacterial infection.[1]

B. H. Thiers, MD

Reference

1. Nickoloff BJ, Schroder JM, von den Driesch P, et al: Is psoriasis a T-cell disease? *Exp Dermatol* 9:359-375, 2000.

Human Keratinocytes Respond to Interleukin-18: Implication for the Course of Chronic Inflammatory Skin Diseases

Wittmann M, Purwar R, Hartmann C, et al (Hannover Med Univ, Germany)
J Invest Dermatol 124:1225-1233, 2005   2–4

Introduction.—Interleukin (IL)-18 has been described to play a role in several inflammatory skin diseases such as eczema and psoriasis. In this study, we aimed to elucidate keratinocytes as potential targets for IL-18 effects. In human primary keratinocytes expression of IL-18Rα as well as responses to IL-18 were determined. In keratinocytes freshly isolated from skin biopsies of lesional atopic dermatitis or psoriasis, we observed a significantly higher expression of the IL-18Rα as compared with keratinocytes from normal donors. A marked upregulation was induced *in vitro* upon stimulation with interferon (IFN)γ+tumor necrosis factor (TNF)α or poly I:C. IL-4 led to downregulation of IL-18Rα. IL-18-induced CXCL10/IP-10 production in freshly isolated keratinocytes from lesional psoriasis as well as in cultured normal keratinocytes. Furthermore, IL-18 upregulated major histocompatibility complex (MHC) class II expression on IFNγ-stimulated keratinocytes. This was of functional significance as verified in coculture experiments with CD4+ T cells in the presence of superantigen. T cells produced significant amounts of IFNγ after coculture with IL-18-induced MHC class II expressing keratinocytes. In conclusion, we have shown that keratinocytes functionally respond to IL-18 with upregulation of MHC II and production of the chemokine CXCL10/IP-10. These findings further support an important role of IL-18 in inflammatory skin diseases in the epidermal compartment.

▶ IL-18 is a pro-inflammatory cytokine that may play an important role in the pathogenesis of T-helper 1–mediated diseases. Indeed, a previous study has demonstrated a significant correlation between IL-18 levels and the Psoriasis Area and Severity Index (PASI) score in patients with psoriasis.[1] Monoclonal antibodies against IL-18 may have significant anti-inflammatory properties. Future studies may test their therapeutic activity in a wide variety of inflammatory disorders.

B. H. Thiers, MD

Reference

1. Pietrzak A, Lecewicz-Torun B, Chodorowska G, et al: Interleukin-18 levels in the plasma of psoriatic patients correlate with the extent of skin lesions and the PASI score. *Acta Derm Venereol* 83:262-265, 2003.

Impact of Obesity and Smoking on Psoriasis Presentation and Management

Herron MD, Hinckley M, Hoffman MS, et al (Univ of Utah, Salt Lake City; Med Univ of South Carolina, Charleston; Univ of Texas, Dallas; et al)
Arch Dermatol 141:1527-1534, 2005

2–5

Objective.—To study the impact of obesity and smoking on psoriasis.

Design.—Cross-sectional study.

Setting.—University of Utah Department of Dermatology clinics.

Patients.—A case series of patients with psoriasis enrolled in the prospective Utah Psoriasis Initiative (UPI) (which carefully performs phenotyping of patients with psoriasis) was compared with 3 population databases: the Behavioral Risk Factor Surveillance System of the Utah population, the 1998 patient-member survey from the National Psoriasis Foundation, and 500 adult patients who attend our clinics and do not have psoriasis (nonpsoriatic population).

Results.—The prevalence of obesity in patients within the UPI population was higher than that in the general Utah population (34% vs 18%; *P*<.001) and higher than that in the nonpsoriatic population attending our clinics. Assessment of body image perception with a standardized diagram in the UPI group resulted in the median body image score of normal weight at 18 years of age and the onset of psoriasis, but it transitioned to overweight at the time of enrollment in the UPI. Thus, obesity appears to be the consequence of psoriasis and not a risk factor for onset of disease. We did not observe an increased risk for psoriatic arthritis in patients with obesity; furthermore, obesity did not positively or negatively affect the response or the adverse effects of topical corticosteroids, light-based treatments, and systemic medications. The prevalence of smoking in the UPI population was higher than in the general Utah population (37% vs 13%; *P*<.001) and higher than in the nonpsoriatic population (37% vs 25%; *P*<.001). We found a higher prevalence of smokers in the obese population within the UPI than in the obese population within the Utah population (25% vs 9%; *P*<.001).

Conclusions.—Patients with psoriasis attending the University of Utah Dermatology Clinics were more likely to be obese and to smoke compared with nonpsoriatic patients and more likely to be obese compared with other large cohorts with psoriasis. Smoking appears to have a role in the onset of psoriasis, but obesity does not. The high prevalence of obesity and smoking in a psoriasis cohort has not been previously noted; if confirmed, it supports the prediction that a significant portion of patients with psoriasis will have the comorbid conditions and public health issues of those with obesity and smoke.

Relationship Between Smoking and the Clinical Severity of Psoriasis

Fortes C, for the IDI Multipurpose Psoriasis Research on Vital Experiences (IMPROVE) Study Group (Istituto di Ricovero e Cura a Carattere Scientifico, Rome; Université de Montréal)
Arch Dermatol 141:1580-1584, 2005   2–6

Objective.—To evaluate the association between different components of smoking history and the clinical severity of psoriasis.

Design.—A hospital-based cross-sectional study.

Setting.—Inpatient wards of a hospital for skin diseases in Rome, Italy.

Patients.—A total of 818 adults with psoriasis.

Main Outcome Measure.—The Psoriasis Area and Severity Index was used to assess the clinical severity of psoriasis between February 21, 2000, and February 19, 2002.

Results.—After adjustment for potential confounders (sex, age, body mass index, psychological distress, family history of psoriasis, duration of psoriasis disease, and alcohol consumption), high intensity of smoking (>20 cigarettes daily) vs a lower level of consumption (≤10 cigarettes daily) was associated with a more than 2-fold increased risk of clinically more severe psoriasis (odds ratio [OR], 2.2; 95% confidence interval [CI], 1.2-4.1). Cigarette-years, measured as the product of the intensity and duration (years) of smoking, significantly increased the risk of clinically more severe psoriasis after adjustment for confounding factors (OR, 1.3; 95% CI, 1.0-1.6, for a 600-U increase in cigarette-years). Separate analyses for men and women showed that the effect of cigarette-years was stronger for women (OR, 1.8; 95% CI, 1.2-2.6, for a 400-U increase in cigarette-years) than for men (OR, 1.2; 95% CI, 0.9-1.6, for a 700-U increase in cigarette-years).

Conclusion.—Smoking is associated with the clinical severity of psoriasis and highlights the importance of smoking cessation in patients with psoriasis.

▶ These studies (Abstracts 2–5 and 2–6) demonstrate that cigarette smoking and obesity can significantly affect the clinical course of psoriasis, especially among women. Counseling on smoking cessation should be considered as an adjunct to any therapeutic protocol for patients with psoriasis.

B. H. Thiers, MD

A Two-Compound Product Containing Calcipotriol and Betamethasone Dipropionate Provides Rapid, Effective Treatment of Psoriasis Vulgaris Regardless of Baseline Disease Severity

van de Kerkhof PCM, Wasel N, Kragballe K, et al (Univ Hosp Nijmegen, The Netherlands; Univ of Alberta, Edmonton, Canada; Dalhousie Univ, Halifax, Canada; et al)
Dermatology 210:294-299, 2005   2–7

Background.—A two-compound product containing calcipotriol and be-tamethasone dipropionate (Daivobet®/Dovobet®) has been evaluated in a large clinical trial programme, providing a wealth of data on the treatment of psoriasis vulgaris.

Objective.—To determine the effectiveness of the two-compound product in patients with mild, moderate and severe psoriasis vulgaris.

Methods.—Data from over 1,534 patients with psoriasis vulgaris who received the two-compound product once daily for at least 4 weeks in four randomised, double-blind studies were pooled. A meta-analysis of the pooled data is presented. Severity of psoriasis at baseline was determined by investigator assessment and Psoriasis Area and Severity Index (PASI) score.

Results.—For patients with severe disease defined by PASI score (PASI baseline ≥ 17), the mean reduction in PASI after up to 4 weeks of treatment was 71.6% compared with 68.9 and 67.2% for those with moderate (PASI baseline 5.1-16.0) and mild disease (PASI baseline ≤ 5). Corresponding reductions for investigator-assessed severity were 72.6, 69.1 and 68.7%, respectively.

Conclusion.—Although the meta-analysis of the data from these four studies was performed post hoc, we may conclude that the two-compound product provided highly effective treatment of psoriasis, regardless of the category of baseline disease severity.

▶ Topical calcipotriol has been available for many years for the treatment of chronic plaque-type psoriasis. It is notable for its slow onset of action and is probably best used as maintenance therapy. I would venture to guess that most of the activity observed in these short-term studies is an effect of the betamethasone dipropionate rather than the calcipotriol.

B. H. Thiers, MD

Topical Tacrolimus in the Treatment of Inverse Psoriasis in Children

Steele JA, Choi C, Kwong PC (Mayo Clinic Jacksonville, Fla; Nemours Children's Clinic, Jacksonville, Fla)
J Am Acad Dermatol 53:713-716, 2005   2–8

Background.—Inverse psoriasis, also known as flexural or intertriginous psoriasis, is common in infants and young children. Topical corticosteroids are the mainstay of treatment. However, the adverse effects of long-term corticosteroid use include atrophy, telangiectasias, and striae. Previous studies have shown that systemic tacrolimus is useful in the treatment of plaque-type psoriasis. More recent studies have shown that topical tacrolimus 0.1% ointment is beneficial in the treatment of psoriasis involving the face and intertriginous areas in adults. The safety and efficacy of topical tacrolimus 0.1% ointment for the treatment of inverse psoriasis in children were investigated.

Methods.—A retrospective review was conducted of the medical records of 13 patients with inverse psoriasis treated with tacrolimus ointment between December 2001 and October 2003. The patients ranged in age from 22 months to 16 years. One patient was treated with tacrolimus 0.03%, and the remaining 12 were treated with tacrolimus 0.1%. The efficacy of treatment was determined by the resolution of symptoms and clearance of skin lesions. Treatment was halted when 100% clearance was achieved and reinitiated when symptoms recurred. Concurrent treatment included topical mupirocin 2% ointment, a mixture of hydrocortisone 2.5% and econazole cream, oral cephalexin, cetirizine, and fluconazole.

Results.—The 12 patients treated with tacrolimus 0.1% had complete clearance of their psoriatic lesions within 2 weeks of initiating treatment. One patient had no improvement in skin lesions; this patient was treated with the lower concentration of 0.03%. The only adverse effect was subjective burning and irritation reported in the patient who used the lower concentration. Recurrence rates ranged from complete sustained resolution to flares within 2 days of discontinuing the medication.

Conclusion.—Tacrolimus ointment 0.1% was effective in the treatment of inverse psoriasis in a group of children age 22 months to 16 years.

▶ As with adults, inverse psoriasis in children appears to clear rapidly with topical tacrolimus. No recurrence of the disease was noted in 5 of the 13 children treated. With intermittent application, topical tacrolimus would be anticipated to be safe and effective for inverse psoriasis in children.

S. Raimer, MD

Treatment of Nail Psoriasis With 8% Clobetasol Nail Lacquer: Positive Experience in 10 Patients

Regaña MS, Ezquerra GM, Millet PU, et al (Univ of Barcelona)
J Eur Acad Dermatol Venereol 19:573-577, 2005   2–9

Background.—Treatment of nail psoriasis is difficult. Several topical therapies have been employed with poor results because drug penetration is limited in this localization. Recently, a new formulation containing 8% clobetasol-17-propionate in a colourless nail lacquer vehicle has shown good results in the control of nail psoriasis.

Objective.—To determine the efficacy and safety of 8% clobetasol-17-propionate in a lacquer vehicle in nail psoriasis.

Methods.—Ten patients with both nail bed and matrix psoriasis were included in the study. They were treated with a colourless nail lacquer contain-

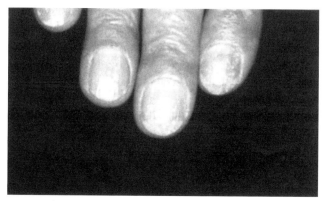

FIGURE 8.—Pitting before treatment. (Courtesy of Regaña MS, Ezquerra GM, Millet PU, et al: Treatment of nail psoriasis with 8% clobetasol nail lacquer: Positive experience in 10 patients. *J Eur Acad Dermatol Venereol* 19:573-577, 2005. Reprinted by permission of Blackwell Publishing.)

ing 8% clobetasol-17-propionate that was applied once daily for 21 days and then twice weekly for 9 months.

Results.—Within 4 weeks of therapy there was a reduction of all the nail alterations, including nail pain. Therapeutic response was directly related to the length of therapy. The nail parameters that responded best to therapy were onycholysis, pitting and salmon patches. Subungual hyperkeratosis and splinter haemorrhages on the other hand had moderate and poor improvement, respectively. The treatment was well tolerated in all of the patients and there were no local (i.e. atrophy and subreinfection) or systemic secondary effects.

Conclusions.—The formulation containing 8% clobetasol-17-propionate is a safe, effective and cosmetically highly acceptable treatment for nail bed and matrix psoriasis (Figs 8 and 9; see color plate VIII).

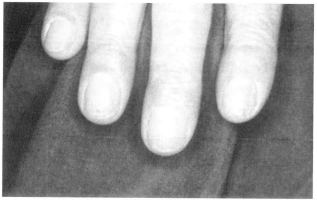

FIGURE 9.—Pitting after 3 months of treatment. (Courtesy of Regaña MS, Ezquerra GM, Millet PU, et al: Treatment of nail psoriasis with 8% clobetasol nail lacquer: Positive experience in 10 patients. *J Eur Acad Dermatol Venereol* 19:573-577, 2005. Reprinted by permission of Blackwell Publishing.)

▶ A larger, double-blind, controlled study will be necessary to confirm these results. Nevertheless, the data presented here are promising, because nail involvement in psoriasis has typically responded poorly to topical therapy. Other reports have described marked improvement of nail bed psoriasis with the use of topical calcipotriol ointment under occlusion, although I have not been able to reproduce these findings among my own patients.[1]

B. H. Thiers, MD

Reference

1. Tosti A, Piraccini BM, Cameli N et al: Calcipotriol ointment in nail psoriasis: A controlled double-blind comparison with betamethasone dipropionate and salicylic acid. *Br J Dermatol* 139:655-659, 1998.

Medication-Related Factors Affecting Health Care Outcomes and Costs for Patients With Psoriasis in the United States

Kulkarni AS, Balkrishnan R, Richmond D, et al (Univ of Texas, Houston; Wake Forest Univ, Winston-Salem, NC)
J Am Acad Dermatol 52:27-31, 2005   2–10

Background.—The impact of psoriasis medication therapy on costs and patient outcomes in large nationally representative samples needs further examination.

Objective.—This study examined the association between factors related to medication use, health status, and health care costs associated with psoriasis in the United States.

Methods.—A cross-sectional cohort study was performed using the 2000 Medical Expenditure Panel Survey database. Information on health care service use, health status (EuroQol-5D instrument), and patient demographics were obtained from the database representing approximately 1.1 million patients with psoriasis. EuroQol was used in the Medical Expenditure Panel Survey.

Results.—Weighted multiple linear regression analysis indicated that use of topical corticosteroid therapy was associated with a decrease in psoriasis-specific health care costs (53.2% lower than average costs vs patients using no medications, $P = .022$) and better health status (34.0% higher than average scores vs patients using no medications, $P = .006$).

Conclusions.—We observed an association with topical corticosteroids for treatment of psoriasis on health care outcomes and costs.

▶ This study examined the effect of topical corticosteroid therapy on psoriasis-specific health care costs and health status. Topical steroids had a beneficial effect on both parameters. However, it might be premature to assume that treatment with topical corticosteroids leads to decreased costs; an alternative explanation might be that patients with less severe (and thus less costly) psoriasis are preferentially treated with these agents.

B. H. Thiers, MD

No Evidence for Increased Skin Cancer Risk in Psoriasis Patients Treated With Broadband or Narrowband UVB Phototherapy: A First Retrospective Study

Weischer M, Blum A, Eberhard F, et al (Eberhard Karls Univ, Tuebingen, Germany)

Acta Derm Venereol 84:370-374, 2004   2–11

Introduction.—Phototherapy of skin diseases such as psoriasis is an effective and safe treatment modality. However, increasing the risk of skin cancer by phototherapy is a serious concern. An increased skin cancer risk occurs after prolonged photochemotherapy (PUVA). In contrast, the role of broadband UVB or narrowband UVB therapy in skin carcinogenesis of humans with psoriasis is less clear. Therefore, we investigated the incidence of skin tumours in a total of 195 psoriasis patients, receiving broadband (n=69) or narrowband (n=126) UVB from 1994 to 2000 with follow-up until 2003. Data were raised from the regional interdisciplinary cancer centre of the University of Tuebingen, Germany and compared with the tumour incidences given for the German population. In this study, with 80% statistical power to detect a 6-7-fold increase in skin cancer with broadband UVB and 83% power to detect a 5-6-fold increase with narrow band UVB at $p=0.05$, only one patient developed skin cancer—an in situ melanoma. The tumour occurred within the same year that phototherapy was initiated. Thus, the present study does not provide evidence for an increased skin cancer risk for patients treated with either broadband or narrowband UVB phototherapy.

The Photocarcinogenic Risk of Narrowband UVB (TL-01) Phototherapy: Early Follow-up Data

Man I, Crombie IK, Dawe RS, et al (Univ of Dundee, Scotland)

Br J Dermatol 152:755-757, 2005   2–12

Background.—Limited information is available on the carcinogenic risk associated with narrowband TL-01 UVB phototherapy in humans.

Objectives.—To determine the skin cancer incidence in a population treated with TL-01 phototherapy.

Patients and methods.—All TL-01-treated patients were identified from the departmental computerized database. Patients with malignant melanoma (MM), squamous cell carcinoma (SCC) and basal cell carcinoma (BCC) were identified by record linkage with the Scottish Cancer Registry. The incidence of each was compared with the normal Scottish population matched for age and sex.

Results.—Data were obtained from 1908 patients. The median follow-up duration was 4 years (range 0.04-13). The median cumulative number of TL-01 treatments and dose were 23 (1-199) and 13 337 (30-284 415) mJ cm^{-2}, respectively. No increased incidence of SCC or MM was observed. Ten patients developed BCC compared with an expected 4.7 in the Scottish population [standardized rate ratio 213 (95% confidence interval 102-391); $P < 0.05$].

Conclusions.—A small but significant increase of BCC was detected in the TL-01 group. This could be explained by a number of factors, including ascertainment bias. To determine the true carcinogenic risk of TL-01 phototherapy, longer follow-up is essential.

▶ These retrospective studies (Abstracts 2–11 and 2–12) attempt to determine the photocarcinogenic risk of narrowband or broadband UVB therapy. The article by Weischer et al (Abstract 2–11) reported no increased risk, whereas the article by Man et al (Abstract 2–12) suggested a possible increase in the incidence of BCC with narrowband exposure. However, both studies had significant limitations. A long-term perspective study would be an ideal, but perhaps not practical, goal.

B. H. Thiers, MD

Topical Aminolaevulinic Acid-based Photodynamic Therapy as a Treatment Option for Psoriasis? Results of a Randomized, Observer-blinded Study

Radakovic-Fijan S, Blecha-Thalhammer U, Schleyer V, et al (Univ of Vienna; Univ of Regensburg, Germany; Estimate GmbH, Augsburg, Germany)
Br J Dermatol 152:279-283, 2005   2–13

Background.—Topical aminolaevulinic acid-based photodynamic therapy (ALA-PDT) has recently been tried in small open studies for several inflammatory dermatoses including psoriasis.

Objectives.—The purpose of this randomized, within patient comparison study was to investigate whether topical ALA-based PDT using a range of light doses can induce a satisfactory response in localized psoriasis.

Patients and Methods.—Twenty-nine patients with chronic plaque type psoriasis were enrolled in the study. After keratolytic pretreatment three psoriatic plaques in each patient were randomly allocated to PDT with 1% ALA and a light dose of 5 J cm^{-2}), 10 J cm^{-2} or 20 J cm^{-2}, respectively. Treatment was performed twice weekly until complete clearance or for a maximum of 12 irradiations. As a measure of clinical response the psoriasis severity index (PSI) of the three target plaques was assessed separately by an observer blinded to the treatment at baseline, before each PDT treatment and 3-4 days after the last irradiation.

Results.—Eight patients withdrew prematurely from the study. Keratolytic pretreatment alone reduced the baseline PSI in all three dose groups by about 25%. Subsequent PDT with 20 J cm^{-2} resulted in a final reduction of PSI by 59%, PDT with the lower doses of 10 J cm^{-2} and 5 J cm^{-2} decreased the baseline PSI by 46% and 49%, respectively. The difference in clinical efficacy between 20 J cm^{-2} and 10 J cm^{-2} or 5 J cm^{-2} was statistically significant ($P = 0.003$; $P = 0.02$), whereas no difference was found between 10 J cm^{-2} and 5 J cm^{-2} ($P = 0.4$). All patients reported some degree of PDT-induced stinging or burning during irradiation.

Conclusions.—The unsatisfactory clinical response and frequent occurrence of pain during and after irradiation renders topical ALA-based PDT an inadequate treatment option for psoriasis.

▶ Although none of us wants to see innovative treatments fail, it is refreshing to find authors willing to report a negative outcome. With the protocol used in their industry-sponsored study, Radakovic-Fijan et al concluded that topical ALA-based PDT is not a viable treatment option for psoriasis. Other regimens might provide a better response, although they have not been tested in controlled studies using large numbers of patients.[1,2]

B. H. Thiers, MD

References

1. Bissonnette R, Zeng H, McLean DI et al: Oral aminolevulinic acid induced IX fluorescence in psoriatic plaques and peripheral blood cells. *Photochem Photobiol* 74:339-345, 2001.
2. Boehncke WH, Elshorst-Schmidt T, Kaufmann R: Systemic photodynamic therapy is a safe and effective treatment for psoriasis (letter). *Arch Dermatol* 136:271-272, 2000.

Methotrexate Reduces Incidence of Vascular Diseases in Veterans With Psoriasis or Rheumatoid Arthritis

Prodanowich S, Ma F, Taylor JR, et al (Univ of Miami, Fla; VA Med Ctr, Miami, Fla)
J Am Acad Dermatol 52:262-267, 2005   2–14

Background.—Methotrexate (MTX) is a folate analogue used in the treatment of moderate to severe psoriasis and rheumatoid arthritis (RA). It oppositely affects inflammation and hyperhomocysteinemia—two independent risk factors for vascular disease. To date, there are no published reports evaluating the impact of these potentially paradoxical actions of MTX.

Objective.—The purpose of this study was to evaluate the effect of MTX therapy on the incidence of vascular disease in patients with psoriasis and RA.

Methods.—We conducted a retrospective cohort study in which we analyzed computerized records of 7,615 outpatients diagnosed with psoriasis and 6,707 with RA at the Veterans Integrated Service Network 8.

Results.—Patients prescribed MTX therapy had a significantly reduced risk of vascular disease compared to those who were not prescribed MTX (psoriasis: RR = 0.73, 95% CI = 0.55-0.98; RA: 0.83, 0.71-0.96). This reduction was most evident for patients prescribed a low cumulative dose of MTX (psoriasis: RR = 0.50, 95% CI = 0.31-0.79; RA = 0.65, 0.52-0.80). Concomitant use of folic acid (FA) with MTX also reduced the incidence of vascular disease in patients prescribed MTX (psoriasis: RR = 0.56, 95% CI = 0.39-0.80; RA: 0.77, 0.38-1.56).

Conclusions.—MTX therapy reduced the incidence of vascular disease in veterans with psoriasis or RA. Low to moderate cumulative dose appears more beneficial than the higher dose. We hypothesize that this effect is caused by its anti-inflammatory properties. In addition, a combination of MTX and FA led to a further reduction in the incidence of vascular disease.

▶ A previous study[1] demonstrated that MTX therapy was associated with a significantly increased survival rate in patients with RA. This included a 70% decrease in the mortality rate from cardiovascular diseases in patients treated with MTX compared with patients who did not receive the drug.

B. H. Thiers, MD

Reference

1. Choi HK, Herman MA, Seeger JD, et al: Methotrexate and mortality in patients with rheumatoid arthritis: A prospective study. *Lancet* 359:1173-1177, 2002.

Folate Supplementation During Methotrexate Therapy for Patients With Psoriasis
Strober BE, Menon K (New York Univ)
J Am Acad Dermatol 53:652-659, 2005   2–15

Introduction.—Methotrexate is a folate antagonist that is a well-established therapy for autoimmune and inflammatory conditions. In some patients, methotrexate is associated with significant side effects and toxicity. Folate supplementation is often used to ameliorate methotrexate-associated side effects and toxicities. We sought to demonstrate that folate supplementation during methotrexate therapy reduces both toxicity and side effects without compromising efficacy. A MEDLINE search of the search terms "methotrexate," "folic acid," "folinic acid," and "leucovorin" was performed and literature relevant to the use of folates as a supplement to methotrexate was reviewed. According to studies reviewed, the use of folate supplements in patients treated with methotrexate reduces the incidence of hepatotoxicity and gastrointestinal intolerance without impairing the efficacy of methotrexate. Both folic acid and folinic acid are equally effective; however, folic acid is more cost effective. It must be noted that there are relatively few studies that have addressed folate supplementation with the use of methotrexate for the treatment of psoriasis. After examining the available data from the literature and drawing from clinical experience, we advise folate supplementation for every patient who receives methotrexate.

▶ I often recommend folic acid to patients on oral methotrexate, especially those intolerant of the drug. My usual approach is to have them take the folic acid on the days that they do not take the methotrexate. The data presented by Strober and Menon seem to support such combination therapy.

B. H. Thiers, MD

Salt Sensitivity of Blood Pressure in Patients With Psoriasis on Ciclosporin Therapy
Magina S, Santos J, Coroas A, et al (Hosp S João, Porto, Portugal; Inst of Pharmacology and Therapeutics, Porto, Portugal)
Br J Dermatol 152:773-776, 2005   2–16

Background.—Cyclosporin has been shown to be effective in the treatment of psoriasis. However, the use of cyclosporin for the treatment of psoriasis is associated with nephrotoxicity and increased blood pressure, and its long-term use is determined by the risk-benefit ratio. It has been suggested that the cyclosporin-induced rise in blood pressure is related to increased vascular resistance in both the systemic and renal circulation, in parallel with renal microvascular and tubulointerstitial damage. Although sodium retention is thought to be a factor in the renal microvascular and tubulointerstitial damage induced by cyclosporin, the influence of salt intake on the 24-hour mean blood pressure of patients with psoriasis treated with cyclosporin is not known. The sodium sensitivity of the cyclosporin-induced rise in blood pressure in these patients was evaluated.

Methods.—Twenty-four hour ambulatory blood pressure was evaluated in 13 patients with psoriasis (mean age, 20-57 years). The blood pressure was measured before (phase 1) and after (phase 2) completion of 4 months of therapy with cyclosporin (3 mg/kg daily). In both phases, the patients were studied in low-sodium and high-sodium intake conditions.

Results.—The 24-hour ambulatory blood pressure (mean ± SD) during low-sodium and high-sodium intake was 86.3 ± 1.6 mm Hg and 85.5 ± 1.8 mm Hg, respectively, during phase 1, and 88.5 ± 1.5 mm Hg and 91.8 ± 2.2 mm Hg during phase 2. The median (interquartile range) sodium sensitivity index was greater during phase 2 than during phase 1. There was no difference in plasma levels and daily urinary excretion of noradrenaline between phases 1 and 2.

Conclusions.—The cyclosporin-induced rise in blood pressure in psoriasis patients is sodium sensitive. It appeared that sympathetic activation is not a factor in the pathogenesis of this cyclosporin-induced rise in blood pressure.

▶ The data suggest that patients commencing cyclosporin therapy should be advised to restrict their salt intake.

B. H. Thiers, MD

A Randomised, Double Blind, Placebo Controlled, Multicentre Trial of Combination Therapy With Methotrexate Plus Ciclosporin in Patients With Active Psoriatic Arthritis
Fraser AD, van Kuijk AWR, Westhovens R, et al (Univ of Leeds, England; VU Med Ctr, Amsterdam; Univ of Leuven, Belgium; et al)
Ann Rheum Dis 64:859-864, 2005   2–17

Objectives.—To evaluate the safety and efficacy of adding ciclosporin A (CSA) to the treatment of patients with psoriatic arthritis (PsA) demonstrating an incomplete response to methotrexate (MTX) monotherapy.

Methods.—In a 12 month, randomised, double blind, placebo controlled trial at five centres in three countries, 72 patients with active PsA with an incomplete response to MTX were randomised to receive either CSA (n=38) or placebo (n=34). Patients underwent full clinical and radiological assessment and, in addition, high resolution ultrasound (HRUS) was performed at one centre. An intention to treat (last observation carried forward) analysis was employed.

Results.—Some significant improvements were noted at 12 months in both groups. However, in the active but not the placebo arm there were significant improvements in swollen joint count, mean (SD), from 11.7 (9.7) to 6.7 (6.5) (p<0.001) and C reactive protein, from 17.4 (14.5) to 12.7 (14.3) mg/l (p<0.05) as compared with baseline. The Psoriasis Area and Severity Index (PASI) score improved in the active group (2 (2.3) to 0.8 (1.3)) as compared with placebo (2.2 (2.7) to 1.9 (2.8)), p<0.001, and synovitis detected by HRUS (33 patients, 285 joints) was reduced by 33% in the active group compared with 6% in the placebo group (p<0.05). No improvement in Health Assessment Questionnaire or pain scores was detected.

Conclusions.—Synovitis detected by HRUS was significantly reduced. Combining CSA and MTX treatment in patients with active PsA, and a partial response to MTX, significantly improves the signs of inflammation but not pain or quality of life.

▶ The authors demonstrate the clinical benefits of combination therapy with CSA and MTX in patients with active PsA and persistent inflammation. Unfortunately, pain and quality of life were not affected. Surprisingly, a marked improvement in clinical outcomes was found in both the placebo group and the group receiving active treatment. The long-term toxicity of combination therapy with CSA and MTX remains to be determined.

B. H. Thiers, MD

TNF Inhibition Rapidly Down-regulates Multiple Proinflammatory Pathways in Psoriasis Plaques

Gottlieb AB, Chamian F, Masud S, et al (Univ of Medicine and Dentistry of New Jersey, New Brunswick; Rockefeller Univ, New York)

J Immunol 175:2721-2729, 2005   2–18

Introduction.—The mechanisms of action of marketed TNF-blocking drugs in lesional tissues are still incompletely understood. Because psoriasis plaques are accessible to repeat biopsy, the effect of TNF/lymphotoxin blockade with etanercept (soluble TNFR) was studied in ten psoriasis patients treated for 6 months. Histological response, inflammatory gene expression, and cellular infiltration in psoriasis plaques were evaluated. There was a rapid and complete reduction of IL-1 and IL-8 (immediate/early genes), followed by progressive reductions in many other inflammation-related genes, and finally somewhat slower reductions in infiltrating myeloid cells (CD11c+ cells) and T lymphocytes. The observed decreases in IL-8, IFN-γ-inducible protein-10 (CXCL10), and MIP-3α (CCL20) mRNA expression may account for decreased infiltration of neutrophils, T cells, and dendritic cells (DCs), respectively. DCs may be less activated with therapy, as suggested by decreased IL-23 mRNA and inducible NO synthase mRNA and protein. Decreases in T cell-inflammatory gene expression (IFN-γ, STAT-1, granzyme B) and T cell numbers may be due to a reduction in DC-mediated T cell activation. Thus, etanercept-induced TNF/lymphotoxin blockade may break the potentially self-sustaining cycle of DC activation and maturation, subsequent T cell activation, and cytokine, growth factor, and chemokine production by multiple cell types including lymphocytes, neutrophils, DCs, and keratinocytes. This results in reversal of the epidermal hyperplasia and cutaneous inflammation characteristic of psoriatic plaques.

▶ Gottlieb et al present data that provide an immunologic basis for the beneficial therapeutic response seen in patients with psoriasis treated with TNF antagonists. The most consistent cellular effects of etanercept were a reduction in keratinocyte hyperplasia and a reduction in myeloid DCs. The authors theorize that etanercept downregulates expression of proinflammatory and proproliferative genes that are induced in keratinocytes and other skin cells by local synthesis of TNF.

B. H. Thiers, MD

Infliximab Induction and Maintenance Therapy for Moderate-to-Severe Psoriasis: A Phase III, Multicentre, Double-blind Trial

Reich K, Nestle FO, Papp K, et al (Georg-August Univ, Göttingen, Germany; Univ of Zurich, Switzerland; Univ of Western Ontario, London, Canada; et al)

Lancet 366:1367-1374, 2005   2–19

Background.—Tumour necrosis factor α (TNFα) is thought to play a part in the pathogenesis of psoriasis. We assessed the efficacy and safety of continuous treatment with infliximab, a monoclonal antibody that binds to and neutralises the activity of TNFα, in patients with psoriasis.

Methods.—In this phase III, multicentre, double-blind trial, 378 patients with moderate-to-severe plaque psoriasis were allocated in a 4:1 ratio to receive infusions of either infliximab 5 mg/kg or placebo at weeks 0, 2, and 6, then every 8 weeks to week 46. At week 24, placebo-treated patients crossed over to infliximab treatment. Skin and nail signs of psoriasis were assessed using the psoriasis area and severity index (PASI) and nail psoriasis severity index (NAPSI), respectively. The primary endpoint, analysed on an intention-to-treat-basis, was the proportion of patients achieving at least a 75% improvement in PASI from baseline to week 10.

Findings.—At week 10, 80% (242/301) of patients treated with infliximab achieved at least a 75% improvement from their baseline PASI (PASI 75) and 57% (172/301) achieved at least a 90% improvement (PASI 90), compared with 3% and 1% in the placebo group, respectively (p<0.0001). At week 24, PASI 75 (82% for infliximab vs 4% for placebo) and PASI 90 (58% vs 1%) were maintained (p<0.0001). At week 50, 61% achieved PASI 75 and 45% achieved PASI 90 in the infliximab group. Infliximab was generally well tolerated in most patients.

Interpretation.—Infliximab is effective in both an induction and maintenance regimen for the treatment of moderate-to-severe psoriasis, with a high percentage of patients achieving sustained PASI 75 and PASI 90 improvement through 1 year.

▶ Reich et al confirm the high level of effectiveness of infliximab for the treatment of moderate to severe psoriasis. In this study, an inverse correlation seemed to occur between the maintenance of PASI 75 improvement at week 50 and the development of antibodies to infliximab.

B. H. Thiers, MD

Sustained Benefits of Infliximab Therapy for Dermatologic and Articular Manifestations of Psoriatic Arthritis: Results From the Infliximab Multinational Psoriatic Arthritis Controlled Trial (IMPACT)

Antoni CE, Kavanaugh A, Kirkham B, et al (Friedrich-Alexander Univ, Erlangen-Nuremberg, Germany; Univ of California, San Diego; Guy's Hosp, London; et al)
Arthritis Rheum 52:1227-1236, 2005   2–20

Objective.—To investigate the efficacy and tolerability of infliximab therapy for the articular and dermatologic manifestations of active psoriatic arthritis (PsA).

Methods.—One hundred four patients with PsA in whom prior therapy with at least 1 disease-modifying antirheumatic drug (DMARD) had failed were recruited into this investigator-initiated, multicenter, randomized, double-blind, placebo-controlled clinical trial. During the initial blinded portion of the study, patients received infusions of infliximab (5 mg/kg) or placebo at weeks 0, 2, 6, and 14. After week 16, patients initially assigned to receive placebo crossed over to receive infliximab 5 mg/kg every 8 weeks through week 50, while patients initially randomized to infliximab continued to receive active treatment at the same dose through week 50. The primary efficacy outcome was achievement of the American College of Rheumatology 20% criteria for improvement in rheumatoid arthritis (ACR20) at week 16. Additional predefined clinical efficacy assessments included the Psoriasis Area and Severity Index (PASI) score, the ACR50 and ACR70 criteria, the Disease Activity Score in 28 joints, the Health Assessment Questionnaire, ratings of enthesitis and dactylitis, and the Psoriatic Arthritis Response Criteria score.

Results.—The proportion of infliximab-treated patients who achieved an ACR20 response at week 16 (65%) was significantly higher than the proportion of placebo-treated patients who achieved this response (10%). In addition, 46% of infliximab-treated patients achieved an ACR50 response, and 29% achieved an ACR70 response; no placebo-treated patient achieved these end points. Among patients who had PASI scores of ≥2.5 at baseline, 68% of infliximab-treated patients achieved improvement of ≥75% in the PASI score at week 16 compared with none of the placebo-treated patients. Continued therapy with infliximab resulted in sustained improvement in articular and dermatologic manifestations of PsA through week 50. The incidence of adverse events was similar between the treatment groups.

Conclusion.—Therapy with infliximab at a dose of 5 mg/kg significantly improved the signs and symptoms of arthritis, psoriasis, dactylitis, and enthesitis in patients with active PsA that had been resistant to DMARD therapy. With continued infliximab treatment, benefits were sustained through 50 weeks. The benefit-to-risk ratio appeared favorable in this study population.

▶ Unlike in most studies purporting to evaluate the efficacy of infliximab for psoriasis alone, in the current study, patients were allowed to continue concomitant therapy with 1 of the following DMARDs: methotrexate, leflunomide, sulfasalazine, hydroxychloroquine, IM gold, penicillamine or azathioprine. Concomitant therapy with oral corticosteroids (10 mg prednisone equivalent per day or less) or nonsteroidal anti-inflammatory drugs was also permitted.

B. H. Thiers, MD

Adalimumab for the Treatment of Patients With Moderately to Severely Active Psoriatic Arthritis: Results of a Double-blind, Randomized, Placebo-controlled Trial

Mease PJ, for the Adalimumab Effectiveness in Psoriatic Arthritis Trial Study Group (Seattle Rheumatology Associates; et al)
Arthritis Rheum 52:3279-3289, 2005   2–21

Objective.—Adalimumab, a fully human, anti–tumor necrosis factor monoclonal antibody, was evaluated for its safety and efficacy compared with placebo in the treatment of active psoriatic arthritis (PsA).

Methods.—Patients with moderately to severely active PsA and a history of inadequate response to nonsteroidal antiinflammatory drugs were randomized to receive 40 mg adalimumab or placebo subcutaneously every other week for 24 weeks. Study visits were at baseline, weeks 2 and 4, and every 4 weeks thereafter. The primary efficacy end points were the American College of Rheumatology 20% improvement (ACR20) response at week 12 and the change in the modified total Sharp score of structural damage at week 24. Secondary end points were measures of joint disease, disability, and quality of life in all patients, as well as the severity of skin disease in those patients with psoriasis involving at least 3% of body surface area.

Results.—At week 12, 58% of the adalimumab-treated patients (87 of 151) achieved an ACR20 response, compared with 14% of the placebo-treated patients (23 of 162) ($P < 0.001$). At week 24, similar ACR20 response rates were maintained and the mean change in the modified total Sharp score was -0.2 in patients receiving adalimumab and 1.0 in those receiving placebo ($P < 0.001$). Among the 69 adalimumab-treated patients evaluated with the Psoriasis Area and Severity Index (PASI), 59% achieved a 75% PASI improvement response at 24 weeks, compared with 1% of the 69 placebo-treated patients evaluated ($P < 0.001$). Disability and quality of life measures were also significantly improved with adalimumab treatment compared with placebo. Adalimumab was generally safe and well-tolerated.

Conclusion.—Adalimumab significantly improved joint and skin manifestations, inhibited structural changes on radiographs, lessened disability due to joint damage, and improved quality of life in patients with moderately to severely active PsA.

▶ In contrast to infliximab, a chimeric anti–tumor necrosis factor monoclonal antibody that must be given IV, adalimumab is a fully human anti–tumor necrosis antibody that can be given subcutaneously. Adalimumab is likely to be a welcome addition to the array of biologic agents available for the treatment of moderate to severe psoriasis, and we all look forward to the publication of data to support its use for that indication.

B. H. Thiers, MD

Etanercept and Clinical Outcomes, Fatigue, and Depression in Psoriasis: Double-blind Placebo-controlled Randomised Phase III Trial

Tyring S, Gottlieb A, Papp K, et al (Univ of Texas, Houston; UMDNJ, New Brunswick; Univ of Western Ontario, London, Canada; et al)
Lancet 367:29-35, 2006   2–22

Background.—Psoriasis has substantial psychological and emotional effects. We assessed the effect of etanercept, an effective treatment for the clinical symptoms of psoriasis, on fatigue and symptoms of depression associated with the condition.

Methods.—618 patients with moderate to severe psoriasis received double-blind treatment with placebo or 50 mg twice-weekly etanercept. The primary efficacy endpoint was a 75% or greater improvement from baseline in psoriasis area and severity index score (PASI 75) at week 12. Secondary and other endpoints included the functional assessment of chronic illness therapy fatigue (FACIT-F) scale, the Hamilton rating scale for depression (Ham-D), the Beck depression inventory (BDI), and adverse events. Efficacy analyses were based on the allocated treatment. Analyses and summaries of safety data were based on the actual treatment received. This study is registered with ClinicalTrials.gov with the identifier NCT00111449.

Findings.—47% (147 of 311) of patients achieved PASI 75 at week 12, compared with 5% (15 of 306) of those receiving placebo (p<0.0001; difference 42%, 95% CI 36-48). Greater proportions of patients receiving etanercept had at least a 50% improvement in Ham-D or BDI at week 12 compared with the placebo group; patients treated with etanercept also had significant and clinically meaningful improvements in fatigue (mean FACIT-F improvement 5.0 vs 1.9; p<0.0001, difference 3.0, 95% CI 1.6-4.5). Improvements in fatigue were correlated with decreasing joint pain, whereas improvements in symptoms of depression were less correlated with objective measures of skin clearance or joint pain.

Interpretation.—Etanercept treatment might relieve fatigue and symptoms of depression associated with this chronic disease.

▶ It is hardly surprising that an improvement in psoriasis is also associated with an improvement in emotional health. However, no strong correlation was found between PASI and depression improvement, as limited lesions in visible areas might have been more psychologically disabling than more extensive lesions in less prominent regions.[1,2] In an accompanying editorial, Bos and De Korte[3] speculate on the possible role of TNFα action in the pathogenesis of fatigue and depression and suggest that further studies are necessary to explore the possible association between increased concentrations of proinflammatory cytokines and major depression.

B. H. Thiers, MD

References

1. Heydendael VM, de Borgie CA, Spuls PI, et al: The burden of psoriasis is not determined by disease severity only. *J Invest Dermatol Symp Proc* 9:131-135, 2004.
2. Kimball AB, Krueger G, Woolley JM: The Dermatology Life Quality Index (DLQI) provides qualitatively different information from the PASI. *J Am Acad Dermatol* 50:156, 2004.
3. Bos JD, De Korte J: Effects of etanercept on quality of life, fatigue, and depression in psoriasis. *Lancet* 367:6-7, 2006.

Psoriasis Induced by Anti–Tumor Necrosis Factor Therapy

Sfikakis PP, Iliopoulos A, Elezoglou A, et al (Athens Univ, Greece; 401 Gen Military Hosp of Athens, Greece)
Arthritis Rheum 52:2513-2518, 2005   2–23

Introduction.—Administration of anti–tumor necrosis factor (anti-TNF) agents is beneficial in a variety of chronic inflammatory conditions, including psoriasis. We describe 5 patients in whom psoriasiform skin lesions developed 6-9 months after the initiation of anti-TNF therapy for longstanding, seropositive rheumatoid arthritis (etanercept or adalimumab), typical ankylosing spondylitis (infliximab), and Adamantiades-Behçet's disease (infliximab). In all 5 patients, the underlying disease had responded well to anti-TNF therapy. Four patients developed a striking pustular eruption on the palms and/or soles accompanied by plaque-type psoriasis at other skin sites, while 1 patient developed thick erythematous scaly plaques localized to the scalp. In 3 patients there was nail involvement with onycholysis, yellow discoloration, and subungual keratosis. Histologic findings from skin biopsies were consistent with psoriasis. None of these patients had a personal or family history of psoriasis. In all patients, skin lesions subsided either with topical treatment alone, or after discontinuation of the responsible anti-TNF agent. The interpretation of this paradoxical side effect of anti-TNF therapy remains unclear but may relate to altered immunity induced by the inhibition of TNF activity in predisposed individuals.

▶ Other similar patients have been described, and I recently have seen a patient who developed rather extensive psoriasis while receiving infliximab therapy for inflammatory bowel disease.

B. H. Thiers, MD

Skin Cancer, Rheumatoid Arthritis, and Tumor Necrosis Factor Inhibitors

Chakravarty EF, Michaud K, Wolfe F (Stanford Univ, Palo Alto, Calif; Natl Data Bank for Rheumatic Diseases, Wichita, Kan; Univ of Kansas, Wichita)
J Rheumatol 32:2130-2135, 2005   2–24

Objective.—To determine the rates of reported non-melanoma skin cancer (NMSC) in a large cohort of patients with rheumatoid arthritis (RA) in comparison to patients with osteoarthritis (OA) and to determine risk factors for the development of NMSC in patients with RA.

Methods.—Self-reported information from 15,789 patients with RA and 3,639 patients with OA were collected through semi-annual questionnaires since 1999. Survival analyses were used to determine incidence rates for NMSC among patients with RA and OA. Multivariate Cox proportional hazard models were used to estimate hazard ratios (HR) for the development of NMSC. Separate analyses were performed for patients with RA to explore associations between use of immunosuppressive medication and development of NMSC.

Results.—The crude (unadjusted) incidence rate for reported NMSC among patients with RA and OA were 18.1 and 20.4 per 1000 patient years, respectively. OA patients were older, more likely to be Caucasian, and had higher past incidence of NMSC. Age, male sex, Caucasian race, and history of NMSC prior to entry into the database were associated with an increased risk of NMSC in multivariate Cox proportional hazard models. After adjustment for covariates, RA was associated with an increased risk of NMSC (HR 1.19, p = 0.042). Among RA patients, the development of NMSC was associated with use of prednisone (HR 1.28, p = 0.014) and tumor necrosis factor (TNF) inhibitors alone or with concomitant methotrexate (HR 1.24, p = 0.89 and HR 1.97, p = 0.001, respectively) in addition to established risk factors including fair skin, age, male sex, and previous history of NMSC. No association was found between use of methotrexate or leflunomide and development of NMSC (HR 1.12, p = 0.471, HR 0.83, p = 0.173, respectively).

Conclusion.—In this large, national cohort, RA was associated with an increased risk for development of NMSC. Among patients with RA, use of TNF inhibitors and prednisone were associated with an increased risk of NMSC.

▶ This series left me with more questions than answers. The findings do suggest at minimum that regular skin cancer screenings should be performed on patients with RA, especially those receiving immunosuppressive therapy. Counseling on sunscreen use and other sun-protective measures would also seem appropriate.

B. H. Thiers, MD

Effector Memory T Cells, Early Metastasis, and Survival in Colorectal Cancer

Pagès F, Berger A, Camus M, et al (Univ Paris 6; Georges Pompidou European Hosp, Paris; Graz Univ of Technology, Austria)
N Engl J Med 353:2654-2666, 2005   2–25

Background.—The role of tumor-infiltrating immune cells in the early metastatic invasion of colorectal cancer is unknown.

Methods.—We studied pathological signs of early metastatic invasion (venous emboli and lymphatic and perineural invasion) in 959 specimens of resected colorectal cancer. The local immune response within the tumor was studied by flow cytometry (39 tumors), low-density-array real-time polymerase-chain-reaction assay (75 tumors), and tissue microarrays (415 tumors).

Results.—Univariate analysis showed significant differences in disease-free and overall survival according to the presence or absence of histologic signs of early metastatic invasion (P<0.001). Multivariate Cox analysis showed that an early conventional pathological tumor–node–metastasis stage (P<0.001) and the absence of early metastatic invasion (P=0.04) were independently associated with increased survival. As compared with tumors with signs of early metastatic invasion, tumors without such signs had increased infiltrates of immune cells and increased levels of messenger RNA (mRNA) for products of type 1 helper effector T cells (CD8, T-BET [T-box transcription factor 21], interferon regulatory factor 1, interferon-γ, granulysin, and granzyme B) but not increased levels of inflammatory mediators or immunosuppressive molecules. The two types of tumors had significant differences in the levels of expression of 65 combinations of T-cell markers, and hierarchical clustering showed that markers of T-cell migration, activation, and differentiation were increased in tumors without signs of early metastatic invasion. The latter type of tumors also had increased numbers of CD8+ T cells, ranging from early memory (CD45RO+CCR7–CD28+CD27+) to effector memory (CD45RO+CCR7–CD28–CD27–) T cells. The presence of high levels of infiltrating memory CD45RO+ cells, evaluated immunohistochemically, correlated with the absence of signs of early metastatic invasion, a less advanced pathological stage, and increased survival.

Conclusions.—Signs of an immune response within colorectal cancers are associated with the absence of pathological evidence of early metastatic invasion and with prolonged survival.

► In an accompanying editorial, Parmiani[1] discusses the implications of these findings on the development of effective immunotherapeutic agents. Of more direct relevance to dermatology is the fact that some of the new biological agents proposed to treat psoriasis (eg, alefacept) selectively reduce memory-effector (CD45RO+) T cells.[2] Are we to feel comfortable prescribing these drugs for patients with a history of malignancy?

B. H. Thiers, MD

References

1. Parmiani G: Tumor-infiltrating T cells: Friend or foe of neoplastic cells? *N Engl J Med* 353:2640-2641, 2005.
2. Gottlieb AB, Casale TB, Frankel E, et al: CD4+ T-cell–directed antibody responses are maintained in patients with psoriasis receiving alefacept: Results of a randomized study. *J Am Acad Dermatol* 49:816-825, 2003.

Oral Lichen Planus in Childhood

Laeijendecker R, Van Joost T, Tank B, et al (Albert Schweitzer Hosp, Dordrecht, The Netherlands; Erasmus Univ, Rotterdam, The Netherlands)
Pediatr Dermatol 22:299-304, 2005   2–26

Introduction.—Oral lichen planus is rare in childhood, and only a few reports on this subject have appeared in the literature. Our objective was to report individual cases of oral lichen planus in childhood from our practice and to review the literature on this subject. We recruited patients younger than 18 years with oral lichen planus and documented several clinical aspects, the histopathology, patch tests, and blood examination findings. Three patients from about 10,000 dermatology patients younger than 18 years seen from 1994 to 2003 were included. Of these three, an Asian girl aged 11 years had an asymptomatic, hyperkeratotic variant of oral lichen planus, which disappeared without any treatment after 1 year. An Asian boy aged 16 years had an erosive oral lichen planus with severe pain, which healed after intensive local and systemic treatment in 2 years. A Caucasian girl aged 14 years had a hyperkeratotic variant with a little soreness, which disappeared with local treatment after 3 months. Our findings indicated that oral lichen planus in childhood is rare and therefore at present it is not possible to draw firm conclusions considering its nature and etiology. Oral lichen planus in childhood seems to occur preferentially in those of Asian race. The clinical features resemble those of oral lichen planus in adults. However, generally the prognosis of oral lichen planus in childhood seems to be more favorable than in adults.

Lichen Planus in 24 Children With Review of the Literature

Luis-Montoya P, Domínguez-Soto L, Vega-Memije E (Gen Hosp "Dr Manuel Gea González," Tlalpan, Mexico)
Pediatr Dermatol 22:295-298, 2005   2–27

Introduction.—Lichen planus is a disease generally considered uncommon in children. Our objective was to obtain epidemiologic data retrospectively and determine the clinical characteristics of lichen planus in Mexican children seen in our dermatology department. We found 235 patients with the clinical and histologic diagnosis of lichen planus seen over a period of 22 years and 7 months. Twenty-four (10.2%) of these patients were children (15 years of age or younger). The ratio of male to female was 1 : 1.2. The main clinical pattern was classic lichen planus (43.5%). Mucous membrane and nail involvement were uncommon. No family history of lichen planus or systemic disease was noted. In the international literature, the frequency of lichen planus varied from 2.1% to 11.2% of the pediatric population. In the majority of studies no significant gender predominance was identified. Most patients had the classic variety of lichen planus. Reported mucosal involvement was rare, except in India and Kuwait. Frequency of nail involvement ranged from 0% to 16.6%. Little evidence of systemic disease or family history was found.

▶ Lichen planus occurs much less commonly in children than in adults, and mucous membrane and nail involvement are uncommon in children. Forty-three percent of children reported in the series of Luis-Montoya et al had chronic lichen planus and 30% had linear lichen planus.

S. Raimer, MD

Pityriasis Lichenoides: A Cytotoxic T-Cell-Mediated Skin Disorder. Evidence of Human Parvovirus B19 DNA in Nine Cases
Tomasini D, Tomasini CF, Cerri A, et al (Hosp of Busto Arsizio, Italy; Univ of Turin, Italy; Univ of Milan, Italy; et al)
J Cutan Pathol 31:531-538, 2004   2–28

Background.—Pityriasis lichenoides et varioliformis acuta (PLEVA) and pityriasis lichenoides chronica (PLC) probably represent the polar ends of the same pathologic process, i.e. pityriasis lichenoides (PL), with intermediate forms in between. Previous studies have demonstrated that the inflammatory infiltrate in PLEVA is composed of cytotoxic suppressor T cells, whereas in PLC the helper/inducer T-cell population drives the immunological answer. Furthermore, monoclonal rearrangement of the T-cell receptor-γ (TCR-γ) genes was repeatedly found both in PLEVA and PLC.

Methods.—Forty-one formalin-fixed, paraffin-embedded tissue specimens of 40 cases of PL were retrieved from the files of the authors. Immunophenotyping for cytotoxic granular proteins (Tia-1/GMP-17 and Granzyme B) and T-cell-related antigens (n = 41), TCR-γ chain gene analysis (n = 30) and molecular investigations for parvovirus B19 (PVB19) DNA (n = 30) were performed.

Results.—Overlapping immunophenotypes were observed in PLEVA and PLC. The dermal and epidermal T cells predominantly expressed CD2, CD3, CD8, and Tia-1 with a variable positivity for CD45RA, CD45RO, and Granzyme B. A monoclonal rearrangement pattern of the TCR-γ genes was detected in three cases (10%). PVB19 DNA was found in nine cases (30%) (Fig 1; see color plate IX). T-cell monoclonality in conjunction with genomic PVB19 DNA was present in one case.

Conclusions.—Our results demonstrate that PL is a skin disorder mediated by the effector cytotoxic T-cell population. The identification of PVB19

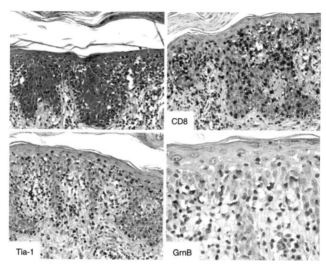

FIGURE 1.—Case no. 23, PVB19-positive. From left to right and from top to bottom: necrotic keratino-cytes, ballooning degeneration, and inflammatory round cells invading the epidermis (hematoxylin and eosin) (×200). CD8 expression of the intraepidermal T cells (×200). Tia-1 positivity of CD8⁺ intraepidermal T cells (×200). Granzyme B-positive T cells in conjunction with cytopathic features, e.g. spongiosis, balloon-ing degeneration, and necrosis of keratinocytes (×200). (Courtesy of Tomasini D, Tomasini CF, Cerri A, et al: Pityriasis lichenoides: A cytotoxic T-cell-mediated skin disorder. Evidence of human parvovirus B19 DNA in nine cases. *J Cutan Pathol* 31:531-538, 2004. Reprinted by permission of Blackwell Publishing.)

DNA in nine cases may be interpreted ambiguously: PVB19 as a true patho-gen or as an innocent bystander.

▶ Erythema multiforme and pityriasis lichenoides share some common histo-pathologic features. Chief among these is the vacuolar interface dermatitis that characterizes both conditions. On a histopathologic basis there is vacuola-tion of the basal layer. Individual necrotic keratinocytes are present in the basal zone and above it, and there is exocytosis of lymphocytes. Ultimately in both conditions there may be full thickness necrosis of the epidermis. The patho-physiology of erythema multiforme has been well studied. There is an immu-nocytotoxic reaction that is mediated by CD8⁺ T lymphocytes. Therefore, it is not unexpected that in pityriasis lichenoides the inflammatory infiltrate also would be rich in CD8⁺ T cells, indicating that the damage to the epidermis is mediated by effector cytotoxic T lymphocytes.

On a clinical basis erythema multiforme and pityriasis lichenoides also share the feature of multiple lesions that appear episodically. Herpesvirus DNA has been detected in the epidermis and lesional skin of erythema multiforme, and it is clear that recurrent erythema multiforme correlates with reactivation of herpes simplex infection. Tomasini et al show that parvovirus B19 DNA local-izes to lesional skin of a high percentage of patients with pityriasis lichenoides. This suggests that parvovirus B19 is one possible etiologic agent for that dis-order. Erythema multiforme may also be caused by a variety of agents, and this may also prove to be true for pityriasis lichenoides.

J. C. Maize, MD

3 Bacterial and Fungal Infections

Ethnic Variations in Sexual Behaviour in Great Britain and Risk of Sexually Transmitted Infections: A Probability Survey
Fenton KA, Mercer CH, McManus S, et al (Univ College, London; Natl Centre for Social Research, London; London School of Hygiene and Tropical Medicine, London)
Lancet 365:1246-1255, 2005   3–1

Background.—Ethnic variations in the rate of diagnosed sexually transmitted infections (STIs) have been reported in many developed countries. We used data from the second British National Survey of Sexual Attitudes and Lifestyles (Natsal 2000) to investigate the frequency of high-risk sexual behaviours and adverse sexual health outcomes in five ethnic groups in Great Britain.

Methods.—We did a stratified probability sample survey of 11 161 men and women aged 16-44 years, resident in Great Britain, using computer-assisted interviews. Additional sampling enabled us to do more detailed analyses for 949 black Caribbean, black African, Indian, and Pakistani respondents. We used logistic regression to assess reporting of STI diagnoses in the past 5 years, after controlling for demographic and behavioural variables.

Findings.—We noted striking variations in number of sexual partnerships by ethnic group and between men and women. Reported numbers of sexual partnerships in a lifetime were highest in black Caribbean (median 9 [IQR 4-20]) and black African (9 [3-20]) men, and in white (5 [2-9]) and black Caribbean (4 [2-7]) women. Indian and Pakistani men and women reported fewer sexual partnerships, later first intercourse, and substantially lower prevalence of diagnosed STIs than did other groups. We recorded a significant association between ethnic origin and reported STIs in the past 5 years with increased risk in sexually active black Caribbean (OR 2.74 [95% CI 1.22-6.15]) and black African (2.95 [1.45-5.99]) men compared with white men, and black Caribbean (2.41 [1.35-4.28]) women compared with white women. Odds ratios changed little after controlling for age, number of sexual partnerships, homosexual and overseas partnerships, and condom use at last sexual intercourse.

Interpretation.—Individual sexual behaviour is a key determinant of STI transmission risk, but alone does not explain the varying risk across ethnic groups. Our findings suggest a need for targeted and culturally competent prevention interventions.

▶ The authors demonstrate that transmission of STIs is dependent on individual sexual behavior. However, this does not explain why risk varies among different ethnic groups.

B. H. Thiers, MD

Single-Dose Azithromycin Versus Penicillin G Benzathine for the Treatment of Early Syphilis

Riedner G, Rusizoka M, Todd J, et al (London School of Hygiene and Tropical Medicine; Regional Med Office, Mbeya, Tanzania; Ludwig-Maximilians-Univ, Munich; et al)

N Engl J Med 353:1236-1244, 2005   3–2

Background.—Pilot studies suggest that a single, 2-g oral dose of azithromycin may be an alternative to a 2.4-MU intramuscular dose of penicillin G benzathine in the prevention and treatment of syphilis. We evaluated the efficacy of treatment with azithromycin in a developing country.

Methods.—A total of 328 subjects, 25 with primary and 303 with high-titer (a titer of at least 1:8 on a rapid plasmin reagin [RPR] test) latent syphilis, were recruited through screening of high-risk populations in Mbeya, Tanzania, and randomly assigned to receive 2 g of azithromycin orally (163 subjects) or 2.4 million units of penicillin G benzathine intramuscularly (165 subjects). The primary outcome was treatment efficacy, with cure defined serologically (a decline in the RPR titer of at least two dilutions by nine months after treatment) and, in primary syphilis, by epithelialization of ulcers within one or two weeks.

Results.—The average age of participants was 27.0 years, 235 (71.6 percent) were female, and 171 (52.1 percent) were seropositive for human immunodeficiency virus. Cure rates were 97.7 percent (95 percent confidence interval, 94.0 to 99.4) in the azithromycin group and 95.0 percent (95 percent confidence interval, 90.6 to 97.8) in the penicillin G benzathine group (95 percent confidence interval for the difference, −1.7 to 7.1 percent), achieving prespecified criteria for equivalence. Cure rates were also similar three and six months after treatment in the two groups and in all subgroups. Cure rates at three months were 59.4 percent (95 percent confidence interval, 51.8 to 67.1) in the azithromycin group and 59.5 percent (95 percent confidence interval, 51.8 to 67.3) in the penicillin G benzathine group and at six months were 85.5 percent (95 percent confidence interval, 79.4 to 90.6) and 81.5 percent (95 percent confidence interval, 74.8 to 87.4), respectively.

Conclusions.—Single-dose oral azithromycin is effective in treating syphilis and may be particularly useful in developing countries in which the use of penicillin G benzathine injections is problematic. However, recent reports of azithromycin-resistant *Treponema pallidum* in the United States indicate the importance of continued monitoring for resistance.

▶ As noted by Holmes in an accompanying editorial, macrolide resistance in *T pallidum* is quite common in homosexual men in North America. Thus, close follow-up of any patients with early syphilis treated with azithromycin is necessary, and data should be gathered on the global prevalence of macrolide resistance in *T pallidum* and its effect on treatment.[1]

B. H. Thiers, MD

Reference

1. Holmes KK: Azithromycin versus penicillin G benzathine for early syphilis. *N Engl J Med* 353:1291-1293, 2005.

Clinical Manifestations of Staphylococcal Scalded-Skin Syndrome Depend on Serotypes of Exfoliative Toxins
Yamasaki O, Yamaguchi T, Sugai M, et al (Hopital E Herriot, Lyon, France; Hiroshima Univ, Japan)
J Clin Microbiol 43:1890-1893, 2005   3–3

Introduction.—We sought a possible correlation between the clinical manifestations of staphylococcal scalded-skin syndrome (SSSS) and the serotype of exfoliative toxins (ET) by PCR screening of the *eta* and *etb* genes in *Staphylococcus aureus* strains isolated from 103 patients with generalized SSSS and 95 patients with bullous impetigo. The *eta* gene and the *etb* gene were detected in, respectively, 31 (30%) and 20 (19%) episodes of generalized SSSS and 57 (60%) and 5 (5%) episodes of bullous impetigo. Both genes were detected in 52 (50%) episodes of generalized SSS and 33 (35%) episodes of bullous impetigo. To explain this link between *etb* and generalized SSSS, we examined the distribution of ETA- and ETB-specific antibodies in the healthy population ($n = 175$) and found that the anti-ETB antibody titer was lower than the anti-ETA titer. Thus, ETA is associated with bullous impetigo and ETB is associated with generalized SSSS, possibly owing to a lower titer of anti-ETB neutralizing antibodies in the general population.

▶ *S aureus* exfoliative toxins cause intraepidermal splitting through the granular layer by specific cleavage of desmoglein 1. In this study, all of the *S aureus* oscillates contained at least 1 exfoliative toxin (*et*) gene. The presence of *eta* was significantly associated with bullous impetigo; *etb* was significantly associated with generalized SSSS. Lower levels of ETB than ETA antibodies were noted in the general population, and the authors postulated that this might explain why SSSS is more frequently associated with *etb*.

S. Raimer, MD

Necrotizing Fasciitis Caused by Community-Associated Methicillin-Resistant *Staphylococcus aureus* in Los Angeles

Miller LG, Perdreau-Remington F, Rieg G, et al (Harbor-UCLA, Torrance, Calif; Univ of California, San Francisco; St Mary Med Ctr, Long Beach, Calif)
N Engl J Med 352:1445-1453, 2005   3–4

Background.—Necrotizing fasciitis is a life-threatening infection requiring urgent surgical and medical therapy. *Staphylococcus aureus* has been a very uncommon cause of necrotizing fasciitis, but we have recently noted an alarming number of these infections caused by community-associated methicillin-resistant *S. aureus* (MRSA).

Methods.—We reviewed the records of 843 patients whose wound cultures grew MRSA at our center from January 15, 2003, to April 15, 2004. Among this cohort, 14 were identified as patients presenting from the community with clinical and intraoperative findings of necrotizing fasciitis, necrotizing myositis, or both.

Results.—The median age of the patients was 46 years (range, 28 to 68), and 71 percent were men. Coexisting conditions or risk factors included current or past injection-drug use (43 percent); previous MRSA infection, diabetes, and chronic hepatitis C (21 percent each); and cancer and human immunodeficiency virus infection or the acquired immunodeficiency syndrome (7 percent each). Four patients (29 percent) had no serious coexisting conditions or risk factors. All patients received combined medical and surgical therapy, and none died, but they had serious complications, including the need for reconstructive surgery and prolonged stay in the intensive care unit. Wound cultures were monomicrobial for MRSA in 86 percent, and 40 percent of patients (4 of 10) for whom blood cultures were obtained had positive results. All MRSA isolates were susceptible in vitro to clindamycin, trimethoprim–sulfamethoxazole, and rifampin. All recovered isolates belonged to the same genotype (multilocus sequence type ST8, pulsed-field type USA300, and staphylococcal cassette chromosome *mec* type IV [SCC*mec*IV]) and carried the Panton–Valentine leukocidin (*pvl*), *lukD*, and *lukE* genes, but no other toxin genes were detected.

Conclusions.—Necrotizing fasciitis caused by community-associated MRSA is an emerging clinical entity. In areas in which community-associated MRSA infection is endemic, empirical treatment of suspected necrotizing fasciitis should include antibiotics predictably active against this pathogen.

Methicillin-Resistant *Staphylococcus aureus* Disease in Three Communities

Fridkin SK, for the Active Bacterial Core Surveillance Program of the Emerging Infections Program Network (Ctrs for Disease Control and Prevention, Atlanta, Ga; et al)
N Engl J Med 352:1436-1444, 2005   3–5

Background.—Methicillin-resistant *Staphylococcus aureus* (MRSA) infection has emerged in patients who do not have the established risk factors. The national burden and clinical effect of this novel presentation of MRSA disease are unclear.

Methods.—We evaluated MRSA infections in patients identified from population-based surveillance in Baltimore and Atlanta and from hospital-laboratory-based sentinel surveillance of 12 hospitals in Minnesota. Information was obtained by interviewing patients and by reviewing their medical records. Infections were classified as community-associated MRSA disease if no established risk factors were identified.

Results.—From 2001 through 2002, 1647 cases of community-associated MRSA infection were reported, representing between 8 and 20 percent of all MRSA isolates. The annual disease incidence varied according to site (25.7 cases per 100,000 population in Atlanta vs. 18.0 per 100,000 in Baltimore) and was significantly higher among persons less than two years old than among those who were two years of age or older (relative risk, 1.51; 95 percent confidence interval, 1.19 to 1.92) and among blacks than among whites in Atlanta (age-adjusted relative risk, 2.74; 95 percent confidence interval, 2.44 to 3.07). Six percent of cases were invasive, and 77 percent involved skin and soft tissue. The infecting strain of MRSA was often (73 percent) resistant to prescribed antimicrobial agents. Among patients with skin or soft-tissue infections, therapy to which the infecting strain was resistant did not appear to be associated with adverse patient-reported outcomes. Overall, 23 percent of patients were hospitalized for the MRSA infection.

Conclusions.—Community-associated MRSA infections are now a common and serious problem. These infections usually involve the skin, especially among children, and hospitalization is common.

▶ In an appropriately titled editorial, Chambers[1] commented on the convergence of resistance and virulence in community-associated MRSA. Clearly, the burden of disease caused by community-associated MRSA is increasing, a phenomenon I now encounter almost daily in my clinic. A high index of suspicion is necessary for early diagnosis of these infections. Although many community-associated MRSA strains are often susceptible in vitro to inexpensive oral agents such as trimethoprim–sulfamethoxazole, doxycycline, and clindamycin, little hard data exist to confirm their clinical effectiveness. Indeed, it is uncertain whether initial therapy with an antibiotic active against MRSA even affects the outcome of skin and soft tissue infections.

B. H. Thiers, MD

Reference

1. Chambers HF: Community-associated MRSA: Resistance and virulence converge (editorial). *N Engl J Med* 352:1485-1487, 2005.

Geographic Information System Localization of Community-Acquired MRSA Soft Tissue Abscesses

Tirabassi MV, Wadie G, Moriarty KP, et al (Tufts Univ, Springfield, Mass)
J Pediatr Surg 40:962-966, 2005   3–6

Background.—Soft tissue infections with methicillin-resistant *Staphylococcus aureus* (MRSA) pose an ever-increasing risk to children in the community. Although historically these infections were limited to children with prolonged hospitalization, the authors have seen an increase in community-acquired infections in children without identifiable risk factors. The goal of this study is to determine the incidence of truly community-acquired MRSA soft tissue infections in our community and geographically map regions of increased risk.

Methods.—After obtaining the institutional review board's approval, a retrospective chart review was conducted on 195 patients records who underwent an incision and drainage of soft tissue infections from January 1, 2000, to December 31, 2003. Thirteen patients were excluded from the study because no cultures were taken at the time of incision and drainage.

Results.—The most common organism isolated from wound culture was *S aureus*, 40% (73/182), of which 45% (33/73) were MRSA. Eighty-one percent (27/33) of MRSA infections were in Springfield, 1 of 18 towns represented in the patient population. Geographic information system analysis identified a significant MRSA cluster 1.96 km in diameter within the city of Springfield.

Conclusions.—Geography proved to be a significant risk factor for presenting with MRSA infection. Geographic maps of antibiotic resistance can be used to guide physician antibiotic selection before culture results are available. This has significant implications for the health care provider in proper antibiotic selection within the community.

▶ Tirabassi et al show that community colonization with MRSA is a significant risk factor for children presenting with soft tissue abscesses caused by the organism. They suggest that geographic coding and mapping of home addresses be used to identify children who are at an increased risk of having an antibiotic-resistant infection.

B. H. Thiers, MD

Isolation of Patients in Single Rooms or Cohorts to Reduce Spread of MRSA in Intensive-Care Units: Prospective Two-Centre Study

Cepeda JA, Whitehouse T, Cooper B, et al (Univ College London; Royal Free Hosp, London; Health Protection Agency, London)
Lancet 365:295-304, 2005   3–7

Background.—Hospital-acquired infection due to meticillin-resistant *Staphylococcus aureus* (MRSA) is common within intensive-care units. Single room or cohort isolation of infected or colonised patients is used to reduce spread, but its benefit over and above other contact precautions is not known. We aimed to assess the effectiveness of moving versus not moving infected or colonised patients in intensive-care units to prevent transmission of MRSA.

Methods.—We undertook a prospective 1-year study in the intensive-care units of two teaching hospitals. Admission and weekly screens were used to ascertain the incidence of MRSA colonisation. In the middle 6 months, MRSA-positive patients were not moved to a single room or cohort nursed unless they were carrying other multiresistant or notifiable pathogens. Standard precautions were practised throughout. Hand hygiene was encouraged and compliance audited.

Findings.—Patients' characteristics and MRSA acquisition rates were similar in the periods when patients were moved and not moved. The crude (unadjusted) Cox proportional-hazards model showed no evidence of increased transmission during the non-move phase (0.73 [95% CI 0.49-1.10], p=0.94 one-sided). There were no changes in transmission of any particular strain of MRSA nor in handwashing frequency between management phases.

Interpretation.—Moving MRSA-positive patients into single rooms or cohorted bays does not reduce crossinfection. Because transfer and isolation of critically ill patients in single rooms carries potential risks, our findings suggest that re-evaluation of isolation policies is required in intensive-care units where MRSA is endemic, and that more effective means of preventing spread of MRSA in such settings need to be found.

▶ The authors demonstrate that in an environment in which MRSA infection is endemic, isolation of ICU patients who are colonized or infected with the organism into single rooms or cohorts does little to reduce its transmission over and above the use of standard precautions. If the findings are confirmed, this will greatly reduce the number of bed moves for this reason and thereby allow better resource use and minimize the inherent risk in transferring and isolating seriously ill patients.

B. H. Thiers, MD

A Clone of Methicillin-Resistant *Staphylococcus aureus* Among Professional Football Players
Kazakova SV, Hageman JC, Matava M, et al (Ctrs for Disease Control and Prevention, Atlanta, Ga; Washington Univ, St Louis; Missouri Dept of Health and Senior Services, St Louis)

N Engl J Med 352:468-475, 2005

3–8

Background.—Methicillin-resistant *Staphylococcus aureus* (MRSA) is an emerging cause of infections outside of health care settings. We investigated an outbreak of abscesses due to MRSA among members of a professional football team and examined the transmission and microbiologic characteristics of the outbreak strain.

Methods.—We conducted a retrospective cohort study and nasal-swab survey of 84 St. Louis Rams football players and staff members. *S. aureus* recovered from wound, nasal, and environmental cultures was analyzed by

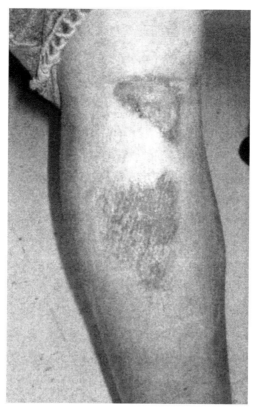

FIGURE 2.—Photograph of an uninfected skin abrasion (turf burn) on a St Louis Rams professional football player in 2003. (Reprinted by permission of *The New England Journal of Medicine* from Kazakova SV, Hageman JC, Matava M, et al: A clone of methicillin-resistant *Staphylococcus aureus* among professional football players. *N Engl J Med* 352:468-475, 2005. Copyright 2005, Massachusetts Medical Society. All rights reserved.)

means of pulsed-field gel electrophoresis (PFGE) and typing for resistance and toxin genes. MRSA from the team was compared with other community isolates and hospital isolates.

Results.—During the 2003 football season, eight MRSA infections occurred among 5 of the 58 Rams players (9 percent); all of the infections developed at turf-abrasion sites. MRSA infection was significantly associated with the lineman or linebacker position and a higher body-mass index. No MRSA was found in nasal or environmental samples; however, methicillin-susceptible *S. aureus* was recovered from whirlpools and taping gel and from 35 of the 84 nasal swabs from players and staff members (42 percent). MRSA from a competing football team and from other community clusters and sporadic cases had PFGE patterns that were indistinguishable from those of the Rams' MRSA; all carried the gene for Panton-Valentine leukocidin and the gene complex for staphylococcal-cassette-chromosome *mec* type IVa resistance (clone USA300-0114).

Conclusions.—We describe a highly conserved, community-associated MRSA clone that caused abscesses among professional football players and that was indistinguishable from isolates from various other regions of the United States (Fig 2).

▶ The Centers for Disease Control and Prevention is working with the National Collegiate Athletic Association to develop guidelines to prevent and control community-associated MRSA infections among college football players. Educational materials to be distributed to athletic trainers will describe infection-control practices and measures for responding to cases or clusters of infections. The community-associated clone described here differs from strains of MRSA observed in health care settings in that it was susceptible to most antimicrobial agents other than β-lactams and macrolides, and it primarily caused skin infections in otherwise healthy persons.

B. H. Thiers, MD

Re-emergence of Early Pandemic *Staphylococcus aureus* as a Community-acquired Meticillin-Resistant Clone
Robinson DA, Kearns AM, Holmes A, et al (Univ of Bath, England; Health Protection Agency, London; Stobhill Hosp, Glasgow, Scotland; et al)
Lancet 365:1256-1258, 2005   3–9

Background.—A penicillin-resistant clone of *Staphylococcus aureus*, known as phage type 80/81, was first isolated from neonatal infections in Australia in 1953. In that same year, similar isolates, designated phage type 81, were isolated in Canada. Both isolates could be lysed by both phages and were thus thought to be members of the same clone, termed phage type 80/81. This type became pandemic in the 1950s and caused a high frequency of skin lesions, sepsis, and pneumonia in children and young adults in both hospitals and the community. The pandemic waned in the 1960s with the introduction and use of methicillin and its derivatives to treat penicillin-resistant staphylococcal infections. Whether early 80/81 isolates had the genes for Panton-Valentine leucocidin, a toxin associated with virulence in healthy young people, was determined.

Method.—Portions of 7 housekeeping genes from 26 isolates of 80/81 isolated between 1955 and 1969 in Australia, England, and the United States were sequenced. These sequences were then compared with more than 1000 isolates in the multilocus sequence typing database. The 80/81 isolates are multilocus sequence type (ST) 30, a common genotype that causes disease in hospital patients and healthy persons. Typing resolution was improved by sequencing portions of 8 genes that are more variable from the 26 isolates of 80/81 and comparing them with sequences from 17 other isolates of ST30 and ST36, which corresponds to the second most common methicillin-resistant *S aureus* (MRSA) clone in hospitals in the United Kingdom.

Results.—Nearly all the early 80/81 isolates were identical at 15 genes to the putative ancestral genotype of ST30. Multilocus sequence analysis suggested that descendants of 80/81 have acquired resistance to methicillin and are reemerging as a community-acquired MRSA clone. It also appeared that descendants of 80/81 are a sister lineage to pandemic, hospital-acquired MRSA.

Conclusions.—The reemergence of the 80/81 clone, which had waned in the 1960s after achieving pandemic proportions in the 1950s, could present a serious challenge to public health in the near future.

▶ The possibility that the virulent clone of *S aureus*, thought to be eliminated in the 1960s, could be reemerging, reequipped, and revitalized, suggests a serious public health challenge in the years to come.

B. H. Thiers, MD

The Evolving Characteristics and Care of Necrotizing Soft-Tissue Infections

Endorf FW, Supple KG, Gamelli RL (Loyola Univ, Maywood, Ill)
Burns 31:269-273, 2005   3–10

Background.—Necrotizing soft-tissue infections such as necrotizing fasciitis and Fournier's gangrene are a source of high morbidity and mortality. These difficult cases are increasingly being referred to burn centers for specialized wound and critical care issues. In this study, we examine our institution's recent experience with a large series of necrotizing soft-tissue infections.

Study Design.—A retrospective chart review was performed of 65 consecutive patients over a 5-year period with necrotizing soft-tissue infections that required radical surgical debridement.

Results.—Overall survival was 83%, with an average length of stay of 32.4 ± 3.32 days for survivors and for the entire group of 29.5 ± 3 days. Time from onset of symptoms to initial presentation to our institution averaged 6.9 ± 1.19 days. Patients averaged 2.9 ± 0.22 surgical procedures, and 46%

of patients required skin grafting with an average graft area of 1554 ± 248 cm². Of the survivors, only 54% were able to return home, with 46% needing further hospitalization or transfer to an inpatient rehabilitation facility.

Conclusions.—There were frequent delays in diagnosis and referrals to and from within our institution, and progress can be made in educating the medical community to identify these patients. Advancements in wound care and critical care have made inroads into the treatment of patients with necrotizing soft-tissue infections. However, these infections continue to be a source of high morbidity and mortality and significant healthcare resource consumption. These challenging patients are best served with prompt diagnosis, immediate radical surgical debridement, and aggressive critical care management. Referral to a major burn center may help provide optimal surgical intervention, wound care, and critical care management.

Idiopathic Necrotizing Fasciitis: Risk Factors and Strategies for Management
Taviloglu K, Cabioglu N, Cagatay A, et al (Istanbul Univ, Turkey)
Am Surg 71:315-320, 2005   3–11

Introduction.—The prognosis of necrotizing fasciitis (NF) depends on early diagnosis and management. Idiopathic NF may be more challenging, because it occurs in the absence of a known causative factor. Therefore, our purpose in this study was to identify the distinct features of idiopathic NF that may be important in early recognition of this disease and determine the factors associated with mortality. A retrospective chart review was performed in patients with a diagnosis of NF between 1988 and 2003. Patients were classified as idiopathic and secondary NF, and data were analyzed in terms of etiological and predisposing factors, causative microbiological organisms, and clinical outcome. The study included 98 patients, 63 men and 35 women, with a diagnosis of NF. The median age was 55.5 years (range, 13-80). Idiopathic NF occurred in 60 of 98 patients (61%). The principal anatomic sites of infection for NF were perineal localisation in 55 patients (66%) and extremities in 31 patients (32%). Characteristics that distinguish patients with idiopathic NF from secondary NF were as follows: age older than 55 years ($P = 0.0001$), presence of comorbid illnesses like DM ($P = 0.007$) or chronic renal failure ($P = 0.041$), and perineal localization ($P = 0.008$). By logistic regression analysis, independent risk factors for idiopathic NF remained age ≥ 55 years and perineal localization as statistically significant factors, when all the significant variables found in univariate analysis were included in the model. The majority of patients (82%) had polymicrobial infections. The mortality rate was 35 per cent. All patients were treated with radical surgical debridement and a combination of antibiotics. Female gender, presence of malignant disease, and diabetes mellitus (DM) were found to be associated with increased mortality as independent factors in logistic regression analysis, when all of these three factors were included in the model. Understanding the distinct clinical characteristics and the factors associated with mortality in patients with NF may lead to rapid diagnosis and improve the survival rates. Therefore, idiopathic NF is a crucial entity that requires serious suspicion for its diagnosis.

▶ As emphasized in articles reviewed in previous editions of the YEAR BOOK OF DERMATOLOGY AND DERMATOLOGIC SURGERY, early diagnosis and surgical debridement are the keys to a successful outcome in patients with necrotizing soft tissue infections. Although they are rare, their incidence is increasing, and they are the sources of significant morbidity and mortality (Abstracts 3–10 and 3–11). Efforts must be made to educate the medical community about the signs and symptoms of these infections to ensure that optimal care is delivered in an appropriate and timely manner.

B. H. Thiers, MD

Predictors of Mortality and Limb Loss in Necrotizing Soft Tissue Infections

Anaya DA, McMahon K, Nathens AB, et al (Harborview Med Ctr, Seattle; Univ of Washington, Seattle)
Arch Surg 140:151-157, 2005   3–12

Hypothesis.—Necrotizing soft tissue infections are associated with a high mortality rate. We hypothesize that specific predictors of limb loss and mortality in patients with necrotizing soft tissue infection can be identified on hospital admission.

Design.—A retrospective cohort study.

Setting.—A tertiary care center.

Patients.—Patients with a diagnosis of necrotizing soft tissue infection during a 5-year period (1996-2001) were included. Patients were identified with *International Classification of Diseases, Ninth Revision* hospital discharge diagnosis codes, and diagnosis was confirmed by medical record review.

Interventions.—Standard current treatment including early and scheduled repeated debridement, broad-spectrum antibiotics, and physiologic and nutritional support was given to all patients.

Main Outcome Measures.—Limb loss and mortality.

Results.—One hundred sixty-six patients were identified and included in the study. The overall mortality rate was 16.9%, and limb loss occurred in 26% of patients with extremity involvement. Independent predictors of mortality included white blood cell count greater than $30\,000 \times 10^3/\mu L$, creatinine level greater than 2 mg/dL (176.8 µmol/L), and heart disease at hospital admission. Independent predictors of limb loss included heart disease and shock (systolic blood pressure <90 mm Hg) at hospital admission. Clostridial infection was an independent predictor for both limb loss (odds ratio, 3.9 [95% confidence interval, 1.1-12.8]) and mortality (odds ratio, 4.1 [95% confidence interval, 1.3-12.3]) and was highly associated with intravenous drug use and a high rate of leukocytosis on hospital admission. The latter was found to be a good variable in estimating the probability of death.

Conclusions.—Clostridial infection is consistently associated with poor outcome. This together with the independent predictors mentioned earlier should aid in identifying patients on hospital admission who may benefit from more aggressive and novel therapeutic approaches.

▶ This retrospective study identified specific criteria associated with a poor outcome in patients with necrotizing soft tissue infections. Although clostridial infection is a powerful predictor of mortality and limb loss, differentiation from nonclostridial infection is difficult at the time of hospital admission, emphasizing the utility of the other parameters cited. Patients at high risk of mortality and limb loss should be considered for aggressive surgical intervention in addition to broad-spectrum antibiotics and physiologic and nutritional support.

B. H. Thiers, MD

Necrotising Fasciitis: Clinical Features in Patients With Liver Cirrhosis
Cheng N-C, Tai H-C, Tang Y-B, et al (Natl Taiwan Univ, Taipei)
Br J Plast Surg 58:702-707, 2005   3–13

Introduction.—Necrotising fasciitis is a fulminant and life-threatening infection. It is associated with a high mortality rate and is often seen in the aged and immunocompromised patients. Liver cirrhosis is regarded as a risk factor of necrotising fasciitis. From January 1995 to December 2003, 17 cirrhotic patients who had been admitted to our hospital for necrotising fasciitis were identified. The infections all developed in the lower extremities. Only six patients survived, and the overall case fatality rate was 64.7%. The cases were divided into two groups: survivors and nonsurvivors. Comparisons were made on age, gender, presenting symptoms, underlying medical diseases, laboratory data and clinical course. Underlying diabetes mellitus and grade C liver cirrhosis were the only statistically significant factors that led to poor prognosis ($p<0.05$).

▶ Necrotizing fasciitis is a life-threatening disease, and an early diagnosis and aggressive debridement are the cornerstones of therapy. Cheng et al show that patients with cirrhosis, especially those with diabetes, have an especially poor prognosis. The diagnosis of necrotizing fasciitis should be considered in any soft tissue infection involving the lower limbs in such patients. Early involvement of experienced surgeons and a low threshold for surgical exploration are mandatory.

B. H. Thiers, MD

Hematogenous Dissemination in Early Lyme Disease

Wormser GP, McKenna D, Carlin J, et al (New York Med College, Valhalla, NY; Vanderbilt Univ, Nashville, Tenn)
Ann Intern Med 142:751-755, 2005

3–14

Background.—Bloodstream invasion in Lyme disease has been difficult to study because until recently blood culture methods were too insensitive to detect spirochetemia.

Objective.—To evaluate the clinical and laboratory features of spirochetemic patients.

Design.—Cross-sectional study.

Setting.—Lyme Disease Diagnostic Center in Valhalla, New York, 1997 to 2002.

Patients.—213 untreated adults with erythema migrans.

Intervention.—Blood culture for *Borrelia burgdorferi*.

Measurements.—Symptom scores and selected laboratory measures.

Results.—Spirochetemia was found in 93 (43.7%) patients. Spirochetemic patients were more often symptomatic (89.2% vs. 74.2%; $P = 0.006$) and more often had multiple erythema migrans lesions (41.9% vs. 15.0%; $P < 0.001$) than patients without spirochetemia. However, 8 (22.9%) of the 35 asymptomatic patients with a single skin lesion nevertheless had a positive blood culture. Risk for spirochetemia was present the day the patient noticed the lesion and continued for more than 2 weeks.

Limitations.—Long-term outcome data were not available.

Conclusions.—The high rate, early onset, and prolonged duration of risk for spirochetemia explain why untreated patients with erythema migrans are at risk for dissemination of *B. burgdorferi* to anatomic sites beyond the lesion site. Differences in the strain of the infecting spirochete, as well as host factors, may be important determinants of hematogenous dissemination.

▶ Until recently, blood culture techniques have been too insensitive to detect spirochetemia in patients with Lyme disease. Thus, clinical and laboratory characteristics of bloodstream invasion in infected patients have not been well studied. Wormser et al show that spirochetemia occurs commonly in patients with erythema migrans and such patients have a higher incidence and greater severity of clinical symptoms than do patients without bloodstream invasion. In untreated patients, spirochetes can be identified in the blood for more than 2 weeks after the onset of the characteristic skin lesion. Thus, the most likely mechanism for the spreading of the spirochete to distant organs is hematogenous dissemination.

B. H. Thiers, MD

Rocky Mountain Spotted Fever From an Unexpected Tick Vector in Arizona

Demma LJ, Traefer MS, Nicholson WL, et al (Ctrs for Disease Control, Atlanta, Ga; Indian Health Service, Whiteriver, Ariz; Indian Health Service, Albuquerque, NM)
N Engl J Med 353:587-594, 2005   3–15

Background.—Rocky Mountain spotted fever is a life-threatening, tick-borne disease caused by *Rickettsia rickettsii*. This disease is rarely reported in Arizona, and the principal vectors, *Dermacentor* species ticks, are uncommon in the state. From 2002 through 2004, a focus of Rocky Mountain spotted fever was investigated in rural eastern Arizona.

Methods.—We obtained blood and tissue specimens from patients with suspected Rocky Mountain spotted fever and ticks from patients' homesites. Serologic, molecular, immunohistochemical, and culture assays were performed to identify the causative agent. On the basis of specific laboratory criteria, patients were classified as having confirmed or probable Rocky Mountain spotted fever infection.

Results.—A total of 16 patients with Rocky Mountain spotted fever infection (11 with confirmed and 5 with probable infection) were identified. Of these patients, 13 (81 percent) were children 12 years of age or younger, 15 (94 percent) were hospitalized, and 2 (12 percent) died. Dense populations of *Rhipicephalus sanguineus* ticks were found on dogs and in the yards of patients' homesites. All patients with confirmed Rocky Mountain spotted fever had contact with tick-infested dogs, and four had a reported history of tick bite preceding the illness. *R. rickettsii* DNA was detected in non-engorged *R. sanguineus* ticks collected at one home, and *R. rickettsii* isolates were cultured from these ticks.

Conclusions.—This investigation documents the presence of Rocky Mountain spotted fever in eastern Arizona, with common brown dog ticks (*R. sanguineus*) implicated as a vector of *R. rickettsii*. The broad distribution of this common tick raises concern about its potential to transmit *R. rickettsii* in other settings.

▶ Demma et al report that a very common type of dog tick can spread Rocky Mountain spotted fever, a serious and occasionally fatal illness whose incidence appears to be increasing in the United States. This is the first time that a tick that routinely infests house pets has been implicated in the transmission of the disease; previously the 2 types of ticks that were known to transmit Rocky Mountain spotted fever were less common and were carried mostly by rodents and dogs that lived near wild or rural areas. The first case of Rocky Mountain spotted fever was recognized a century ago in Idaho but has now been observed throughout much of the United States, with more than half the cases being reported from the South Atlantic states. *R sanguineus* is present worldwide and may be the vector in many unexplained cases of the disease throughout the United States.[1]

B. H. Thiers, MD

Reference

1. Dumler JS, Walker DH: Rocky Mountain spotted fever—Changing ecology and persisting virulence. *N Eng J Med* 353:551-553, 2005.

Infection With *Chlamydia trachomatis* After Mass Treatment of a Trachoma Hyperendemic Community in Tanzania: A Longitudinal Study

West SK, Munoz B, Mkocha H, et al (Johns Hopkins Univ, Baltimore, Md; Kongwa Trachoma Project, Tanzania; London School of Hygiene and Tropical Medicine; et al)

Lancet 366:1296-1300, 2005   3–16

Background.—Data from studies done in communities where trachoma is mesoendemic suggest that ocular infection with *Chlamydia trachomatis* can be eliminated after one mass treatment with antibiotics. However, there are no comparable long-term data from trachoma hyperendemic communities. Our aim, therefore, was two-fold: first, to ascertain the disease pattern of trachoma and ocular infection with *C trachomatis* in a trachoma hyperendemic community after mass treatment; and, second, to ascertain the risk factors for incident infection.

Methods.—We did a longitudinal study of a trachoma hyperendemic community (n=1017) in Tanzania. We did surveys, including ocular swabs, at baseline, 2, 6, 12, and 18 months to identify the presence, and quantity, of *C trachomatis* after single mass treatment of all individuals aged 6 months or older with azithromycin 20 mg per kg; pregnant women without clinical disease received topical tetracycline.

Findings.—Mass treatment (coverage 86%) significantly reduced the prevalence of infection from 57% (495 of 871) to 12% (85 of 705) at 2 months. Infection remained fairly constant to 12 months, with evidence of increasing numbers and load of infection by 18 months post-treatment. Incident infection at 6 months was 3.5-times more likely if another member of the household had more than 19 organisms per swab at 2 months. Travel outside the village, and visitors to the household, did not increase the risk of infection within households up to 12 months.

Interpretation.—In this trachoma hyperendemic community, infection levels after high antibiotic coverage persisted at a low level to 18 months, with evidence for re-emergence after 1 year. Fairly light loads of infection were associated with household transmission. Yearly mass treatment over a few years could be sufficient to eliminate infection.

Re-emergence of *Chlamydia trachomatis* Infection After Mass Antibiotic Treatment of a Trachoma-Endemic Gambian Community: A Longitudinal Study

Burton MJ, Holland MJ, Makalo P, et al (London School of Hygiene and Tropical Medicine; Med Research Council Labs, Fajara, The Gambia; Natl Eye Care Programme, Banjul, The Gambia; et al)
Lancet 365:1321-1328, 2005   3–17

Background.—Community-wide mass antibiotic treatment is a central component of trachoma control. The optimum frequency and duration of treatment are unknown. We measured the effect of mass treatment on the conjunctival burden of *Chlamydia trachomatis* in a Gambian community with low to medium trachoma prevalence and investigated the rate, route, and determinants of re-emergent infection.

Methods.—14 trachoma-endemic villages in rural Gambia were examined and conjunctival swabs obtained at baseline, 2, 6, 12, and 17 months. Mass antibiotic treatment with azithromycin was given to the community at baseline. *C trachomatis* was detected by qualitative PCR and individual infection load then estimated by real-time quantitative PCR.

Findings.—*C trachomatis* was detected in 95 (7%) of 1319 individuals at baseline. Treatment coverage was 83% of the population (1328 of 1595 people). The effect of mass treatment was heterogeneous. In 12 villages all baseline infections (34 [3%] of 1062 individuals) resolved, and prevalence (three [0.3%]) and infection load remained low throughout the study. Two villages (baseline infection: 61 [24%] of 257 individuals) had increased infection 2 months after treatment (74 [30%]), after extensive contact with other untreated communities. Subsequently, this value reduced to less than half of that before treatment (25 [11%]).

Interpretation.—Mass antibiotic treatment generally results in effective, longlasting control of *C trachomatis* in this environment. For low prevalence regions, one treatment episode might be sufficient. Infection can be re-introduced through contact with untreated populations. Communities need to be monitored for treatment failure and control measures implemented over wide geographical areas.

▶ Infection with *C trachomatis* is an important cause of blindness worldwide. It affects some of the world's poorest regions, in which 146 million people are estimated to have active disease. A single dose of azithromycin, as administered in this study, would seem to be a very small price to pay for long-lasting control of the disease.

B. H. Thiers, MD

Interactions Between Bacteria and *Candida* in the Burn Wound

Gupta N, Haque A, Mukhopadhyay G, et al (Jawaharlal Nehru Univ, New Delhi, India; Safdarjung Hosp, New Delhi, India)
Burns 31:375-378, 2005

3–18

Background.—Bacterial-fungal interactions may have an important role in clinical situations in which a patient suffers from mixed infections of both bacterial and fungal origins. A classic example of such a scenario is the burn wound. The susceptibility of the burn wound to such infections is the result of several factors, including the presence of coagulated proteins, the absence of blood-borne immune factors and antibiotics, and the avascularity of the burn. In addition, the indiscriminate use of antibiotics promotes fungal growth, particularly colonization of the burn wound by yeast.

Among the pathogenic yeasts, *Candida* species is the one most frequently isolated in burn wounds. In developing countries such as India, thermal and electric burns are a national problem. The majority of burn patients in India suffer from mixed bacterial and fungal infections that result in complex interactions between these organisms. These interactions may completely alter the clinical scenario of the patient. Whether the presence of some bacterial species affects the growth of *Candida* species in the wounds of burn patients was investigated.

Methods.—A retrospective analysis was conducted of fungal (*Candida* species) and bacterial isolates obtained from the wound swabs of 300 burn patients. Four swabs were collected from each patient. Two swabs were subjected to mycologic analysis and 2 were subjected to bacteriologic analysis.

Results.—*Pseudomonas* species, when present alone or in combination with other bacterial species, invariably inhibited the growth of *Candida* species. A significant growth inhibition of *Candida* species in the presence of bacterial combinations such as *Klebsiella* species plus others, others alone, or *Staphylococcus aureus* alone was also observed, but these results were not consistent when either *Klebsiella* species or *S aureus* were present in the burn wound in isolation or in different bacterial combinations.

Conclusion.—The absence of *Candida* species in burn wounds where *Pseudomonas* species is present is a result of the inhibition of *Candida* growth by *Pseudomonas*.

▶ The presumed inhibitory effect of *Pseudomonas* species on *Candida* species is an interesting finding with therapeutic implications.

B. H. Thiers, MD

Chronic Dermatomycoses of the Foot as Risk Factors for Acute Bacterial Cellulitis of the Leg: A Case-Control Study

Roujeau J-C, Sigurgeirsson B, Korting H-C, et al (Hôpital Henri-Mondor, Créteil, France; Landspitali Univ, Reykjavik, Iceland; Univ of Munich; et al)
Dermatology 209:301-307, 2004   3–19

Background.—Erysipelas, or acute non-necrotizing bacterial cellulitis of the leg, is a common infection of the skin and subcutaneous tissue and a cause of significant morbidity. Foot dermatomycosis (tinea pedis and onychomycosis) may be an important, treatable risk factor for bacterial cellulitis of the leg. In the absence of other predisposing factors, clinical signs suggestive of ipsilateral athlete's foot (tinea pedis interdigitalis) have been observed in up to 80% of patients with cellulitis of the leg. The role of foot dermatomycosis and other potential risk factors in the development of acute bacterial cellulitis of the leg was determined.

Methods.—A case-control study was conducted, consisting of 243 patients with acute bacterial cellulitis of the leg and 467 control subjects matched for gender, age (±5 years), hospital, and admission date (±2 months). The mean age of the patients and control subjects was 59 and 61 years, respectively.

Results.—Overall, mycology-proved foot dermatomycosis was a significant risk factor for acute bacterial cellulitis. Tinea pedis interdigitalis, tinea pedis plantaris, and onychomycosis were also significant individual risk factors for acute bacterial cellulitis. Other risk factors included a disruption of the cutaneous barrier, a history of bacterial cellulitis, chronic venous insufficiency, and leg edema.

Conclusions.—Tinea pedis and onychomycosis were significant risk factors for acute bacterial cellulitis of the leg. These risk factors can be treated effectively with pharmacologic therapy. Careful screening and treatment of foot dermatomycoses can help to eliminate these specific risk factors, particularly in patients with other risk factors, such as a history of acute bacterial cellulitis, chronic venous insufficiency, and being overweight.

▶ The message is clear: patients with bacterial cellulitis of the leg should be investigated for coincident tinea pedis and onychomycosis and, if these conditions are present, they should be treated aggressively. Clearly, the same can be said for other risk factors for cellulitis such as obesity and venous insufficiency.

B. H. Thiers, MD

Venous Insufficiency in Patients With Toenail Onychomycosis

Kulac M, Acar M, Karaca S, et al (Afyon Kocatepe Univ, Turkey)
J Ultrasound Med 24:1085-1089, 2005   3–20

Objective.—Onychomycosis is a common fungal infection of the toenails and can originate secondary to vascular abnormalities. The aim of this study was to evaluate the relationship between onychomycosis and venous insufficiency.

Methods.—Forty-two patients with onychomycosis and 39 healthy control subjects who had normal toenails were enrolled in the study. Doppler examinations were performed with a commercially available scanner and a 7.5-MHz linear probe. Major superficial and deep veins of the lower limb, including long and short saphenous, femoral, and popliteal veins, were examined. Venous insufficiency was assessed with the Valsalva test. With the Doppler examination, retrograde flow of more than 1 second was accepted as venous insufficiency.

Results.—Venous insufficiency was detected more frequently in patients with onychomycosis than in the control group (15 [35.7%] of 42 and 6 [15.4%] of 39, respectively; $P = .037$). Reflux was bilateral in 4 (26.7%) of 15 patients with onychomycosis, and in those 4 patients the onychomycosis was also bilateral. In 7 (46.7%) of 15 patients, onychomycosis and venous insufficiency were detected ipsilaterally, whereas there were no onychopathic features contralaterally. Although unilateral insufficiency was present in 4 (26.7%) of 15 patients, these patients had bilateral onychomycosis.

Conclusions.—We found a significant relationship between onychomycosis and venous insufficiency; therefore, we recommend a routine venous Doppler examination for patients with onychomycosis to diagnose or rule out venous insufficiency.

▶ Although the authors' suggestion that patients with onychomycosis undergo routine venous Doppler examination to rule out venous insufficiency is somewhat extreme, it would be interesting to study the effect of compromised venous return on the response to systemic therapy. Presumably, the response rates reported in the literature were derived from patients without any such comorbidities that might compromise their response to treatment.[1]

B. H. Thiers, MD

Reference

1. Evans EG, Sigurgeirsson B: Double blind, randomised study of continuous terbinafine compared with intermittent itraconazole in treatment of toenail onychomycosis: The LION Study Group. *BMJ* 318:1031-1035, 1999.

Pulse Versus Continuous Terbinafine for Onychomycosis: A Randomized, Double-blind, Controlled Trial
Warshaw EM, Fett DD, Bloomfield HE, et al (Minneapolis Veterans Affairs Med Ctr; Univ of Minnesota, Minneapolis; Palm Harbor, Fla; et al)
J Am Acad Dermatol 53:578-584, 2005   3–21

Background.—Effective treatments for onychomycosis are expensive. Previous studies suggest that less costly, pulsed doses of antifungal medications may be as effective as standard, continuous doses. Terbinafine is the current treatment of choice for toenail onychomycosis.

Objective.—Our purpose was to determine whether pulse-dose terbinafine is as effective as standard continuous-dose terbinafine for treatment of toenail onychomycosis.

Methods.—We conducted a double-blind, randomized, noninferiority, clinical intervention trial in the Minneapolis Veterans Affairs Medical Center. The main inclusion criteria for participants were a positive dermatophyte culture and at least 25% distal subungual clinical involvement. Six hundred eighteen volunteers were screened; 306 were randomized. Terbinafine, 250 mg daily for 3 months (continuous) or terbinafine, 500 mg daily for 1 week per month for 3 months (pulse) was administered. The primary outcome measure was mycological cure of the target toenail at 18 months. Secondary outcome measures included clinical cure and complete (clinical plus mycological) cure of the target toenail and complete cure of all 10 toenails.

Results.—Results of an intent-to-treat analysis did not meet the prespecified criterion for noninferiority but did demonstrate the superiority of continuous-dose terbinafine for: mycological cure of the target toenail (70.9% [105/148] vs 58.7% [84/143]; $P = .03$, relative risk [RR] of 1.21 [95% confidence interval (CI), 1.02-1.43]); clinical cure of the target toenail (44.6% [66/148] vs 29.3% [42/143]; $P = .007$, RR = 1.52 [95% CI, 1.11-2.07); complete cure of the target toenail (40.5% [60/148] vs 28.0% [40/143]; $P = .02$, RR = 1.45 [95% CI, 1.04-2.01); and complete cure of all 10 toenails (25.2% [36/143] vs 14.7% [21/143]; $P = .03$, RR = 1.71 [95% CI, 1.05-2.79). Tolerability of the regimens did not differ significantly between the groups ($\chi^2 = 1.63$; $P = .65$).

Limitations.—The study population primarily consisted of older men with severe onychomycosis.

Conclusions.—This study demonstrated the superiority of continuous- over pulse-dose terbinafine. We also found this expensive therapy to be much less effective than previously believed, particularly for achieving complete cure of all 10 toenails.

▶ The authors demonstrate that continuous terbinafine therapy is more effective than pulse dosing. They also present interesting data to show that in patients with extensive onychomycosis (eg, involvement of all 10 toenails), treatment with either of these regimens may be an exercise in futility.

B. H. Thiers, MD

Prevention of Onychomycosis Reinfection for Patients With Complete Cure of All 10 Toenails: Results of a Double-blind, Placebo-controlled, Pilot Study of Prophylactic Miconazole Powder 2%
Warshaw EM, St Clair KR (Univ of Minnesota, Minneapolis; Colby College, Waterville, Maine)
J Am Acad Dermatol 53:717-720, 2005   3–22

Background.—Onychomycosis, the most common nail disease in adults, was considered an incurable disease by many practitioners until recently.

However, the view has changed with the development of effective oral antifungal agents. The challenge for physicians now is to prevent reinfection after successful treatment. Reinfection rates after a successful cure have ranged from 9% to 53% during a period of up to 5 years. Several studies have addressed the use of topical agents for prophylaxis of tinea pedis, but none have evaluated treatments for prophylaxis of onychomycosis. Whether biweekly miconazole powder can prevent an onychomycosis recurrence was determined.

Methods.—A double-blind placebo-controlled study was conducted to determine whether the biweekly use of 2% miconazole powder in shoes and on feet would prevent reinfection in patients who have been successfully treated for onychomycosis. The study group consisted of 48 patients with a mycologic and clinical cure of all 10 toenails at least 12 months but no more than 36 months after treatment with terbinafine or itraconazole for culture-proved onychomycosis. No statistically significant differences were present between the placebo and treatment groups in terms of sex, age, height, weight, diabetic status, duration of infection before treatment, or culture results before treatment. Analysis was by intention-to-treat.

Results.—No significant differences were found between the treatment and placebo groups in mycologic, clinical, or complete onychomycosis reinfection rates or time to reinfection. The rate of reinfection in the treatment group was 17.4% (4 patients) compared with a rate of 27.3% (6 patients) in the placebo group.

Conclusions.—The study was limited by a small sample size and an arbitrarily chosen dosing regimen, but it found no significant association between the use of clotrimazole and a mycologic, clinical, or complete recurrence of toenail onychomycosis. Larger studies are needed to determine whether different dosing regimens of topical prophylactic antifungals, oral antifungals, or a combination of both are effective in preventing onychomycosis reinfection.

▶ I often ask patients to continue topical antifungal treatment to the toes after systemic therapy has been completed, under the assumption that, if reinfection occurs, it would result from spreading of the infection to the nail from the periungual skin. The data presented here suggest that this approach may be in vain.

B. H. Thiers, MD

A Randomized Controlled Trial Assessing the Efficacy of Fluconazole in the Treatment of Pediatric Tinea Capitis
Foster KW, Friedlander SF, Panzer H, et al (Univ of Alabama at Birmingham; University of California, San Diego; Pfizer, New York; et al)
J Am Acad Dermatol 53:798-809, 2005   3–23

Background.—Griseofulvin is considered first-line therapy for tinea capitis, and the Physician's Desk Reference currently recommends 11 mg/kg per day microsize formulation for use in children. Diverse selective pressures have resulted in waning clinical efficacy of griseofulvin, such that higher doses and longer courses of treatment are required. These events have prompted the search for therapeutic alternatives. Fluconazole is one such treatment option, and a variety of studies using this drug have shown promise in the treatment of pediatric tinea capitis.

Objective.—We sought to assess the efficacy, safety, and optimal dose and duration of fluconazole therapy compared with standard-dose griseofulvin (11 mg/kg per day microsize formulation) in the treatment of pediatric tinea capitis.

Methods.—This randomized, multicenter, third-party-blind, 3-arm trial was designed as a superiority study to identify a therapeutically superior agent/regimen from the 3 treatment arms: (1) fluconazole 6 mg/kg per day for 3 weeks followed by 3 weeks of placebo, (2) fluconazole 6 mg/kg per day for 6 weeks, and (3) griseofulvin 11 mg/kg per day for 6 weeks. Efficacy variables included mycological, clinical, and combined outcomes. The primary efficacy variable was the combined outcome of the modified intent-to-treat population at week 6. Patient safety was assessed throughout the study. Statistical analysis of the efficacy variables was conducted by means of the Cochran-Mantel-Haenszel test.

Results.—At the end of treatment, mycological cures were present in 44.5%, 49.6%, and 52.2% of the fluconazole 3-week, fluconazole 6-week, and griseofulvin groups, respectively. Analysis of the primary efficacy variable failed to identify any superior agent, and differences between the combined outcomes of the fluconazole 6-week and griseofulvin groups at week 6 were not significant ($P = .32$). Regarding mycological, clinical, and combined outcomes, no significant differences between the fluconazole 6-week and griseofulvin groups were detected at any time point in the study. No new safety concerns were raised by this trial, and the incidence of treatment-related adverse events noted in this study is concordant with previous reports. Patients in the fluconazole arms of the study fared similarly. At the end of the trial, the difference in mycological cures between the fluconazole arms was only 7.5%, and increases in the incidence of certain treatment-related adverse events were observed in the fluconazole 6-week group.

Limitations.—Adjunctive topical therapies and the impact of infected contacts were not assessed in this trial.

Conclusion.—Systemic therapy with fluconazole 6 mg/kg per day and standard-dose griseofulvin produces comparable but low mycological and clinical cure rates. The limited efficacy of standard-dose griseofulvin and the lack of consensus regarding dose and duration of griseofulvin therapy in tinea capitis emphasize the need for controlled trials to identify optimal treatment parameters. Although the efficacy of fluconazole is no better than that of standard-dose griseofulvin, it may still be useful in select patients with a contraindication or intolerance to high-dose griseofulvin. The outcomes observed in this trial highlight the need to more clearly define the relative importance of adjunctive topical therapies and the evaluation and treatment of infected contacts as factors affecting cure rates.

▶ Although it is convenient that fluconazole comes in a liquid form, cure rates were poor in this study. Fluconazole is more expensive than griseofulvin or terbinafine for the treatment of tinea capitis.

S. Raimer, MD

Primary Cutaneous Opportunistic Mold Infections in a Pediatric Population

Katta R, Bogle MA, Levy ML (Baylor College of Medicine, Houston; Univ of Texas at Houston)

J Am Acad Dermatol 53:213-219, 2005   3–24

Objective.—We sought to describe the features of cutaneous opportunistic mold infections in a general pediatric population.

Methods.—Computerized pathology records from Texas Children's Hospital in Houston during the years 1991 to 2000 were used to identify any biopsy specimens of skin diagnosed as having fungus or mold. The corresponding medical records were reviewed to identify cases of cutaneous opportunistic mold infections. Cases were limited to those with histologic confirmation of hyphae within the dermis or extending to the dermis.

Results.—A total of 11 cases in neonates and 22 cases in children and adolescents were identified. Prematurity and low birth weight were the major risk factors in the neonatal population. The nonneonatal cases mainly occurred in those with malignancies or undergoing transplantation. Mortality in neonates was 64%, but decreased to 18% in the nonneonatal population.

Conclusion.—Our overview of cutaneous infection by opportunistic molds in a pediatric population highlights the risk factors, causative organisms, and outcome of this group of infections. Even in the presence of severe compromise of the immune system, children with primary cutaneous mold infections had a favorable outcome with appropriate diagnosis and therapy.

▶ The incidence of opportunistic mold infections in children has increased as more low birth weight premature infants survive and as there are greater numbers of immunosuppressed children in the population. In this study from Houston, the most common organisms isolated were *Aspergillus*, *Mucor* species, and *Fusarium*. Ninety-one percent of the cases found in children were primary cutaneous infections, typically occurring at a venous access site or as the result of trauma. Necrotic or purpuric lesions were the most common cutaneous finding. Almost all were treated with amphotericin or liposomal amphotericin, with almost half receiving surgical therapy as well. With early recognition and treatment, the survival rate in the nonneonatal group was an impressive 82%.

S. Raimer, MD

Multifocal Cutaneous Mucormycosis Complicating Polymicrobial Wound Infections in a Tsunami Survivor From Sri Lanka

Andresen D, Donaldson A, Choo L, et al (St George Hosp, Sydney, Australia)
Lancet 365:876-878, 2005   3–25

Introduction.—A man injured in the tsunami of Dec 26, 2004, returned to Sydney for management of his soft-tissue injuries. Despite broad-spectrum antibiotics, surgical wound debridement, and vigilant wound care, his condition worsened. Muscle and fat necrosis developed in a previously debrided thigh wound, and necrotising lesions arose from previous abrasions. Histological analysis showed mucormycosis in three non-contiguous sites, and *Apophysomyces elegans* was isolated from excised wound tissue. Wound infections, both bacterial and fungal, will undoubtedly add to the morbidity and mortality already recorded in tsunami-affected areas. Other causes of cutaneous mucormycosis might develop in survivors, but this disease can be difficult to diagnose and even harder to treat, particularly in those remaining in affected regions.

Cutaneous Mucormycosis of the Upper Extremity: A Series of Patients and Review of the Literature

Chun JK, Christy M, Rudikoff D, et al (Mount Sinai Med Ctr, New York)
Eur J Plast Surg 27:291-294, 2004   3–26

Background.—Zygomycosis, a fungal infectious disease, is cause by Zygomycetes species and the orders Mucorales and Entomophthorales, all of which are common in the environment. Human exposure to these organisms is common, as they release a large number of airborne spores; however, clinical infection is usually limited to immunocompromised patients. Three cases of cutaneous mucormycosis of the upper extremity were reported.

> *Case 1.*—Man, 71, presented with a chief complaint of diffuse rashes for 1 month. He had polymyalgia rheumatica and myelodysplastic syndrome and had been receiving corticosteroid therapy for 18 months. On hospital day 15, a small skin lesion was noted on his right wrist near a previous IV site. Examination revealed a 2 × 2-cm, tender, purple-black eschar on the ulnar side of the right wrist, surrounded by a 4 × 5-cm area of induration and erythema (Fig 3; see color plate IX). The rest of the hand was normal. Initial biopsy of the lesion and potassium hydroxide preparation showed fungal nonseptate hyphae consistent with mucormycosis.
>
> *Case 2.*—Woman, 46, who was HIV positive and had a medical history of thrush, idiopathic thrombocytopenic purpura, multiple episodes of bacterial pneumonia, pulmonary tuberculosis, and syphilis, was admitted with recurrent pneumococcal pneumonia requiring intubation for 3 weeks. After transfer to the floor, an eschar appeared on the forearm around a previous IV site on the left fore-

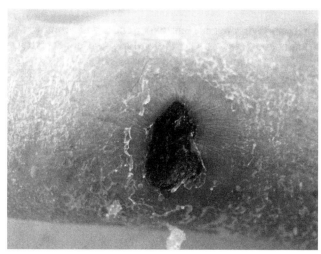

FIGURE 3.—Case 1. Well-demarcated eschar with surrounding erythema and induration at presentation. (Courtesy of Chun JK, Christy M, Rudikoff D, et al: Cutaneous mucormycosis of the upper extremity: A series of patients and review of the literature. *Eur J Plast Surg* 27:291-294, 2004. Copyright Springer-Verlag.)

arm. Biopsy results and cultures were positive for cutaneous mucormycosis.

Case 3.—Woman, 64, with a past medical history of insulin-dependent diabetes mellitus and end-stage renal disease, received an orthotopic renal transplant. The patient returned 2 weeks after discharge with a lesion on her right distal forearm. The patient was receiving immunosuppressive therapy to prevent transplant rejection. Biopsy of the site was found to be positive for mucormycosis.

Conclusions.—In all 3 cases, the patients underwent wide local excision of the eschar and skin graft as immediate coverage or as a delayed reconstruction. Systemic amphotericin B treatment was administered per recommendations of the infectious disease service. In all cases, the skin grafts healed with full resolution of the infectious process; however, 1 patient died of pneumonia.

▶ Any hospital-based physician would agree that mucormycosis is by no means a rare condition in immunosuppressed patients. Awareness of its presentation is necessary for early diagnosis and treatment. Cutaneous mucormycosis appears to have a propensity to affect areas of minor trauma; thus, the hand and the wrist are favored areas.

B. H. Thiers, MD

4 Viral Infections (Excluding HIV Infections)

Imiquimod Cream 5% for Recalcitrant Cutaneous Warts in Immunosuppressed Individuals

Harwood CA, Perrett CM, Brown VL, et al (Univ of London)
Br J Dermatol 152:122-129, 2005   4–1

Background.—Viral warts may cause significant morbidity in individuals unable to mount an adequate T-helper 1 cell-mediated immune response to human papillomavirus. Imiquimod is a potent inducer of antiviral cytokine activity which has shown significant efficacy in the treatment of genital warts. Similar efficacy in cutaneous warts is not yet established.

Objectives.—To assess the response of persistent cutaneous warts to 5% imiquimod cream in immunosuppressed individuals.

Methods.—Fifteen immunosuppressed patients with warts on the hands and/or feet present for more than 18 months, which had failed to respond to a minimum of 12 weeks of topical salicylic acid and four cycles of cryotherapy, were recruited. Imiquimod 5% cream was applied in an open label, right vs. left comparison study for 24 weeks (three times weekly for 8 weeks, daily for 8 weeks, then daily with occlusion for 8 weeks).

Results.—Twelve (80%) patients completed the study protocol. Benefit was seen in five patients [36% in the intent-to-treat analysis (14 patients)], including more than 30% clearance of warts in three patients and reduction in overall size of warts in two further cases. Local skin reactions occurred in four (29%) patients and were usually mild. A transient rise in creatinine (11-29% above baseline) was measured in three renal transplant recipients, but we did not consider that this was related to imiquimod exposure.

Conclusions.—This is the first controlled study to assess therapeutic efficacy of topical 5% imiquimod cream in persistent warts associated with immunosuppression. It provides preliminary evidence that topical imiquimod may benefit a subgroup of immunosuppressed patients with recalcitrant cutaneous warts.

▶ Imiquimod stimulates the immune response in otherwise healthy individuals. One unanswered question is how effectively the drug might work in patients who are immunosuppressed. Moreover, are there adverse consequences to stimulating the immune response in patients who are therapeutically immunosuppressed (eg, to prevent rejection of a transplanted organ)? Unfortunately, the study by Harwood et al leaves many questions unanswered.

B. H. Thiers, MD

Intralesional Immunotherapy of Warts With Mumps, *Candida*, and *Trichophyton* Skin Test Antigens: A Single-blinded, Randomized, and Controlled Trial

Horn TD, Johnson SM, Helm RM, et al (Univ of Arkansas for Medical Sciences, Little Rock)

Arch Dermatol 141:589-594, 2005   4–2

Background.—Warts occur commonly in humans. Destructive modalities are generally the first physician-administered therapy. Other treatment options include immunotherapy. Intralesional immunotherapy using mumps, *Candida*, or *Trichophyton* skin test antigens has proved efficacy in the treatment of warts.

Objectives.—To determine rates of wart resolution in response to injection of antigen alone, antigen plus interferon alfa-2b, interferon alfa-2b alone, and normal saline; and to compare response according to viral type, major histocompatibility complex antigens, and peripheral blood mononuclear cell proliferation to autologous human papillomavirus antigen before and after injection.

Design.—Randomized, single-blinded, placebo-controlled, clinical trial.

Setting.—Medical school–based dermatology department.

Patients.—Two hundred thirty-three patients clinically diagnosed as having 1 or more warts.

Main Outcome Measure.—Clinical resolution of warts in response to intralesional immunotherapy.

Results.—Responders were observed in all treatment arms, but were significantly more likely to have received antigen ($P<.001$). Resolution of distant untreated warts was observed, and was significantly more likely in subjects receiving antigen ($P<.001$). Interferon did not significantly enhance the response rate ($P=.20$) and did not differ from normal saline ($P=.65$). No viral type or major histocompatibility complex antigen correlated with response or lack of response ($P>.99$ and $P=.86$, respectively). A positive peripheral blood mononuclear cell proliferation assay result (2 times pretreatment levels) was significantly more likely among responders

(P=.002). While there was no significant difference in response based on sex (P=.56), older subjects (>40 years) were less likely to respond (P=.01).

Conclusions.—Intralesional immunotherapy using injection of *Candida*, mumps, or *Trichophyton* skin test antigens is an effective treatment for warts, as indicated by significantly higher response rates and distant response rates in subjects receiving antigen. Viral type and major histocompatibility complex antigens did not seem to influence treatment response. Response is accompanied by proliferation of peripheral blood mononuclear cells to human papillomavirus antigens, suggesting that a human papillomavirus-directed cell-mediated immune response plays a role in wart resolution.

▶ This continues to be an interesting approach for the treatment of warts. Unfortunately, any known successful therapy for warts may be quite effective in some patients and totally devoid of efficacy in others. Moreover, to my knowledge, one cannot easily predict which patients will respond to different therapies.

Nevertheless, I have had significant success using serial injections of *Candida* antigen in a subgroup of patients with recalcitrant warts. The best responders typically are women with a prior history of vaginal yeast infections. These patients typically have a significant degree of local tissue edema and discomfort, not only in injected warts but in noninjected warts as well.

Occasionally, patients with multiple warts may clear with 1 or a few injections. These individuals may experience a significant flu-like reaction, likely attributable to cytokine release after injection of the *Candida* antigen. Certainly, this approach should be considered before proceeding with more complicated and disabling destructive therapies.

J. Cook, MD

Photodynamic Therapy: New Treatment for Therapy-Resistant Plantar Warts

Schroeter CA, Pleunis J, van Nispen tot Pannerden C, et al (Med Centre Maastricht, The Netherlands; Student Universiteit Maastricht, The Netherlands; Univ of Cologne, Germany; et al)
Dermatol Surg 31:71-75, 2005   4–3

Background.—Plantar wart treatment remains a challenging one. Various treatment modalities have been previously used and are still in current use. The problem remains in the degree of response to these treatments and the side effects associated with them.

Objective.—The aim of this study was to test a new treatment modality for therapy-resistant plantar warts.

Methods.—Thirty-one patients with 48 plantar warts were randomly selected from the Department of Laser Therapy, Medical Centre Maastricht, The Netherlands. The mean age of the patients was 29 years (range 6–74 years). The mean incubation time was 6.8 hours, and the mean treatment time was 18.7 minutes per wart. Each wart was treated an average of 2.3 times, with a median fluence of 100 cm².

Results.—Forty-two of 48 (88%) warts showed a complete response. A trend was found between total clearance and size of the warts, age of the patient, and the mean treatment time. No significant side effects were seen postoperatively.

Conclusion.—This study showed that recalcitrant plantar warts were successfully treated with no significant side effects; however, the user needs sufficient experience for this new effective treatment application.

▶ The perfect treatment for plantar warts has yet to be discovered. Current treatments that are painless are often ineffective, and those that may be more effective can be associated with pain, prolonged healing, disability, and sometimes scarring. In this report the authors describe yet another treatment for plantar warts: topical photodynamic therapy. The results are almost too good to be true; the treatments were well tolerated and 88% effective. However, before we become too excited, we should await the results of other studies to confirm these findings. It should be noted that the investigators used a red light source that penetrates more deeply than the blue light commonly used for photodynamic therapy.

P. G. Lang, Jr, MD

Application of Viable Bacille Calmette-Guérin Topically as a Potential Therapeutic Modality in Condylomata Acuminata: A Placebo-controlled Study

Metawea B, El-Nashar A-R, Kamel I, et al (Cairo Univ Hosp; Kobri-Elkobba Military Hosp, Cairo)
Urology 65:247-250, 2005   4–4

Objectives.—To evaluate the efficacy of topical application of viable bacille Calmette-Guérin (BCG) as a primary line of treatment in patients with condylomata acuminata.

Methods.—We recruited 50 patients from the Department of Andrology and Sexually Transmitted Diseases, Cairo University Hospital complaining of genital warts. Patients were divided into two groups. Group 1 consisted of 25 patients who received BCG as a weekly topical treatment for 6 consecutive weeks. If still resistant, another intensive three-times-a-week course for 3 consecutive weeks was given. Group 2 consisted of 25 patients who received 0.9% saline solution as a placebo solution with the same procedure and follow-up as for group 1. All patients were followed up for 6 consecutive months. During the treatment course, the local response, wart state and size, and any side effects were reported.

Results.—A complete response with the disappearance of all condylomata acuminata was achieved in 20 (80%) of the 25 patients after a maximum of six BCG applications. Three patients (12%) needed another, more extensive, course, resulting in complete clearance 3 weeks later. Only 2 patients (8%) did not achieve a full response even after application of the intensified BCG course. No response was detected in the placebo group, with no improvement during follow-up. No recurrence developed in any responder. Minimal side effects, such as transient erythema and fever, were recorded during the study.

Conclusions.—Topical BCG in the treatment of genital warts attained a high success rate in our study compared with the placebo solution, with insignificant side effects and no recurrence.

▶ The authors present yet another approach to harness the immune response to combat genital human papillomavirus infection. Although the results are quite impressive and the reported side effects minimal, larger controlled studies will be necessary to confirm the results reported here. Additionally, BCG is a relatively expensive immunomodulatory agent.

B. H. Thiers, MD

Clinic-Initiated, Twice-Daily Oral Famciclovir for Treatment of Recurrent Genital Herpes: A Randomized, Double-blind, Controlled Trial

Sacks SL, Aoki FY, Martel AY, et al (Univ of British Columbia, Vancouver, Canada; Basic Med Sciences Bldg, Winnipeg, Manitoba, Canada; Université de Montréal; et al)

Clin Infect Dis 41:1097-1104, 2005   4–5

Background.—Famciclovir, the oral prodrug of penciclovir, is effective for the treatment of recurrent genital herpes. This randomized, clinic-initiated, double-blind trial compared the therapeutic efficacy and safety of treatment with famciclovir at dosages of 125 mg, 250 mg, and 500 mg twice daily for 5 days with placebo in immunocompetent adults with a recurrent episode of genital herpes.

Methods.—Efficacy and tolerability were assessed in 308 patients with lesions present for no more than 6.5 h at the time of the first dose. Two assessments per day were performed to increase the precision of the determination of study end points.

Results.—All doses of famciclovir were significantly more effective than placebo in reducing the time to cessation of viral shedding, complete lesion healing, and loss of all lesion-associated symptoms, particularly lesion tenderness, pain, and itching. Patients receiving treatment with famciclovir were significantly less likely to experience new lesions than were patients receiving placebo. All doses of famciclovir were tolerated as well as placebo was. There was no difference in efficacy or tolerability among the different doses of famciclovir; the lowest effective dose was 125 mg twice per day.

Conclusions.—In immunocompetent adults with recurrent genital herpes, a 5-day course of famciclovir at a dosage of 125 mg, 250 mg, or 500 mg twice per day was significantly more effective than was placebo in reducing the duration of viral shedding and symptoms and in accelerating lesion healing. These results support the use of treatment with famciclovir at a dosage of 125 mg for 5 days as an effective, well-tolerated treatment for episodes of recurrent genital herpes.

▶ Improved oral bioavailability allows for less frequent dosing of valacyclovir and famciclovir than is necessary with acyclovir, which is prescribed at a frequency of 5 times per day. This study compared twice daily administration of 3 different doses of famciclovir, 125 mg, 250 mg, and 500 mg, in the treatment of recurrent genital herpesvirus infection. A visit to some online pharmacy Web sites showed that the presumed cost savings may be illusory. The 125-mg and 250-mg tablets are virtually identically priced, although the 500-mg tablet is substantially more expensive.

B. H. Thiers, MD

Herpes Zoster in Immunocompromised Patients: Incidence, Timing, and Risk Factors
Wung PK, for the WGET Research Group (Johns Hopkins Univ, Baltimore, Md; Cleveland Clinic Found, Ohio; Mayo Clinic, Rochester, Minn; et al)
Am J Med 118:1416.e9-1416.e18, 2005   4–6

Purpose.—To evaluate the risk factors for herpes zoster as well as the incidence and timing of this complication in patients who were treated with immunosuppression because of active Wegener's granulomatosis.

Subjects and Methods.—We studied the 180 Wegener's granulomatosis patients in the Wegener's Granulomatosis Etanercept Trial (WGET). Herpes zoster events during WGET were documented prospectively. Follow-up questionnaires were employed to describe the location, treatment, and complication(s) of herpes zoster and its therapy. Univariate and multivariate analyses were performed to evaluate risk factors, including history of herpes zoster, for the occurrence of herpes zoster during the trial. All analyses were based on the time to first occurrence of herpes zoster.

Results.—Eighteen patients (10% of the WGET cohort) suffered a total of 19 herpes zoster episodes over a mean follow-up period of 27 months. The annual incidence of herpes zoster in the WGET cohort was 45 cases/1000 patient-years (95% confidence interval [CI]: 27, 70). The median time from enrollment to the occurrence of herpes zoster in the subgroup of patients with that complication was 16.5 months (± 9.4). Fifteen of the 19 herpes zoster events (79%) occurred between months 6 and 36, many months after the period of most intensive immunosuppression. In univariate analyses, history of serum creatinine ≥ 1.5 mg/dL before enrollment was associated with a relative risk (RR) of 3.0 (95% CI: 1.1, 7.8) for herpes zoster during WGET ($P = .03$). In multivariate analyses, serum creatinine ≥ 1.5 mg/dL was associated with an RR of 6.3 (95% CI: 2.0, 19.8; $P = .002$), and female sex with an RR of 4.6 (95% CI: 1.6, 13.2; $P = .004$).

Conclusion.—Renal dysfunction and female sex were consistently strong risk factors for herpes zoster events in this population. Contrary to expectation, most herpes zoster events did not occur during periods of most intensive immunosuppression. These data may inform studies of interventions designed to prevent herpes zoster in patients on treatment for immune-mediated diseases.

▶ The authors identify 2 major risk factors for herpes zoster in their population of immunocompromised patients with Wegener's granulomatosis: renal compromise and female sex. Surprisingly, the timing of zoster had little direct temporal relationship to the period of most intensive immunosuppression. Prophylactic antiviral agents or, perhaps, vaccines may be indicated in patients at highest risk.

B. H. Thiers, MD

The PINE Study of Epidural Steroids and Local Anaesthetics to Prevent Postherpetic Neuralgia: A Randomised Controlled Trial
van Wijck AJM, Opstelten W, Moons KGM, et al (Univ Med Ctr, Utrecht, The Netherlands; Catharina Hosp, Eindhoven, The Netherlands)
Lancet 367:219-224, 2006   4–7

Background.—Postherpetic neuralgia is the most frequent complication of herpes zoster. Treatment of this neuropathic pain syndrome is difficult and often disappointing. We assessed the effectiveness of a single epidural injection of steroids and local anaesthetics for prevention of postherpetic neuralgia in older patients with herpes zoster.

Methods.—We randomly assigned 598 patients older than 50 years, with acute herpes zoster (rash <7 days) below dermatome C6, to receive either standard therapy (oral antivirals and analgesics) or standard therapy with one additional epidural injection of 80 mg methylprednisolone acetate and 10 mg bupivacaine. The primary endpoint was the proportion of patients with zoster-associated pain 1 month after inclusion. Analyses were by intention-to-treat. This study is registered as an International Standard Randomised Controlled Trial, number ISRCTN32866390.

Findings.—At 1 month, 137 (48%) patients in the epidural group reported pain compared with 164 (58%) in the control group (relative risk [RR] 0.83, 95% CI 0.71–0.97, p=0.02). After 3 months these values were 58 (21%) and 63 (24%) respectively (0.89, 0.65–1.21, p=0.47) and, at 6 months, 39 (15%) and 44 (17%; 0.85, 0.57–1.13, p=0.43). We detected no subgroups in which the relative risk for pain 1 month after inclusion substantially differed from the overall estimate. No patient had major adverse events related to epidural injection.

Interpretation.—A single epidural injection of steroids and local anaesthetics in the acute phase of herpes zoster has a modest effect in reducing zoster-associated pain for 1 month. This treatment is not effective for prevention of long-term postherpetic neuralgia.

▶ A previous study demonstrated the efficacy of methylprednisolone and bupivacaine, delivered by an epidural catheter for 7 to 21 days, in the relief of severe zoster pain.[1] However, such treatment requires hospitalization and thus must be reserved for selected patients. The single epidural injection reported in this open, randomized, multicenter trial, although not dramatically effective, can be done in an outpatient setting.

B. H. Thiers, MD

Reference

1. Pasqualucci A, Pasqualucci V, Galla F et al: Prevention of post-herpetic neuralgia: Acyclovir and prednisolone versus epidural local anesthetic and methylprednisolone. *Acta Anaesthesiol Scand* 44:910-918, 2000.

A Vaccine to Prevent Herpes Zoster and Postherpetic Neuralgia in Older Adults

Oxman MN, for the Shingles Prevention Study Group (VA San Diego Healthcare System, Calif; et al)
N Engl J Med 352:2271-2284, 2005   4–8

Background.—The incidence and severity of herpes zoster and postherpetic neuralgia increase with age in association with a progressive decline in cell-mediated immunity to varicella-zoster virus (VZV). We tested the hypothesis that vaccination against VZV would decrease the incidence, severity, or both of herpes zoster and postherpetic neuralgia among older adults.

Methods.—We enrolled 38,546 adults 60 years of age or older in a randomized, double-blind, placebo-controlled trial of an investigational live attenuated Oka/Merck VZV vaccine ("zoster vaccine"). Herpes zoster was diagnosed according to clinical and laboratory criteria. The pain and discomfort associated with herpes zoster were measured repeatedly for six months. The primary end point was the burden of illness due to herpes zoster, a measure affected by the incidence, severity, and duration of the associated pain and discomfort. The secondary end point was the incidence of postherpetic neuralgia.

Results.—More than 95 percent of the subjects continued in the study to its completion, with a median of 3.12 years of surveillance for herpes zoster. A total of 957 confirmed cases of herpes zoster (315 among vaccine recipients and 642 among placebo recipients) and 107 cases of postherpetic neuralgia (27 among vaccine recipients and 80 among placebo recipients) were included in the efficacy analysis. The use of the zoster vaccine reduced the burden of illness due to herpes zoster by 61.1 percent (P<0.001), reduced the incidence of postherpetic neuralgia by 66.5 percent (P<0.001), and reduced the incidence of herpes zoster by 51.3 percent (P<0.001). Reactions at the injection site were more frequent among vaccine recipients but were generally mild.

Conclusions.—The zoster vaccine markedly reduced morbidity from herpes zoster and postherpetic neuralgia among older adults.

▶ Resolution of primary varicella is associated with the induction of VZV-specific memory T cells, which protect against reactivation of or reinfection by the virus. It is likely that the cell-mediated immune response to VZV may be boosted periodically by exposure to other infected individuals. However, VZV-specific memory T cells decline with age, and a reduction below some theoretically critical level might correlate with an increased risk of zoster. The zoster vaccine reported here likely prevents VZV-specific T cells from dropping below that critical level. As stated by Arvin and Gilden in accompanying essays,[1,2] the possibility that a feared consequence of aging may be minimized or avoided by use of this vaccine is an important advance.

B. H. Thiers, MD

References

1. Arvin A: Aging, immunity, and the varicella-zoster virus. *N Engl J Med* 352:2266-2267, 2005.
2. Gilden DH: Varicella-zoster virus vaccine: Grown-ups need it, too. *N Engl J Med* 352:2344-2346, 2005.

Decline in Mortality Due to Varicella After Implementation of Varicella Vaccination in the United States

Nguyen HQ, Jumaan AO, Seward JF (Ctrs for Disease Control and Prevention, Atlanta, Ga)
N Engl J Med 352:450-458, 2005   4–9

Background.—Varicella disease has been preventable in the United States since 1995. Starting in 1999, active and passive surveillance data showed sharp decreases in varicella disease. We reviewed national death records to assess the effect of the vaccination program on mortality associated with varicella.

Methods.—Data on deaths for which varicella was listed as an underlying or contributing cause were obtained from National Center for Health Statistics Multiple Cause-of-Death Mortality Data for 1990 through 2001. We calculated the numbers and rates of death due to varicella according to age, sex, race, ethnic background, and birthplace.

Results.—The rate of death due to varicella fluctuated from 1990 through 1998 and then declined sharply. For the interval from 1990 through 1994, the average number of varicella-related deaths was 145 per year (varicella was listed as the underlying cause in 105 deaths and as a contributing cause in 40); it then declined to 66 per year during 1999 through 2001. For deaths for which varicella was listed as the underlying cause, age-adjusted mortality rates dropped by 66 percent, from an average of 0.41 death per 1 million population during 1990 through 1994 to 0.14 during 1999 through 2001 (P<0.001). This decline was observed in all age groups under 50 years, with the greatest reduction (92 percent) among children 1 to 4 years of age. In addition, by the period from 1999 through 2001, the average rates of mortality due to varicella among all racial and ethnic groups were below 0.15 per 1 million population, as compared with rates ranging from 0.37 per 1 million for whites to 0.66 per 1 million for other races in the period from 1990 through 1994.

Conclusions.—The program of universal childhood vaccination against varicella in the United States has resulted in a sharp decline in the rate of death due to varicella.

▶ In the short time since its introduction, the varicella vaccine has significantly reduced varicella-related morbidity and mortality.[1]. As shown elsewhere in this edition (Abstract 4–8), the vaccine may also play a key role in preventing or ameliorating zoster in older individuals.[2]

B. H. Thiers, MD

References

1. Vázquez M, Shapiro ED: Varicella vaccine and infection with varicella-zoster virus. *N Engl J Med* 352:439-440, 2005.
2. Oxman MN, Levin MJ, Johnson GR, et al: A vaccine to prevent herpes zoster and postherpetic neuralgia in older adults. *N Engl J Med* 352:2271-2284, 2005.

Additional Evidence That Pityriasis Rosea Is Associated With Reactivation of Human Herpesvirus-6 and -7

Broccolo F, Drago F, Careddu AM, et al (DIBIT San Raffaele Scientific Inst, Milan, Italy; Univ of Genoa, Italy; Ospedale Maggiore, Milan, Italy; et al)

J Invest Dermatol 124:1234-1240, 2005   4–10

Introduction.—To elucidate the role of human herpesvirus (HHV)-6 and -7 (HHV-7) in pityriasis rosea (PR), we measured their DNA load in plasma, peripheral blood mononuclear cells (PBMC), and tissues using a calibrated quantitative real-time PCR assay. We also studied HHV-6- and HHV-7-specific antigens in skin by immunohistochemistry and anti-HHV-7 neutralizing activity using a syncytia-inhibition test. Plasma and PBMC were obtained from 31 PR patients (14 children, 17 adults), 12 patients with other dermatites, and 36 blood donors. Skin biopsies were obtained from 15 adults with PR and 12 with other dermatites. HHV-6 and HHV-7 DNA were detected in 17% and in 39% of PR plasmas, respectively, but in no controls. HHV-7 viremia was associated with a higher PBMC load and, in adults, with systemic symptoms. HHV-7, but not HHV-6, levels in PBMC were higher in PR patients than in controls. HHV-6 and HHV-7 antigens were found only in PR skin (17% and 67% of patients analyzed, respectively), indicating a productive infection. Syncytia-neutralizing antibodies were found in PR patients and controls, but their titers were lower in patients with HHV-7 viremia. These data confirm the causal association between PR and active HHV-7 or, to a lesser extent, HHV-6 infection.

▶ The authors developed a sensitive and accurate, calibrated, quantitative real-time PCR approach to assess the HHV-6 and HHV-7 DNA load in PBMCs, plasma, and skin lesions of different cohorts of individuals. They also studied the expression of specific HHV-6 and HHV-7 antigens in skin lesions and the presence of anti–HHV-7 neutralizing antibodies in the sera of patients and controls. They concluded that PR may result from the endogenous reactivation of HHV-7 or HHV-6 infection.

These Italian investigators first postulated such an association in 1997, but several subsequent studies done by others failed to confirm the original findings. A report from India claims that PR may respond to erythromycin, suggesting that a bacterium may be involved.[1] Is it possible that PR-like eruptions can be caused by different infectious agents in different parts of the world?

B. H. Thiers, MD

Reference

1. Sharma PK, Yadav TP, Gautam RK, et al: Erythromycin in pityriasis rosea: A double-blind, placebo-controlled clinical trial. *J Am Acad Dermatol* 24:241-244, 2000.

Antiviral Medications to Prevent Cytomegalovirus Disease and Early Death in Recipients of Solid-Organ Transplants: A Systematic Review of Randomised Controlled Trials
Hodson EM, Jones CA, Webster AC, et al (Child Hosp of Westmead, Sydney, Australia; Westmead Hosp, Sydney, Australia; Univ of Sydney, Australia; et al)
Lancet 365:2105-2115, 2005   4–11

Background.—Antiviral prophylaxis is commonly used in recipients of solid-organ transplants with the aim of preventing the clinical syndrome associated with cytomegalovirus infection. We undertook a systematic review to investigate whether this approach affects risks of cytomegalovirus disease and death.

Methods.—Randomised controlled trials of prophylaxis with antiviral medications for cytomegalovirus disease in solid-organ-transplant recipients were identified. Data were combined in meta-analyses by a random-effects model.

Findings.—Compared with placebo or no treatment, prophylaxis with aciclovir, ganciclovir, or valaciclovir significantly reduced the risks of cytomegalovirus disease (19 trials, 1981 patients; relative risk 0.42 [95% CI 0.34-0.52]), cytomegalovirus infection (17 trials, 1786 patients; 0.61 [0.48-0.77]), and all-cause mortality (17 trials, 1838 patients; 0.63 [0.43-0.92]), mainly owing to lower mortality from cytomegalovirus disease (seven trials, 1300 patients; 0.26 [0.08-0.78]). Prophylaxis also lowered the risks of disease caused by herpes simplex or zoster virus, bacterial infections, and protozoal infections, but not fungal infection, acute rejection, or graft loss. Meta-regression showed no significant difference in the risk of cytomegalovirus disease or all-cause mortality by organ transplanted or cytomegalovirus serostatus; no conclusions were possible for cytomegalovirus-negative recipients of negative organs. In trials of direct comparisons, ganciclovir was more effective than aciclovir in preventing cytomegalovirus disease. Valganciclovir and intravenous ganciclovir were as effective as oral ganciclovir.

Interpretation.—Prophylaxis with antiviral medications reduces the risk of cytomegalovirus disease and associated mortality in recipients of solid-organ transplants. This approach should be used routinely in cytomegalovirus-positive recipients and in cytomegalovirus-negative recipients of organs positive for the virus.

▶ Those of us who see organ transplant patients in consultation occasionally encounter patients with systemic cytomegalovirus (CMV) disease. Although the kidneys, liver, heart, and lungs are most often affected, skin lesions can occur. More than 50% of transplant recipients have laboratory evidence of primary or reactivated CMV infection in the first year after solid-organ transplantation. Primary infections are associated with the highest risk of symptomatic disease. Before prophylaxis was widely available, CMV disease occurred in 7% to 32% of recipients of solid-organ transplants, with the highest risk in heart-lung recipients and the lowest risk in kidney recipients. The analysis by Hodson et al confirms the beneficial effects of antiviral prophylaxis.

B. H. Thiers, MD

Public-Health Impact of Accelerated Measles Control in the WHO African Region 2000-03

Otten M, Kezaala R, Fall A, et al (Centers for Disease Control and Prevention, Atlanta, Ga; WHO Regional Office for Africa, Harare, Zimbabwe; WHO Regional Office for Africa, Abidjan, Côte d'Ivoire; et al)
Lancet 366:832-839, 2005   4–12

Background.—In 2000, the WHO African Region adopted a plan to accelerate efforts to lower measles mortality with the goal of decreasing the number of measles deaths to near zero. By June, 2003, 19 African countries had completed measles supplemental immunisation activities (SIA) in children aged 9 months to 14 years as part of a comprehensive measles-control strategy. We assessed the public-health impact of these control measures by use of available surveillance data.

Methods.—We calculated percentage decline in reported measles cases during 1-2 years after SIA, compared with 6 years before SIA. On the basis of data from 13 of the 19 countries, we assumed that the percentage decline in measles deaths equalled that in measles cases. We also examined data on routine and SIA measles vaccine coverage, measles case-based surveillance, and suspected measles outbreaks.

Findings.—Between 2000 and June, 2003, 82.1 million children were targeted for vaccination during initial SIA in 12 countries and follow-up SIA in seven countries. The average decline in the number of reported measles cases was 91%. In 17 of the 19 countries, measles case-based surveillance confirmed that transmission of measles virus, and therefore measles deaths, had been reduced to low or very low rates. The total estimated number of deaths averted in the year 2003 was 90,043. Between 2000 and 2003 in the African Region as a whole, we estimated that the percentage decline in annual measles deaths was around 20% (90,043 of 454,000).

Interpretation.—The burden of measles in sub-Saharan Africa can be reduced to very low levels by means of appropriate strategies, resources, and personnel.

▶ The article by Otten et al demonstrates the dramatic success achieved in reducing measles mortality in Africa. Measles causes 1% to 9% of the nearly 11 million deaths in children younger than 5 years every year,[1] and of the preventable causes of death, measles is perhaps the disease for which we have the most cost-effective and most readily available intervention.[2] The cost of delivering measles vaccine in underdeveloped countries is about $0.60 to $1.00 per child, and overall cost savings is attained by averting the disease and death.

B. H. Thiers, MD

References

1. de Quadros CA, Hersh BS, Nogueira AC, et al: Measles eradication: Experience in the Americas. *Bull World Health Organ* 76(suppl 2):47-52, 1998.
2. Salama P, McFarland J, Mulholland K: Reaching the unreached with measles vaccination. *Lancet* 366:787-788, 2005.

Necrolytic Acral Erythema: A Cutaneous Sign of Hepatitis C Virus Infection
Abdallah MA, Ghozzi MY, Monib HA, et al (Ain Shams Univ, Cairo; Univ of Arkansas, Little Rock)
J Am Acad Dermatol 53:247-251, 2005   4–13

Background.—Hepatitis C virus (HCV) infection is globally epidemic. Several mucocutaneous diseases are well established in association with HCV infection. Few case reports describe the recently recognized HCV-related skin disorder termed *necrolytic acral erythema* (NAE).

Methods.—Thirty patients with NAE were identified in a university-based dermatology clinic in Cairo, Egypt. These patients were observed over time to document the clinical and histologic findings of this disorder.

Results.—All patients were infected with HCV. Erythematous papules arose most commonly on the dorsal aspect of the feet, particularly the dorsal surface of the great toe. Progression resulted in confluence into erythematous dusky plaques with adherent scale and central erosion. The eruption extended to involve the lower leg and other regions in some patients but never affected palms or soles, the nail bed, nail plate, or mucous membranes. Skin biopsy specimens from fully evolved lesions displayed psoriasiform changes in association with more characteristic findings of keratinocyte necrosis and papillomatosis.

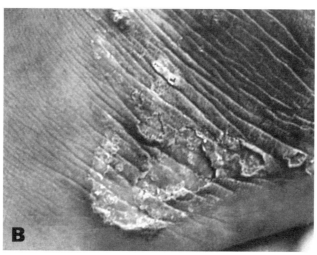

FIGURE 1.—B, This sharply marginated hyperpigmented and erythematous plaque displays focal erosion. (Reprinted by permission of the publisher from Abdallah MA, Ghozzi MY, Monib HA, et al: Necrolytic acral erythema: A cutaneous sign of hepatitis C virus infection. *J Am Acad Dermatol* 53:247-251, 2005. Copyright 2005 by Elsevier.)

Limitations.—We did not perform a prospective review of patients known to be infected with HCV. Patients were identified from a general clinic population and then assayed for HCV serology.

Conclusions.—NAE is a distinctive skin disorder associated with HCV infection in all cases reported to date. Recognition of this disease should alert practitioners to the need for viral testing and appropriate counseling of patients (Fig 1; see color plate X).

▶ Clinically, NAE most closely resembles psoriasis, although acrodermatitis enteropathica and necrolytic migratory erythema share clinical and histologic similarities. The exact incidence of NAE and its specificity for underlying HCV infection can only be determined by prospective studies.

B. H. Thiers, MD

5 HIV Infection

Cost-Effectiveness of Screening for HIV in the Era of Highly Active Anti-retroviral Therapy
Sanders GD, Bayoumi AM, Sundaram V, et al (Duke Univ, Durham, NC; Stanford Univ, Calif; Univ of Toronto; et al)
N Engl J Med 352:570-585, 2005   5–1

Background.—The costs, benefits, and cost-effectiveness of screening for human immunodeficiency virus (HIV) in health care settings during the era of highly active antiretroviral therapy (HAART) have not been determined.

Methods.—We developed a Markov model of costs, quality of life, and survival associated with an HIV-screening program as compared with current practice. In both strategies, symptomatic patients were identified through symptom-based case finding. Identified patients started treatment when their CD4 count dropped to 350 cells per cubic millimeter. Disease progression was defined on the basis of CD4 levels and viral load. The likelihood of sexual transmission was based on viral load, knowledge of HIV status, and efficacy of counseling.

Results.—Given a 1 percent prevalence of unidentified HIV infection, screening increased life expectancy by 5.48 days, or 4.70 quality-adjusted days, at an estimated cost of $194 per screened patient, for a cost-effectiveness ratio of $15,078 per quality-adjusted life-year. Screening cost less than $50,000 per quality-adjusted life-year if the prevalence of unidentified HIV infection exceeded 0.05 percent. Excluding HIV transmission, the cost-effectiveness of screening was $41,736 per quality-adjusted life-year. Screening every five years, as compared with a one-time screening program, cost $57,138 per quality-adjusted life-year, but was more attractive in settings with a high incidence of infection. Our results were sensitive to the efficacy of behavior modification, the benefit of early identification and therapy, and the prevalence and incidence of HIV infection.

Conclusions.—The cost-effectiveness of routine HIV screening in health care settings, even in relatively low-prevalence populations, is similar to that of commonly accepted interventions, and such programs should be expanded.

Expanded Screening for HIV in the United States—An Analysis of Cost-Effectiveness

Paltiel AD, Weinstein MC, Kimmel AD, et al (Yale School of Medicine, New Haven, Conn; Harvard School of Public Health, Boston; Harvard Med School, Boston; et al)

N Engl J Med 352:586-595, 2005

5–2

Background.—Although the Centers for Disease Control and Prevention (CDC) recommend routine HIV counseling, testing, and referral (HIVCTR) in settings with at least a 1 percent prevalence of HIV, roughly 280,000 Americans are unaware of their human immunodeficiency virus (HIV) infection. The effect of expanded screening for HIV is unknown in the era of effective antiretroviral therapy.

Methods.—We developed a computer simulation model of HIV screening and treatment to compare routine, voluntary HIVCTR with current practice in three target populations: "high-risk" (3.0 percent prevalence of undiagnosed HIV infection; 1.2 percent annual incidence); "CDC threshold" (1.0 percent and 0.12 percent, respectively); and "U.S. general" (0.1 percent and 0.01 percent). Input data were derived from clinical trials and observational cohorts. Outcomes included quality-adjusted survival, cost, and cost-effectiveness.

Results.—In the high-risk population, the addition of one-time screening for HIV antibodies with an enzyme-linked immunosorbent assay (ELISA) to current practice was associated with earlier diagnosis of HIV (mean CD4 cell count at diagnosis, 210 vs. 154 per cubic millimeter). One-time screening also improved average survival time among HIV-infected patients (quality-adjusted survival, 220.7 months vs. 219.8 months). The incremental cost-effectiveness was $36,000 per quality-adjusted life-year gained. Testing every five years cost $50,000 per quality-adjusted life-year gained, and testing every three years cost $63,000 per quality-adjusted life-year gained. In the CDC threshold population, the cost-effectiveness ratio for one-time screening with ELISA was $38,000 per quality-adjusted life-year gained, whereas testing every five years cost $71,000 per quality-adjusted life-year gained, and testing every three years cost $85,000 per quality-adjusted life-year gained. In the U.S. general population, one-time screening cost $113,000 per quality-adjusted life-year gained.

Conclusions.—In all but the lowest-risk populations, routine, voluntary screening for HIV once every three to five years is justified on both clinical and cost-effectiveness grounds. One-time screening in the general population may also be cost-effective.

▶ Unfortunately, in the United States, most patients with HIV infection are diagnosed at an advanced stage. Early diagnosis would be preferable as it could speed access to appropriate care and increase the proportion of HIV-infected patients who receive care. The articles by Sanders et al (Abstract 5–1) and

Paltiel et al (Abstract 5–2) suggest that widespread use of routine screening could yield substantial benefits in this regard.[1]

B. H. Thiers, MD

Reference

1. Bozzette SA: Routine screening for HIV infection—Timely and cost-effective. *N Engl J Med* 352:620-621, 2005.

Detection of Acute Infections During HIV Testing in North Carolina
Pilcher CD, Fiscus SA, Nguyen TQ, et al (Univ of North Carolina at Chapel Hill; North Carolina Dept of Health and Human Services, Raleigh)
N Engl J Med 352:1873-1883, 2005   5–3

Background.—North Carolina has added nucleic acid amplification testing for the human immunodeficiency virus (HIV) to standard HIV antibody tests to detect persons with acute HIV infection who are viremic but antibody-negative.

Methods.—To determine the effect of nucleic acid amplification testing on the yield and accuracy of HIV detection in public health practice, we conducted a 12-month observational study of methods for state-funded HIV testing. We compared the diagnostic performance of standard HIV antibody tests (i.e., enzyme immunoassay and Western blot analysis) with an algorithm whereby serum samples that yielded negative results on standard antibody tests were tested again with the use of nucleic acid amplification. A surveillance algorithm with repeated sensitive–less-sensitive enzyme immunoassay tests was also evaluated. HIV infection was defined as a confirmed positive result on a nucleic acid amplification test or as HIV antibody seroconversion.

Results.—Between November 1, 2002, and October 31, 2003, 109,250 persons at risk for HIV infection who had consented to HIV testing presented at state-funded sites. There were 606 HIV-positive results. Established infection, as identified by standard enzyme immunoassay or Western blot analysis, appeared in 583 participants; of these, 107 were identified, with the use of sensitive–less-sensitive enzyme immunoassay tests, as recent infections. A total of 23 acutely infected persons were identified only with the use of the nucleic acid amplification algorithm. With all detectable infections taken into account, the sensitivity of standard antibody testing was 0.962 (95 percent confidence interval, 0.944 to 0.976). There were two false positive results on nucleic acid amplification tests. The specificity and positive predictive value of the algorithm that included nucleic acid amplification testing were greater than 0.999 (95 percent confidence interval, 0.999 to >0.999) and 0.997 (95 percent confidence interval, 0.988 to >0.999), respectively. Of the 23 acute HIV infections, 16 were detected at sexually transmitted disease clinics. Emergency measures for HIV prevention protected 48 sex partners and one fetus from high-risk exposure to HIV.

Conclusions.—The addition of nucleic acid amplification testing to an HIV testing algorithm significantly increases the identification of cases of infection without impairing the performance of diagnostic testing. The detection of highly contagious, acutely infected persons creates new opportunities for HIV surveillance and prevention.

▶ The authors found that compared with a diagnostic panel that includes nucleic acid amplification tests, standard antibody tests alone detect only 96% of HIV infections. The detection of acute HIV infection by nucleic acid amplification, which is relatively inexpensive, allows for early clinical intervention and may delay progression of the disease.[1]

B. H. Thiers, MD

Reference

1. Rosenberg ES, Altfeld M, Poon SH, et al: Immune control of HIV-1 after early treatment of acute infection. *Nature* 407:523-526, 2000.

Newly Diagnosed HIV Infections: Review in UK and Ireland
Sullivan AK, Curtis H, Sabin CA, et al (Chelsea and Westminster Healthcare NHS Trust, London; British HIV Association, London; Royal Free and Univ College Med School, London; et al)
BMJ 330:1301-1302, 2005   5–4

Background.—In 2001, more than half (59%) of persons in the United Kingdom with HIV who were starting treatment had CD4 lymphocyte counts of less then 200 cells/μL. In most cases, these low counts were attributable to late diagnosis. New HIV diagnoses in the United Kingdom and Ireland were investigated to assess the incidence of late diagnosis (CD4 lymphocyte count <200 cells/μL) and associated features, and to determine whether patients had prior presentations that may have been related to HIV infection.

Methods.—A national case review was conducted through structured questionnaire forms sent to adult HIV care providers in the United Kingdom and Ireland for patients presenting with a new diagnosis of HIV infection in the first 3 months of 2003. Data were collected on clinical and immune status, hospital admissions, and symptoms or conditions in the previous 12 months that could have been related to the presence of HIV infection.

Results.—Data were obtained on 977 patients. Overall, 301 patients (33%) presented late, and late presentation was more common in older patients and in black African patients. Late presentation was less likely in homosexual men, independent of age and ethnicity. Overall, 41% had HIV diagnosed via routine screening, which was associated with being young, female, black African, and heterosexual; 68% had the diagnosis established in a genitourinary, sexual health, or HIV clinic, which was associated with being young, male, and homosexual and was less commonly associated with being black African. After adjustment for demographic factors, diagnosis as part of a routine screen and testing at a genitourinary, sexual health, or HIV clinic were both independently associated with a lower chance of late diagnosis.

Conclusions.—There were a significant number of missed opportunities for earlier diagnosis of HIV infection in 17% of patients who sought medical care with symptoms in the previous 12 months, but were not diagnosed. There is a need to increase the proportion of patients who have HIV diagnosed as part of routine screening.

▶ The authors demonstrate many missed opportunities in the early diagnosis of HIV. While increasing the proportion of patients subjected to routine screening remains an option, heightened clinical awareness is also important. The cutaneous manifestations of HIV are many and are often the presenting clinical manifestation. Dermatologists should question the patient regarding HIV risk factors when indicated by the clinical examination.

B. H. Thiers, MD

Infection With Multidrug Resistant, Dual-Tropic HIV-1 and Rapid Progression to AIDS: A Case Report

Markowitz M, Mohri H, Mehandru S, et al (Rockefeller Univ, New York; ViroLogic, San Francisco; Cabrini Med Ctr, New York)
Lancet 365:1031-1038, 2005   5–5

Background.—Rapid progression to AIDS after acute HIV-1 infection, though uncommon, has been noted, as has the transmission of multidrug resistant viruses. Here, we describe a patient in whom these two factors arose concomitantly and assess the effects.

Methods.—We did a case study of a patient with HIV-1 seroconversion. We genotyped the virus and host genetic markers by PCR and nucleotide sequencing. To ascertain the drug susceptibility of our patient's HIV-1 we did phenotypic studies with the PhenoSense assay. We assessed viral coreceptor use via syncytium formation in vitro and with a modified PhenoSense assay.

Findings.—Our patient seems to have been recently infected by a viral variant of HIV-1 resistant to multiple classes of antiretroviral drugs. Furthermore, his virus population is dual tropic for cells that express CCR5 or CXCR4 coreceptor. The infection has resulted in progression to symptomatic AIDS in 4-20 months.

Interpretation.—The intersection of multidrug resistance and rapid development of AIDS in this patient is of concern, especially in view of his case history, which includes high-risk sexual contacts and use of metamfetamine. The public health ramifications of such a case are great.

▶ The possibility of a "super" strain of HIV is frightening, and only time will tell whether this case merely represents an isolated phenomenon or has more ominous connotations.

B. H. Thiers, MD

Time Trends in Primary Resistance to HIV Drugs in the United Kingdom: Multicentre Observational Study

Dunn D, for the UK Group on Transmitted HIV Drug Resistance (Med Research Centre Clinical Trials Unit, London)
BMJ 331:1364-1368, 2005   5–6

Objective.—To examine whether the level of primary resistance to HIV drugs is increasing in the United Kingdom.

Design.—Multicentre observational study.

Setting.—All virology laboratories in the United Kingdom carrying out tests for HIV resistance as part of routine clinical care.

Participants.—2357 people infected with HIV who were tested for resistance before receiving antiretroviral therapy.

Main Outcome Measure.—Prevalence of drug resistance on basis of the Stanford genotypic interpretation system.

Results.—Over the study period (February 1996 to May 2003), 335 (14.2%, 95% confidence interval 12.8% to 15.7%) samples had mutations that conferred resistance to one or more antiretroviral drugs (9.3% high level resistance, 5.9% medium level resistance). The prevalence of primary resistance has increased markedly over time, although patterns are specific to drug class; the largest increase was for non-nucleoside reverse transcriptase inhibitors. In 2002-3, the prevalence of resistance to any antiretroviral drug to nucleoside or nucleotide reverse transcriptase inhibitors, to non-nucleoside reverse transcriptase inhibitors, or to protease inhibitors was 19.2% (15.7% to 23.2%), 12.4% (9.5% to 15.9%), 8.1% (5.8% to 11.1%), and 6.6% (4.4% to 9.3%), respectively. The risk of primary resistance was only weakly related to most demographic and clinical factors, including ethnicity and viral subtype.

Conclusions.—The United Kingdom has one of the highest reported rates of primary resistance to HIV drugs worldwide. Prevalence seems still to be increasing and is high in all demographic subgroups.

▶ It is well known that primary HIV drug resistance limits therapeutic options. The spread of such resistance could negate the large reductions in morbidity and mortality since combination antiviral therapy was introduced. This study confirms the high rates of primary HIV drug resistance in the United Kingdom and documents its increasing prevalence in all demographic subgroups.

B. H. Thiers, MD

Long-term Effectiveness of Potent Antiretroviral Therapy in Preventing AIDS and Death: A Prospective Cohort Study

Sterne JAC, for the Swiss HIV Cohort Study (Univ of Bristol, England; et al)
Lancet 366:378-384, 2005   5–7

Background.—Evidence on the effectiveness of highly active antiretroviral therapy (HAART) for HIV-infected individuals is limited. Most clinical trials examined surrogate endpoints over short periods of follow-up and there has been no placebo-controlled randomised trial of HAART. Estimation of treatment effects in observational studies is problematic, because of confounding by indication. We aimed to use novel methodology to overcome this problem in the Swiss HIV Cohort Study.

Methods.—Patients were included if they had been examined after January 1996, when HAART became available in Switzerland, were not on HAART, and were free of AIDS at baseline. Cox regression models were weighted to create a statistical population in which the probability of being treated at each time point was unrelated to prognostic factors.

Results.—Low CD4 counts and increasing HIV-1 viral load were associated with increased probability of starting HAART. Overall hazard ratios were 0.14 (95% CI 0.07-0.29) for HAART compared with no treatment, and 0.49 (0.31-0.79) compared with dual therapy. Compared with no treatment, HAART became more beneficial with increasing time since initiation but was less beneficial for patients whose presumed mode of transmission was via intravenous drug use (hazard ratio 0.27, 0.12-0.61) than for other patients (0.08, 0.03-0.19).

Interpretation.—Our results, which are appropriately controlled for confounding by indication, are consistent with reported declines in rates of AIDS and death in developed countries, and provide a context in which to consider adverse effects of HAART.

▶ Sterne et al found that HAART reduced the rate of progression to AIDS or death by 86%, and compared with the figure for no treatment, the efficacy of HAART increased with the time since initiation. The results are not unexpected, as evidenced by the improved outcome of HIV-infected patients since HAART became available. The beneficial effects of HAART do not vary greatly according to patient characteristics, other than a somewhat reduced efficacy in patients who have been infected via IV drug use. This may be explained by a number of factors including reduced adherence to HAART in the IV drug group, an increased risk of death from overdose or violent causes, or coinfection with the hepatitis C virus.

B. H. Thiers, MD

Treatment Exhaustion of Highly Active Antiretroviral Therapy (HAART) Among Individuals Infected With HIV in the United Kingdom: Multicentre Cohort Study

Sabin CA, for the Steering Committee of the UK Collaborative HIV Cohort (UK CHIC) Study Group (Royal Free and UC Med School, London; MRC Clinical Trials Unit, London; Brighton and Sussex Univ Hosp Trust, England; et al)
BMJ 330:695-699, 2005   5–8

Objectives.—To investigate whether there is evidence that an increasing proportion of HIV infected patients is starting to experience increases in viral load and decreases in CD4 cell count that are consistent with exhaustion of available treatment options.

Design.—Multicentre cohort study.

Setting.—Six large HIV treatment centres in southeast England.

Participants.—All individuals seen for care between 1 January 1996 and 31 December 2002.

Main Outcome Measures.—Exposure to individual antiretroviral drugs and drug classes, CD4 count, plasma HIV RNA burden.

Results.—Information is available on 16,593 individuals 13,378 (80.6%) male patients, 10,340 (62.3%) infected via homosexual or bisexual sex, 4426 (26.7%) infected via heterosexual sex, median age 34 years). Overall, 10,207 of the 16,593 patients (61.5%) have been exposed to any antiretroviral therapy. This proportion increased from 41.2% of patients under follow up at the end of 1996 to 71.3% of those under follow up in 2002. The median CD4 count and HIV RNA burden of patients under follow up in each year changed from 270 cells/mm^3 and 4.34 log$_{10}$ copies/ml in 1996 to 408 cells/mm^3 and 1.89 log$_{10}$ copies/ml, respectively, in 2002. By 2002, 3060 (38%) of patients who had ever been treated with antiretroviral therapy had experienced all three main classes. Of these, around one quarter had evidence of "viral load failure" with all these three classes. Patients with three class failure were more likely to have an HIV RNA burden > 2.7 log$_{10}$ copies/ml and a CD4 count < 200 cells/mm^3.

Conclusions.—The proportion of individuals with HIV infection in the United Kingdom who have been treated has increased gradually over time. A substantial proportion of these patients seem to be in danger of exhausting their options for antiretroviral treatment. New drugs with low toxicity, which are not associated with cross resistance to existing drugs, are urgently needed for such patients.

▶ HAART has had a dramatic impact on HIV-infected patients. Nevertheless, many patients cannot tolerate treatment or experience virologic failure while undergoing the regimen. This may require altering their antiretroviral approach. This leads to an improvement in many patients, but a small number of patients eventually exhaust their treatment options.

B. H. Thiers, MD

Depletion of Latent HIV-1 Infection In Vivo: A Proof-of-Concept Study

Lehrman G, Hogue IB, Palmer S, et al (Univ of Texas, Dallas; NIH, Frederick, Mass; Rush-Presbyterian-St Luke's Med Ctr, Chicago; et al)

Lancet 366:549-555, 2005   5–9

Background.—Persistent infection in resting CD4+ T cells prevents eradication of HIV-1. Since the chromatin remodeling enzyme histone deacetylase 1 (HDAC1) maintains latency of integrated HIV, we tested the ability of the HDAC inhibitor valproic acid to deplete persistent, latent infection in resting CD4+ T cells.

Procedures.—We did a proof-of-concept study in four volunteers infected with HIV and on highly-active antiretroviral therapy (HAART). After intensifying the effect of HAART with subcutaneous enfuvirtide 90 μg twice daily for 4-6 weeks to prevent the spread of HIV, we added oral valproic acid 500-750 mg twice daily to their treatment regimen for 3 months. We quantified latent infection of resting CD4+ T cells before and after augmented treatment by limiting-dilution culture of resting CD4+ T cells after ex-vivo activation.

Findings.—The frequency of resting cell infection was stable before addition of enfuvirtide and valproic acid, but declined thereafter. This decline was significant in three of four patients (mean reduction 75%, range 68% to >84%). Patients had slight reactions to enfuvirtide at the injection site, but otherwise tolerated treatment well.

Interpretation.—Combination therapy with an HDAC inhibitor and intensified HAART safely accelerates clearance of HIV from resting CD4+ T cells in vivo, suggesting a new and practical approach to eliminate HIV infection in this persistent reservoir. This finding, though not definitive, suggests that new approaches will allow the cure of HIV in the future.

▶ Although HAART has dramatically improved treatment outcomes in HIV-infected patients, low levels of viral replication often remain and the HIV genome can persist silently in some infected cells. The study by Lehrman et al demonstrates that drugs, in this case valproic acid, might selectively induce the expression of latent proviral genomes and potentially deplete these reservoirs. If confirmed in larger, randomized trials, this new therapeutic approach might represent a possible step towards making HIV infection a curable condition rather than a chronic disease.[1]

B. H. Thiers, MD

Reference

1. Routy J-P: Valproic acid: A potential role in treating latent HIV infection. *Lancet* 366:523-524, 2005.

6 Parasitic Infections, Bites, and Infestations

Treatment of Head Louse Infection With 4% Dimeticone Lotion: Randomised Controlled Equivalence Trial
Burgess IF, Brown CM, Lee PN (Insect Research Development, Royston, UK; P N Lee Statistics and Computing, Sutton, Surrey, England)
BMJ 330:1423-1425, 2005   6–1

Objective.—To evaluate the efficacy and safety of 4% dimeticone lotion for treatment of head louse infestation.

Design.—Randomised controlled equivalence trial.

Setting.—Community, with home visits.

Participants.—214 young people aged 4 to 18 years and 39 adults with active head louse infestation.

Interventions.—Two applications seven days apart of either 4.0% dimeticone lotion, applied for eight hours or overnight, or 0.5% phenothrin liquid, applied for 12 hours or overnight.

Outcome Measures.—Cure of infestation (no evidence of head lice after second treatment) or reinfestation after cure.

Results.—Cure or reinfestation after cure occurred in 89 of 127 (70%) participants treated with dimeticone and 94 of 125 (75%) treated with phenothrin (difference −5%, 95% confidence interval −16% to 6%). Per protocol analysis showed that 84 of 121 (69%) participants were cured with dimeticone and 90 of 116 (78%) were cured with phenothrin. Irritant reactions occurred significantly less with dimeticone (3/127, 2%) than with phenothrin (11/125, 9%; difference −6%, −12% to −1%). Per protocol this was 3 of 121 (3%) participants treated with dimeticone and 10 of 116 (9%) treated with phenothrin (difference −6%, −12% to −0.3%).

Conclusion.—Dimeticone lotion cures head louse infestation. Dimeticone seems less irritant than existing treatments and has a physical action on lice that should not be affected by resistance to neurotoxic insecticides.

▶ Dimeticone lotion is a new product that contains 4% long-chain linear silicone (dimeticone) in a volatile silicone base (cyclomethicone). Dimeticone is a clear odorless liquid that is applied by coating the scalp and full length of the hair. The product dries by evaporation of the cyclomethicone solvent. In vitro studies found that dimeticone universally immobilized lice within 5 minutes of application. In some cases, especially in girls with thick hair, it may be difficult to ensure that the hair and scalp have been thoroughly covered, but additional treatment, if needed, would be safe. Agents such as this, if found effective, would seem preferable to treatment with insecticides to which the lice readily become resistant and which could potentially be toxic to some patients.

S. Raimer, MD

Macrofilaricidal Activity After Doxycycline Treatment of *Wuchereria bancrofti*: A Double-blind, Randomised Placebo-controlled Trial

Taylor MJ, Makunde WH, McGarry HF, et al (Liverpool School of Tropical Medicine, England; Natl Inst for Med Research, Tanga, Tanzania; Univ of Bonn, Germany; et al)

Lancet 365:2116-2121, 2005

6–2

Background.—*Wolbachia* endosymbionts of filarial nematodes are vital for larval development and adult-worm fertility and viability. This essential dependency on the bacterium for survival of the parasites has provided a new approach to treat filariasis with antibiotics. We used this strategy to investigate the effects of doxycycline treatment on the major cause of lymphatic filariasis, *Wuchereria bancrofti*.

Methods.—We undertook a double-blind, randomised, placebo-controlled field trial of doxycycline (200 mg per day) for 8 weeks in 72 individuals infected with W *bancrofti* from Kimang'a village, Pangani, Tanzania. Participants were randomly assigned by block randomisation to receive capsules of doxycycline (n=34) or placebo (n=38). We assessed treatment efficacy by monitoring microfilaraemia, antigenaemia, and ultrasound detection of adult worms. Follow-up assessments were done at 5, 8, 11, and 14 months after the start of treatment. Analysis was per protocol.

Findings.—One person from the doxycycline group died from HIV infection. Five (doxycycline) and 11 (placebo) individuals were absent at the time of ultrasound analysis. Doxycycline treatment almost completely eliminated microfilaraemia at 8-14 months' follow-up (for all timepoints p<0.001). Ultrasonography detected adult worms in only six (22%) of 27 individuals treated with doxycycline compared with 24 (88%) of 27 with placebo at 14 months after the start of treatment (p<0.0001). At the same timepoint, filarial antigenaemia in the doxycycline group fell to about half of that before treatment (p=0.015). Adverse events were few and mild.

Interpretation.—An 8-week course of doxycycline is a safe and well-tolerated treatment for lymphatic filariasis with significant activity against adult worms and microfilaraemia.

▶ Currently available treatments for filariasis, including diethylcarbamazine or ivermectin (both of which are usually given with albendazole), effectively kill the microfilariae (the larval offspring of the parasite) but are less effective against the macrofilariae (adult worms). Taylor et al suggest a novel macrofilaricidal approach using a treatment directed at *Wolbachia*, the intracellular bacterial symbiont of filarial parasites. They provide convincing evidence that depletion of *Wolbachia* by doxycycline kills most adult worms, without causing severe side effects. The significant reduction in the number of worm nests in the scrotum and the reduced levels of filarial antigen in the blood 14 months after treatment suggest that the antibiotic indirectly kills the adult worm.[1]

B. H. Thiers, MD

Reference

1. Stolk WA, de Vlas SJ, Habbema JDF: Anti-*Wolbachia* treatment of lymphatic filariasis. *Lancet* 365:2067-2068, 2005.

Reassessment of the Cost of Chronic Helmintic Infection: A Meta-analysis of Disability-Related Outcomes in Endemic Schistosomiasis

King CH, Dickman K, Tisch DJ (Case Western Reserve Univ, Cleveland, Ohio)
Lancet 365:1561-1569, 2005   6–3

Background.—Schistosomiasis is one of the world's most prevalent infections, yet its effect on the global burden of disease is controversial. Published disability-adjusted life-year (DALY) estimates suggest that the average effect of schistosome infection is quite small, although this is disputed. To develop an evidenced-based reassessment of schistosomiasis-related disability, we did a systematic review of data on disability-associated outcomes for all forms of schistosomiasis.

Methods.—We did structured searches using EMBASE, PUBMED, and Cochrane electronic databases. Published bibliographies were manually searched, and unpublished studies were obtained by contacting research groups. Reports were reviewed and abstracted independently by two trained readers. All randomised and observational studies of schistosomiasis morbidity were eligible for inclusion. We calculated pooled estimates of reported disability-related effects using weighted odds ratios for categorical outcomes and standardised mean differences for continuous data.

Findings.—482 published or unpublished reports (March, 1921, to July, 2002) were screened. Of 135 selected for inclusion, 51 provided data for performance-related symptoms, whereas 109 reported observed measures of disability-linked morbidities. Schistosomiasis was significantly associated with anaemia, chronic pain, diarrhoea, exercise intolerance, and undernutrition.

Interpretation.—By contrast with WHO estimates of 0.5% disability weight assigned to schistosomiasis, 2-15% disability seems evident in different functional domains of a person with schistosomiasis. This raised estimate, if confirmed in formal patient-preference studies, indicates a need to reassess our priorities for treating this silent pandemic of schistosomiasis.

▶ It is estimated that more than 200 million people worldwide, most of whom live in sub-Saharan Africa, are infected with chronic schistosomiasis. The disease is associated with chronic tissue inflammation; the range and potential severity of symptoms and pathologic changes associated with the disease have been well described. This report helps quantify the disabling effects of these clinical manifestations and provides an estimate of the effects of chronic schistosomiasis on quality of life. Schistosomiasis clearly represents a substantial public health burden because of the large number of individuals affected and the chronicity of infection.

B. H. Thiers, MD

Artesunate Versus Quinine for Treatment of Severe Falciparum Malaria: A Randomised Trial

White NJ, for the South East Asian Quinine Artesunate Malaria Trial (SEAQUAMAT) group (Mahidol Univ, Bangkok, Thailand; et al)
Lancet 366:717-725, 2005   6–4

Background.—In the treatment of severe malaria, intravenous artesunate is more rapidly acting than intravenous quinine in terms of parasite clearance, is safer, and is simpler to administer, but whether it can reduce mortality is uncertain.

Methods.—We did an open-label randomised controlled trial in patients admitted to hospital with severe falciparum malaria in Bangladesh, India, Indonesia, and Myanmar. We assigned individuals intravenous artesunate 2.4 mg/kg bodyweight given as a bolus (n=730) at 0, 12, and 24 h, and then daily, or intravenous quinine (20 mg salt per kg loading dose infused over 4 h then 10 mg/kg infused over 2-8 h three times a day; n=731). Oral medication was substituted when possible to complete treatment. Our primary endpoint was death from severe malaria, and analysis was by intention to treat.

Findings.—We assessed all patients randomised for the primary endpoint. Mortality in artesunate recipients was 15% (107 of 730) compared with 22% (164 of 731) in quinine recipients; an absolute reduction of 34.7% (95% CI 18.5-47.6%; p=0.0002). Treatment with artesunate was well tolerated, whereas quinine was associated with hypoglycaemia (relative risk 3.2, 1.3-7.8; p=0.009).

Interpretation.—Artesunate should become the treatment of choice for severe falciparum malaria in adults.

▶ The findings from this large, multicenter trial showed that parenteral artesunate reduces the mortality rate for patients with severe malaria by more than one third compared with quinine. This large reduction in the mortality rate was consistent across countries and in all prospectively defined subgroups.

Thus, the authors conclude that artesunate should be the treatment of choice for adults with severe malaria. It appears to be safe (although rarely linked to a type I hypersensitivity reaction in about 1 in 3000 treated patients[1]), simple to administer, and more effective than quinine.

B. H. Thiers, MD

Reference

1. Leonardi-Nield E, Gilvary G, White NJ, et al: Severe allergic reactions to oral artesunate: A report of two cases. *Trans R Soc Trop Med Hyg* 95:182-183, 2001.

Resistance of *Plasmodium falciparum* Field Isolates to In-Vitro Artemether and Point Mutations of the SERCA-Type PfATPase6

Jambou R, Legrand E, Niang M, et al (Institut Pasteur de Dakar, Senegal; Institut Pasteur de Guyane Française, Cayenne, French Guiana; Institut Pasteur du Cambodge, Phnom Penh, Cambodia; et al)
Lancet 366:1960-1963, 2005   6–5

Introduction.—Artemisinin derivatives are an essential component of treatment against multidrug-resistant *Plasmodium falciparum* malaria. We aimed to investigate in-vitro resistance to artemisinin derivatives in field isolates. In-vitro susceptibility of 530 *P falciparum* isolates from three countries (Cambodia, French Guiana, and Senegal) with different artemisinin use was assessed with an isotopic microtest. Artemether IC_{50} up to 117 and 45 nmol/L was seen in French Guiana and Senegal, respectively. DNA sequencing in a subsample of 60 isolates lends support to SERCA-*PfATPase6* as the target for artemisinins. The S769N *PfATPase6* mutation, noted exclusively in French Guiana, was associated with raised (>30 nmol/L) artemether IC_{50}s (p<0.0001, Mann-Whitney). All resistant isolates came from areas with uncontrolled use of artemisinin derivatives. This rise in resistance indicates the need for increased vigilance and a coordinated and rapid deployment of drug combinations.

▶ Widespread multidrug-resistant *P falciparum* malaria has been associated with a sharp rise in mortality due to the disease in Africa. Current World Health Organization guidelines recommend combination drug therapy as first-line treatment, with formulations containing an artemisinin compound as one component. The combination of artesunate (an artemisinin derivative) and mefloquine has been used in Thailand for about 10 years with no apparent decrease in efficacy. Unfortunately, as indicated in the report by Jambou et al, the expectation that all combinations with artemisinins will have a long therapeutic life may be overly optimistic. In fact, indiscriminate use of artemisinins may create conditions favorable for the selection of resistant mutants. In short, resistance to artemisinins may be accelerated by their uncontrolled use as monotherapy or in combination with ineffective partner drugs.[1]

B. H. Thiers, MD

Reference

1. Duffy PE, Sibley CH: Are we losing artemisinin combination therapy already? Lancet 366:1908-1909, 2005.

7 Disorders of the Pilosebaceous Apparatus

Elevated 17-Hydroxyprogesterone Serum Values in Male Patients With Acne
Placzek M, Arnold B, Schmidt H, et al (Ludwig-Maximilian-Univ, Munich)
J Am Acad Dermatol 53:955-958, 2005   7–1

Background.—Androgen excess may provoke or aggravate acne by inducing seborrhea. In women, androgen disorders are frequently suspected when acne is accompanied by hirsutism or irregularities of the menstrual cycle. In men, however, acne may be the only sign of androgen excess.

Objective.—Our aim was to investigate whether male patients with acne display pathologic androgen blood values.

Methods.—This case-control study at a university dermatology department with referred and unreferred patients investigated male acne patients (n = 82, consecutive sample) in whom the diagnosis of mild to severe acne was made, as well as a control group of men without acne (n = 38). The main outcome measures were androgen parameters including morning values of testosterone, luteinizing hormone, follicle-stimulating hormone, dehydroepiandrosterone sulfate, androstenedione, and 17-hydroxyprogesterone; as well as a corticotropin stimulation test.

Results.—17-Hydroxyprogesterone levels were significantly higher ($P = .01$) in acne patients than in the control group, whereas the other parameters did not differ significantly. In addition, the corticotropin stimulation test revealed abnormal 17-hydroxyprogesterone induction values in 10 of 82 patients.

Limitations.—The analysis is limited to a selection of androgen parameters.

Conclusion.—The results suggest that in men irregularities of adrenal steroid metabolism may be a factor contributing to acne.

Acne in Adolescence and Cause-Specific Mortality: Lower Coronary Heart Disease but Higher Prostate Cancer Mortality: The Glasgow Alumni Cohort Study

Galobardes B, Smith GD, Jeffreys M, et al (Univ of Bristol, England; Massey Univ, Wellington, New Zealand; Queen's Univ of Belfast, United Kingdom)
Am J Epidemiol 161:1094-1101, 2005   7–2

Introduction.—Androgen level or androgen activity is implicated in several health outcomes, but its independent role remains controversial. This study investigated the association between history of acne in young adulthood, a marker of hormone activity, and cause-specific mortality in the Glasgow Alumni Cohort Study. Male students who attended Glasgow University between 1948 and 1968 and participated in voluntary health checks reported history of acne ($n = 11,232$). Vital status has been traced, and risk factors in adulthood are known for about 50% of the participants. Those with a history of acne were more often nonsmokers while university students and tended to be from a lower socioeconomic position. The two groups did not differ in other adolescent (height, body mass index, blood pressure, and number of siblings) or in most adult risk factors. Students who reported a history of acne had a lower risk of all-cause (hazard ratio = 0.89, 95% confidence interval (CI): 0.76, 1.04) and coronary heart disease (hazard ratio = 0.67, 95% CI: 0.48, 0.94) mortality but had some evidence of a higher risk of prostate cancer mortality (hazard ratio = 1.67, 95% CI: 0.79, 3.55). This study shows that androgen activity during adolescence may protect against coronary heart disease but confer a higher risk of prostate cancer mortality.

▶ Without actual measurements of androgen levels, the authors' conclusion ("that androgen activity during adolescence may protect against coronary heart disease but confer a higher risk of prostate cancer mortality") remains questionable. Most dermatologists are well aware that the vast majority of our acne patients have no measurable abnormality of androgen metabolism.

B. H. Thiers, MD

High School Dietary Dairy Intake and Teenage Acne

Adebamowo CA, Spiegelman D, Danby FW, et al (Harvard Med School, Boston)
J Am Acad Dermatol 52:207-214, 2005   7–3

Background.—Previous studies suggest possible associations between Western diet and acne. We examined data from the Nurses Health Study II to retrospectively evaluate whether intakes of dairy foods during high school were associated with physician-diagnosed severe teenage acne.

Methods.—We studied 47,355 women who completed questionnaires on high school diet in 1998 and physician-diagnosed severe teenage acne in 1989. We estimated the prevalence ratios and 95% confidence intervals of acne history across categories of intakes.

Results.—After accounting for age, age at menarche, body mass index, and energy intake, the multivariate prevalence ratio (95% confidence intervals; *P* value for test of trend) of acne, comparing extreme categories of intake, were: 1.22 (1.03, 1.44; .002) for total milk; 1.12 (1.00, 1.25; .56) for whole milk; 1.16 (1.01, 1.34; .25) for low-fat milk; and 1.44 (1.21, 1.72; .003) for skim milk. Instant breakfast drink, sherbet, cottage cheese, and cream cheese were also positively associated with acne.

Conclusion.—We found a positive association with acne for intake of total milk and skim milk. We hypothesize that the association with milk may be because of the presence of hormones and bioactive molecules in milk.

▶ This retrospective study found a correlation between milk intake, particularly skim milk, and the presence of severe teenage acne. The problems with this study are (1) it is retrospective, and participants were expected to remember the amount of dairy products consumed at least 9 years before the study; (2) only the participants were asked whether they had ever had physicians diagnose their acne, but there may have been individuals in the control group who had severe acne that was never physician-diagnosed; and (3) it was basically left to the participants to grade the severity of their acne. Obviously, there is much variation in what young women consider severe acne. Individuals in the severe acne group may, in reality, not have had severe acne. Some treatment-resistant cases of acne may warrant a trial off of dairy products. However, dairy products are an important source of calcium in this age group. It would seem prudent to conduct prospective studies in which the intake of dairy products could be more accurately quantified, and the severity of acne could be more accurately judged. Only then could general recommendations be made to all acne patients about the avoidance of milk and other dairy products.

S. Raimer, MD

Antibiotic Treatment of Acne May Be Associated With Upper Respiratory Tract Infections
Margolis DJ, Bowe WP, Hoffstad O, et al (Univ of Pennsylvania, Philadelphia)
Arch Dermatol 141:1132-1136, 2005   7–4

Objective.—To determine if the long-term use of antibiotics for the treatment of acne results in an increase in either of 2 common infectious illnesses: upper respiratory tract infections (URTIs) or urinary tract infections.

Design.—Retrospective cohort study.

Setting.—General Practice Research Database of the United Kingdom, London, England, from 1987 to 2002.

Patients.—Patients with a diagnosis of acne.

Main Outcome Measure.—The onset of either a URTI or a urinary tract infection.

Results.—Of 118 496 individuals with acne (age range, 15-35 years) who were identified in the General Practice Research Database, 84 977 (71.7%)

received a topical or oral antibiotic (tetracyclines, erythromycin, or clindamycin) for treatment of their acne and 33 519 (28.3%) did not. Within the first year of observation, 18 281 (15.4%) of the patients with acne had at least 1 URTI, and within that year, the odds of a URTI developing among those receiving antibiotic treatment were 2.15 (95% confidence interval, 2.05-2.23; $P<.001$) times greater than among those who were not receiving antibiotic treatment. Multiple additional analyses, which were conducted to show that this effect was not an artifact of increased health care-seeking behavior among our cohorts, included comparing the cohorts of patients with acne with a cohort of patients with hypertension and the likelihood of developing a urinary tract infection.

Conclusions.—Patients with acne who were receiving antibiotic treatment for acne were more likely to develop a URTI than those with acne who were not receiving such treatment. The true clinical importance of our findings will require further investigation.

▶ Larger randomized trials are necessary to confirm the apparent association between antibiotics and URTIs and to elucidate the relevant mechanisms.[1]

B. H. Thiers, MD

Reference

1. Chan A-W, Shaw JC: Acne, antibiotics, and upper respiratory tract infections. *Arch Dermatol* 141:1157-1158, 2005.

Effects and Side-effects of Spironolactone Therapy in Women With Acne

Yemisci A, Gorgulu A, Piskin S (Kesan State Hosp, Edirne, Turkey; Trakya Univ, Edirne, Turkey)

J Eur Acad Dermatol Venereol 19:163-166, 2005   7–5

Background and aims.—Androgen hormones play an important role in the pathogenesis of acne. Despite the demonstrated effects, spironolactone, an androgen receptor blocker, is not commonly used to treat acne. We planned an open-labelled, prospective study to evaluate the effects and side-effects of spironolactone therapy in women with acne.

Materials and methods.—Thirty-five consecutive patients with acne were treated with spironolactone 100 mg/day, 16 days each month for 3 months. The patients were divided according to the clinical severity of the lesions as having mild, moderate and severe acne. Serum total testosterone and dehydroepiandrosterone sulfate (DHEAS) levels were measured before and after treatment. Lesion numbers and hormone levels before and after treatment were compared with one-sampled t-test.

Results.—The mean age of the patients was 21.4 ± 3.5 years. Two patients discontinued the study due to side-effects. Five patients were lost in the follow-up. Clinically significant improvement was noted in 24 patients (85.71%). No response was seen in four patients. All of the nonresponding patients had received previous unsuccessful therapies. Mean number of lesions and mean DHEAS levels of the 24 patients with clinical improvement decreased significantly after treatment ($P < 0.01$ and $P < 0.05$, respectively). There was no change in the mean total testosterone levels before and after treatment ($P > 0.05$).

Conclusion.—Spironolactone is a safe and effective medication for women with acne vulgaris. Although its side-effects seem to be high, they are in the majority of cases not a reason to stop treatment.

▶ Patients took 50 mg spironolactone twice daily, starting on the fifth day of the menstrual cycle and continuing for 16 days. Menstrual irregularities occurred in 50% of patients. Although certainly not a first-line therapy, spironolactone may be a reasonable alternative for patients with acne vulgaris that does not respond to other therapies. Because of side effects such as decreased libido and gynecomastia, which have been reported in men, its use has been restricted mainly to women.

B. H. Thiers, MD

Isotretinoin Therapy and Mood Changes in Adolescents With Moderate to Severe Acne: A Cohort Study

Chia CY, Lane W, Chibnall J, et al (Saint Louis Univ; Univ of Missouri, Columbia)
Arch Dermatol 141:557-560, 2005   7–6

Objective.—To determine whether patients with moderate to severe acne who were treated with isotretinoin experienced significant increases in depressive symptoms over a 3- to 4-month period compared with patients who received conservative acne therapy.

Design.—Cohort study.

Setting.—Hospital-affiliated and community-based clinics in St Louis, Mo.

Participants.—One hundred thirty-two subjects aged 12 to 19 years with moderate to severe acne.

Main Outcome Measures.—Depressive symptoms were assessed using the Center for Epidemiological Studies Depression Scale (CES-D), a standardized self-reported instrument. Mean CES-D scores were compared between treatment groups, as were the prevalence and incidence of scores suggestive of clinically significant depression (CES-D score >16).

Results.—A total of 101 subjects completed the study. At follow-up, CES-D scores (adjusted for baseline CES-D score and sex of patient) suggestive of clinically significant depression were no more prevalent in the isotretinoin group than in the conservative therapy group. Similarly, the incidence (new onset) of depressive symptoms suggestive of clinical significance also was not significantly different between the treatment groups.

Conclusions.—The use of isotretinoin in the treatment of moderate-severe acne in adolescents did not increase symptoms of depression. On the contrary, treatment of acne either with conservative therapy or with isotretinoin was associated with a decrease in depressive symptoms.

Functional Brain Imaging Alterations in Acne Patients Treated with Isotretinoin

Bremner JD, Fani N, Ashraf A, et al (Emory Univ, Atlanta, Ga; Atlanta Dept of Veterans Affairs Med Ctr, Decatur, Ga)

Am J Psychiatry 162:983-991, 2005   7–7

Objective.—Although there have been case reports suggesting a relationship between treatment with the acne medication isotretinoin and the development of depression and suicide, this topic remains controversial. In order for isotretinoin to cause depression, it must have an effect on the brain; however, the effects of isotretinoin on brain functioning in acne patients have not been established. The purpose of this study was to assess the effects of isotretinoin on brain functioning in acne patients.

Method.—Brain functioning in adults was measured with [^{18}F]fluorodeoxyglucose positron emission tomography before and after 4 months of treatment with isotretinoin (N=13) or an antibiotic (N=15).

Results.—Isotretinoin but not antibiotic treatment was associated with decreased brain metabolism in the orbitofrontal cortex (-21% change versus 2% change for antibiotic), a brain area known to mediate symptoms of depression. There were no differences in the severity of depressive symptoms between the isotretinoin and antibiotic treatment groups before or after treatment.

Conclusions.—This study suggests that isotretinoin treatment is associated with changes in brain functioning.

▶ Chia et al (Abstract 7–6) found no increase in the incidence of new depressive symptoms or the prevalence of clinically significant depression in acne patients treated with either conservative therapy or isotretinoin; in fact, there was a decrease in depressive symptoms in both groups. Similarly, Bremner et al (Abstract 7–7) found no difference in the severity of depression in patients treated with either isotretinoin or antibiotics. However, they did note an alteration in metabolism in the part of the brain thought to mediate the symptoms of depression. The failure to correlate this with clinical symptomology casts doubt on the significance of the findings. Perhaps the most significant bit of information came from the conflict of interest statement published with this article, which noted funding from "lawyers involved in Accutane litigation!"

B. H. Thiers, MD

Trends in Adherence to a Revised Risk Management Program Designed to Decrease or Eliminate Isotretinoin-Exposed Pregnancies: Evaluation of the Accutane SMART Program

Brinker A, Kornegay C, Nourjah P (Food and Drug Administration, Rockville, Md)
Arch Dermatol 141:563-569, 2005   7–8

Objective.—To review adherence to selected procedures outlined in the System to Manage Accutane-Related Teratogenicity (SMART) program during the first year of implementation vs the procedures in effect in the year prior to initiation of the SMART program.

Design.—Observational.

Setting.—A novel pharmacy compliance survey and an ongoing, voluntary survey.

Patients.—Female recipients of isotretinoin.

Intervention.—In April 2002, Hoffmann-La Roche Inc, Nutley, NJ, manufacturer of Accutane brand isotretinoin and at that time the sole source of isotretinoin, revised earlier guidelines and instituted the SMART risk management program, which included the use of qualification stickers to affix to all prescriptions for Accutane to indicate, among other things, a negative pregnancy test just before the prescription was written. The goal of the SMART program was to decrease or eliminate isotretinoin-exposed pregnancies.

Main Outcome Measures.—Use and completion of prescription qualification stickers; changes in pretherapy pregnancy testing and birth control use.

Results.—The results of the pharmacy compliance survey indicated high (>90%) use of prescription qualification stickers. Results of the patient survey suggested that 9% of prescription qualification stickers within the observed user cohort were issued without a pregnancy test. Furthermore, the pregnancy rate for patients participating in the survey was similar to that reported for cohorts recruited before the SMART program.

Conclusions.—The usefulness of the results derived from 2 surveys designed to evaluate the SMART program is limited by the lack of reliability and validity of the survey instruments and by questionable generalizability to all female recipients of isotretinoin. The presence of a qualification sticker may not have an impact on pregnancy testing or compliance with effective birth control behavior as outlined in the SMART program.

▶ Although compliance with the qualification sticker was high, it did not appear to have any impact on the performance of pregnancy testing or compliance with birth control use. As a result, a new, stricter (although not necessarily more effective) program (iPLEDGE) is now in place.

B. H. Thiers, MD

Prescription of Teratogenic Medications in United States Ambulatory Practices

Schwarz EB, Maselli J, Norton M, et al (Univ of Pittsburgh, Pa; Univ of California, San Francisco)

Am J Med 118:1240-1249, 2005   7–9

Purpose.—The purpose of this study was to identify the potentially teratogenic medications most frequently prescribed to women of childbearing age and the specialty of physicians who provide ambulatory care to women who use such medications. In addition, we evaluated rates of contraceptive counseling to explore awareness of the risks associated with teratogenic medication use.

TABLE 1.—Volume of Prescriptions for Potentially Teratogenic (US Food and Drug Administration Class D or X) Medications Given to Women of Childbearing Age, by Medication

Medication Class	Annual Prescriptions for Class D or X* Drugs, in Millions (95% CI)	Proportion of Prescription for Class D or X* Drugs
Anxiolytics	4.06 (3.88-4.23)	35%
Alprazolam	1.46	
Clonazepam	0.99	
Lorazepam	0.76	
Diazepam	0.69	
Temazepam	0.12	
Chlordiazepoxide	0.03	
Anticonvulsants	1.42 (1.33-1.51)	12%
Divalproex sodium	0.71	
Carbamazepine	0.44	
Phenytoin	0.18	
Valproate	0.05	
Phenobarbital	0.04	
Primidone	0.01	
Antibiotics	1.38 (1.29-1.47)	12%
Doxycycline	0.90	
Tetracycline	0.38	
Tobramycin	0.10	
Statins	0.76 (0.69-0.83)	6%
Atorvastatin	0.45	
Pravastatin	0.16	
Simvastatin	0.11	
Fluvastatin	0.02	
Lovastatin	0.01	
Isotretinoin	0.54 (0.49-0.59)	5%
Methotrexate	0.40 (0.35-0.45)	3%
Lithium	0.40 (0.35-0.45)	3%
Warfarin	0.21 (0.18-0.24)	2%
Others	1.67 (1.57-1.77)	14%
Total	11.7 (11.3-12.1)	100%†

*Potentially teratogenic class D or X medications.
†Proportions listed do not total 100% as a result of rounding.
(Reprinted from Schwarz EB, Maselli J, Norton M, et al: Prescription of teratogenic medications in United States ambulatory practices. *Am J Med* 118:1240-1249, 2005. Copyright 2005, with permission from Elsevier Science.)

Subjects and Methods.—The prescription of teratogenic medications and provision of contraceptive counseling on 12,681 visits made by nonpregnant women, 14 to 44 years of age, to 1880 physicians in US ambulatory practice (National Ambulatory Medical Care Survey) between 1998 and 2000 was analyzed.

Results.—Use of a potentially teratogenic, class D or X, medication by a woman of childbearing age is documented on 1 of every 13 visits made to US ambulatory practices. These include anxiolytics (4.1 million annual prescriptions), anticonvulsant medications (1.4 million annual prescriptions), antibiotics like doxycycline (1.4 million annual prescriptions), and statins (0.8 million annual prescriptions). Isotretinoin accounts for less than 5% of potentially teratogenic prescriptions (0.5 million annual prescriptions). Internists and family/general practitioners provide ambulatory care to 45% of women prescribed potentially teratogenic medications, psychiatrists provide ambulatory care to 20% of women prescribed potentially teratogenic medications, and dermatologists provide ambulatory care to 20% of women prescribed potentially teratogenic medications. Contraceptive counseling was provided on less than 20% of visits that documented use of a potential teratogen by a woman of childbearing age. Women using low-risk (class A or B) drugs received contraceptive counseling as frequently as women using potential teratogens ($P = .24$).

Conclusion.—Potentially teratogenic medications are prescribed to millions of women of childbearing age each year. Physician awareness of the teratogenic risk associated with class D or X medications seems low (Table 1).

▶ So what's next: iPLEDGE for doxycycline?

B. H. Thiers, MD

Subcision for Acne Scarring: Technique and Outcomes in 40 Patients
Alam M, Omura N, Kaminer MS (SkinCare Physicians, Chestnut Hill, Mass; Northwestern Univ, Chicago; Dartmouth Med School, Hanover, Mass; et al)
Dermatol Surg 31:310-317, 2005   7–10

Background.—Treatment of acne scars is a therapeutic challenge that may require multiple modalities. Subcision is a technique that has been anecdotally reported to be of value in treating so-called "rolling scars."

Objectives.—To assess the efficacy of subcision in the treatment of "rolling" acne scars.

Methods.—A standard technique was developed for subcision. This was then applied to the treatment of rolling scars in patients, 40 of whom completed treatment and the prescribed follow-up. Six-month follow-up data were obtained from both patients and investigators.

Results.—Subcision is associated with patient and investigator reports of approximately 50% improvement. Ninety percent of treated patients reported that subcision improved their appearance. The side effects of swelling, bruising, and pain are transient, but patients may have persistent firm bumps at the treatment site.

Conclusions.—Subcision appears to be a safe technique that may provide significant long-term improvement in the "rolling scars" of selected patients. When complete resolution of such scars does not occur, combining subcision with other scar revision procedures or repeat subcision may be beneficial.

▶ How nice to see this simple and successful technique reintroduced into the dermatologic surgical literature! I use subcision frequently for acne scarring and iatrogenic scarring. The procedure is simple and reasonably risk free. In my experience, patient satisfaction is quite high. The dermatologist needs to consider this technique, especially given its modest benefits and demonstrated safety compared with alternative treatment methods for scarring.

J. Cook, MD

Critical Appraisal of Reports on the Treatment of Perioral Dermatitis
Weber K, Thurmayr R (Krankenhaus der Missionsbenediktiner, Tutzing, Germany; Technical Univ of Munich)
Dermatology 210:300-307, 2005   7–11

Background.—Presently, problems exist with the rationale of oral therapy and the nature and indication of topical and accompanying treatment of perioral dermatitis.

Objective.—Providing the basis to overcome these problems by a quality evaluation of treatment reports and assessment of the consistency of treatment experience.

Methods.—Sources were Medline (1964-2004), Embase (1966-2004), the Cochrane Central (1971-2004) and 526 references of 3 textbooks, 2 recent reviews and 30 papers on perioral dermatitis. Thirty English and German articles were selected. These studies were evaluated according to principles of evidence-based medicine and related criteria. Evaluation of 28 papers was carried out by the authors and of our own 2 papers by 2 other reviewers. Consistency of results was qualitatively assessed by the authors.

Results.—There were only 2 therapeutic trials of medium-range quality. The other studies were of low quality. Consistency was noted concerning treatment with oral tetracycline (with 1 exception), discontinuation of topical corticosteroids and cosmetics and, to a lesser extent, regarding no therapy. There was inconsistency in respect to topical therapy.

Conclusion.—The presented data help to interpret and conduct studies on the treatment of perioral dermatitis.

▶ Treatment initiatives designed to control perioral dermatitis are hindered by the lack of consensus regarding the cause of this disorder. Weber and Thurmayr decry the poor quality of studies to assess the effectiveness of available therapies, although they do note that discontinuation of topical steroids and cosmetics often has a beneficial effect on the condition.

B. H. Thiers, MD

Hairless Triggers Reactivation of Hair Growth by Promoting Wnt Signaling
Beaudoin GMJ III, Sisk JM, Coulombe PA, et al (Johns Hopkins Univ, Baltimore, Md)
Proc Natl Acad Sci U S A 102:14653-14658, 2005   7–12

Background.—Maintenance of hair is accomplished through a cyclic process that includes periodic regeneration of hair follicles in a stem cell–dependent manner. This process is composed of 3 defined stages: growth (anagen), regression (catagen), and rest (telogen). New hair growth is dependent on reentry into anagen. Multiple signaling pathways, including Wnts, Sonic hedgehog, and TGF-β family members have been shown to promote anagen initiation. However, the exact mechanism by which hair follicles regenerate has not been elucidated.

Disruption of Hairless (Hr) gene function is responsible for a complex skin phenotype that includes a specific defect in hair follicle regeneration in both humans and mice. The role of a nuclear receptor corepressor (HR) in follicle regeneration was investigated.

Methods.—$Hr^{-/-}$ mice and TOP-Gal mice were used in this study. In addition, K14-rHr mice were made by cloning the coding sequence of the rHr cDNA downstream of a human K14 promoter. The promoter of the Wise gene was isolated through cell culture and transfection assays. Nuclear HR protein was localized throughout the hair cycle using HR-specific antisera to determine where and when HR acts in hair follicles.

Results.—Follicles actively growing hair in anagen did not contain detectable HR. HR protein was detected as follicles entered catagen, which coincided with the onset of phenotypic alterations in hair follicles of Hr mutant mice. Within the follicles, HR protein was found in the nuclei of keratin 14-positive cells in the outer root sheath, which includes the bulb region. Expression of HR was maintained in the outer root sheath through late catagen into telogen and the early part of the next anagen phase. After reformation of the hair bulb in mid anagen, HR protein was again undetectable. Thus, the transgenic expression of HR in progenitor keratinocytes was shown to rescue follicle regeneration in $Hr^{-/-}$ mice. The expression of Wise, a modulator of Wnt signaling, was repressed by HR in these cells, coincident with the timing of follicle regeneration.

Conclusion.—A link between HR (the Hairless protein) and Wnt function was established, providing a model in which HR regulates the timing of Wnt signaling required for hair follicle regeneration.

Long-term Renewal of Hair Follicles From Clonogenic Multipotent Stem Cells

Caludinot S, Nicolas M, Oshima H, et al (Ecole Polytechnique Fédérale de Lausanne, Switzerland; Lausanne Univ, Switzerland)
Proc Natl Acad Sci U S A 102:14677-14682, 2005   7–13

Background.—Adult stem cells are essential for tissue renewal, regeneration, and repair in mammals, and their expansion in culture is vital to regenerative medicine. Skin stem cells, like other stem cells, are thought to reside at precise locations, or niches, where they benefit from a unique environment favoring self-renewal through symmetric or asymmetric divisions. Hair follicles and epidermis contain keratinocytes that are clonogenic, some of which (homoclones) can be serially propagated in culture for more than 180 doublings. Thus, in theory, it is possible to generate the entire epithelial compartment of the epidermis of an adult human with the progeny of a single homoclone.

Opposing views of the nature of the clonogenic keratinocytes have been advanced, with some viewing them as progenitor cells incapable of sustaining long-term hair follicle renewal and others viewing them as stem cells. The fact that clonogenic keratinocytes are bona fide multipotent stem cells was demonstrated.

Methods.—Rat whisker follicles were obtained from Fischer 344 rats, and single cells were isolated and individually cultivated on a feeder layer of lethally irradiated 3T3-J2 cells. Retroviral infection was introduced to the keratinocytes, and no recombinant viruses were produced by the transduced keratinocytes. Donor cells were injected into the dermo-epidermal junction of newborn mouse or rat skin, and grafts were transplanted on the backs of athymic mice with their dermal side facing the mouse fascia. The grafts were then covered with a mouse skin flap to prevent drying.

Results.—Flap necrosis usually occurred a few days after transplantation, and the graft became air exposed. Dense hairs covered the graft within days. Histologic examination, RT-PCR, and FISH analysis showed that clonogenicity is an intrinsic property of the adult stem cells of the hair follicle. After cultivation for more than 140 doublings, these transplanted stem cells formed part or all of the developing follicles at the dermo-epidermal junction of newborn mouse skin.

Conclusion.—The stem cells incorporated into follicles are multipotent because they generate all of the lineages of a hair follicle and sebaceous gland. Thousands of hair follicles can be generated from the progeny of a single cultivated stem cell. This study found that cultured stem cells express the self-renewal genes Bmi1 and Zfp145 and that several stem cells participate in the formation of a single hair bulb.

▶ These articles (Abstracts 7–12 and 7–13) present data that elucidate the many complex factors underlying the genetic and molecular control of stem cell trafficking and hair growth. Knowledge of the various modulators and signaling pathways involved will lead not only to a better understanding of the process but also to better treatments for conditions involving hair loss.

B. H. Thiers, MD

Modulation of Hair Growth With Small Molecule Agonists of the Hedgehog Signaling Pathway

Paladini RD, Saleh J, Qian C, et al (Curis Inc, Cambridge, Mass)
J Invest Dermatol 125:638-646, 2005   7–14

Introduction.—The hedgehog (Hh) family of intercellular signaling proteins is intricately linked to the development and patterning of almost every major vertebrate organ system. In the skin, sonic hedgehog (Shh) is required for hair follicle morphogenesis during embryogenesis and for regulating follicular growth and cycling in the adult. We recently described the identification and characterization of synthetic, non-peptidyl small molecule agonists of the Hh pathway. In this study, we examined the ability of a topically applied Hh-agonist to modulate follicular cycling in adult mouse skin. We report that the Hh-agonist can stimulate the transition from the resting (telogen) to the growth (anagen) stage of the hair cycle in adult mouse skin. Hh-agonist-induced hair growth caused no detectable differences in epidermal proliferation, differentiation, or in the endogenous Hh-signaling pathway as measured by *Gli1*, *Shh*, *Ptc1*, and *Gli2* gene expression when compared with a normal hair cycle. In addition, we demonstrate that Hh-agonist is active in human scalp in vitro as measured by *Gli1* gene expression. These results suggest that the topical application of Hh-agonist could be effective in treating conditions of decreased proliferation and aberrant follicular cycling in the scalp including androgenetic alopecia (pattern hair loss).

▶ Paladini et al propose that small molecule agonists of the Hh pathway may be effective in the treatment of male and female pattern alopecia. These are clearly preliminary observations that will require confirmation both in the laboratory and in the clinic.

B. H. Thiers, MD

Mechanisms of Hair Graying: Incomplete Melanocyte Stem Cell Maintenance in the Niche

Nishimura EK, Granter SR, Fisher DE (Harvard Med School, Boston)
Science 307:720-724, 2005   7–15

Background.—One of the most obvious signs of aging in humans is graying of the hair. However, the mechanism of hair graying has not been clearly elucidated. Qualitative and quantitative changes in stem and progenitor cells have been implicated in physiologic aging, but these changes are poorly understood, and the process of aging in stem cells has not been visually observed. The involvement of stem and progenitor cells in aging of multiple organ systems has been suggested in mice defective in DNA damage repair and telomere maintenance, but melanocytes may be unique because the oxidative chemistry of melanin biosynthesis can be cytotoxic. This observation led to a suggestion that differentiated, pigmented melanocytes are specifically targeted in hair graying. The recent discovery of unpigmented melanocyte cells located distinctly within the hair follicle has provided an opportunity to determine whether the process of hair graying is initiated specifically from changes in differentiated melanocytes or the stem-cell pool that provides them.

Methods and Results.—Melanocyte-tagged transgenic mice and aging human hair follicles were used to demonstrate that hair graying is caused by defective self-maintenance of melanocyte stem cells. The graying process was accelerated with *Bc12* deficiency, which causes selective apoptosis of melanocyte stem cells, but not of differentiated melanocytes, within the niche at their entry into the dominant state. It was also observed that physiologic aging of melanocyte stem cells was associated with ectopic pigmentation or differentiation within the niche, which was accelerated by mutation of the melanocyte master transcriptional regulator *Mitf*.

Conclusions.—A previously unknown pathophysiologic mechanism for hair graying was identified. Incomplete maintenance of melanocyte stem cells appears to cause physiologic hair graying through loss of the differentiated progeny with aging. The specific roles for stem-cell apoptosis versus ectopic differentiation have not been determined but may similarly contribute to stem-cell loss in other aging organ systems.

▶ The authors describe a previously unknown pathophysiologic mechanism for hair graying involving loss of melanocyte stem cells. This leads to physiologic hair graying related to loss of their differentiated progeny with aging. Acceleration of this process appears to be genetically determined. Can gene therapy for graying hair be far behind?

B. H. Thiers, MD

Distinguishing Androgenetic Alopecia From Chronic Telogen Effluvium When Associated in the Same Patient: A Simple Noninvasive Method

Rebora A, Guarrera M, Baldari M, et al (Univ of Genoa, Italy)
Arch Dermatol 141:1243-1245, 2005   7–16

Background.—Distinguishing chronic telogen effluvium (CTE) from androgenetic alopecia (AGA) may be difficult especially when associated in the same patient.

Observations.—One hundred consecutive patients with hair loss were clinically diagnosed as having CTE, AGA, AGA + CTE, or remitting CTE. Patients washed their hair in the sink in a standardized way. All shed hairs were counted and divided "blindly" into 5 cm or longer, intermediate length (>3 to <5 cm), and 3 cm or shorter. The latter were considered telogen vellus hairs, and patients having at least 10% of them were classified as having

AGA. We assumed that patients shedding 200 hairs or more had CTE. The κ statistic revealed, however, that the best concordance between clinical and numerical diagnosis (κ = 0.527) was obtained by setting the cutoff shedding value at 100 hairs or more. Of the 100 patients, 18 with 10% or more of hairs that were 3 cm or shorter and who shed fewer than 100 hairs were diagnosed as having AGA; 34 with fewer than 10% of hairs that were 3 cm or shorter and who shed at least 100 hairs were diagnosed as having CTE; 34 with 10% or more of hairs that were 3 cm or shorter and who shed at least 100 hairs were diagnosed as having AGA + CTE; and 14 with fewer than 10% of hairs that were 3 cm or shorter and who shed fewer than 100 hairs were diagnosed as having CTE in remission.

Conclusion.—This method is simple, noninvasive, and suitable for office evaluation.

▶ This is an interesting observation of uncertain utility. Is this more useful as a classification scheme or as a diagnostic tool? In any case, who among us has the time to count and measure hairs in the context of a busy practice?

B. H. Thiers, MD

A Comparison of Vertical Versus Transverse Sections in the Evaluation of Alopecia Biopsy Specimens

Elston DM, Ferringer T, Dalton S, et al (Geisinger Med Ctr, Danville, Pa; Brooke Army Med Ctr, San Antonio, Tex)
J Am Acad Dermatol 53:267-272, 2005   7–17

Background.—Both vertical and transverse sections are used in the histologic interpretation of alopecia biopsy specimens. Although a combination of the two may be optimal, the pathologist is frequently only provided with a single specimen. Even though the trend in recent years has been toward transverse sections in this setting, we are not aware of any published data directly comparing the two methods.

Methods.—One hundred two consecutive archived hair biopsy accessions that demonstrated comparable vertical and transverse sections were examined twice, each time in a random order. The pathologist's interpretation based only on the vertical sections and an interpretation based only on the transverse sections were compared with the original biopsy report, which had been based on the combination of vertical and transverse sections.

Results.—In 76 cases, all 3 diagnoses were concordant (ie, the diagnosis made with vertical sections alone, the diagnosis made with transverse sections alone, and the original diagnosis were all in agreement). In 2 cases, neither the diagnosis made with vertical sections alone nor the diagnosis made with transverse sections alone were in full agreement with the original diagnosis. In 20 cases, only the diagnosis made with vertical sections was concordant with the original diagnosis. In 4 cases, only the diagnosis made with transverse sections alone was concordant with the original diagnosis.

Limitations.—Our practice is heavily weighted toward scarring alopecia, and the results of our study may not be applicable to practices weighted toward other forms of alopecia. Because the cases had been signed out over a period of several years, the nomenclature for some entities changed. For the purposes of our study, we counted the diagnoses of follicular degeneration syndrome and idiopathic pseudopelade to be subtypes of (and concordant with) a diagnosis of central centrifugal cicatricial alopecia. In some cases, a definitive diagnosis was not possible at the time of the original diagnosis, but rather the pathologist had provided a histologic description and a differential diagnosis. For purposes of this study, an interpretation was considered to be concordant with the original descriptive diagnosis if all of the important histologic features were identified that had been described in the original report. Sampling error could have contributed to discordant diagnoses, but would be expected to affect both vertical and transverse samples in a random manner.

Conclusion.—The combination of vertical and transverse sections is superior to either alone. Although transverse sections have revolutionized the evaluation of alopecia, in this study, the diagnosis made with vertical sections alone had a higher concordance rate with the combination than did transverse sections alone. As there are advantages and disadvantages inherent in either method, when only a single biopsy specimen is submitted, it may be sectioned either vertically or transversely, at the discretion of the pathologist. With either method, serial step sections should be obtained to reduce the risk of missing important histologic findings.

▶ The value of transverse sections in the evaluation of alopecia biopsy specimens has been emphasized in recent years. More follicles can be evaluated, and the relative sizes of follicles at any level of the dermis or subcutaneous tissue can be assessed, as can the relative size of the sebaceous glands compared with the hair follicles. The proportions of anagen, telogen, and catagen follicles can be more accurately assessed than in vertical sections. The major disadvantage of this technique is the inability in some instances to assess changes in the epidermis, as may occur in lupus erythematosus. It is, therefore, surprising that these authors found that the results from vertical sections had a higher rate of concordance with the original biopsy report, which had been based on a combination of vertical and transverse sections. In the cases that were not concordant, the critical diagnostic features that were missed with transverse sections were, as would be expected, in the epidermis, at the dermal-epidermal junction, or in the superficial dermis. Since these areas are not sometimes well represented in the transverse sections, the ideal situation is that the clinician would submit two biopsy specimens so that one may be sectioned vertically and the other transversely. It is important that the biopsy specimens extend through the adipose tissue. A 4-mm punch specimen when cut in cross section has almost 75% more area than a 3-mm punch specimen. Therefore, many more hair follicles can be evaluated with no increased risk or discomfort to the patient. If only one specimen is submitted, then it should be sectioned transversely if the physician suspects a nonscarring alopecia. If the physician suspects a scarring alopecia then sectioning in the vertical plane may be more informative because the epidermis and superficial dermis will be present in the histologic sections.

J. C. Maize, MD

Value of Direct Immunofluorescence for Differential Diagnosis of Cicatricial Alopecia

Trachsler S, Trüeb RM (Univ Hosp of Zurich, Switzerland)
Dermatology 211:98-102, 2005   7–18

Background.—There are diverse causes of cicatricial alopecia characterized by lack of follicular ostia and irreversible loss of hair. While clinical differentiation between the causes may be difficult, particularly with regard to lichen planus (LP), lupus erythematosus (LE) and pseudopelade of Brocq (PB), it has been suggested that both histopathologic examination and direct immunofluorescence studies (DIF) are necessary for an accurate diagnosis.

Objective.—The aim of this study was to evaluate the diagnostic value of DIF studies in addition to histopathology in patients with cicatricial alopecia as a clinical feature.

Methods.—136 scalp biopsy specimens received for histopathology and DIF during a 5-year period were reviewed.

Results.—Definitive diagnosis was achieved by careful evaluation of scalp biopsies. The most prevalent diagnoses in order of frequency were LP (26%), LE (21%) and folliculitis decalvans (20%). PB was diagnosed in 10%. In most cases, the diagnosis could be made on the basis of histopathology and independently of DIF. Characteristic DIF patterns showed high specificity, but low sensitivity for LP, and high specificity and sensitivity for LE. The DIF pattern in PB showed no difference to LP.

Conclusions.—Histopathology permits diagnosis in the majority of cicatricial alopecias. DIF is of value in histopathologically inconclusive cases, particularly when LE is in question.

▶ The differential diagnosis of cicatricial alopecia is often a challenge to the clinician and to the dermatopathologist. The clinician may wonder whether DIF examination of a biopsy specimen in addition to clinical examination and histopathologic analysis would be helpful in the differential diagnosis of scarring alopecia. The authors of this study found that in 126 (93%) of 136 biopsy specimens, a definitive diagnosis of the cause of the scarring alopecia could be made on the basis of histopathology and DIF examination. However, on the basis of histopathology alone and independent of DIF examination, an accurate diagnosis could be made in 97% of diagnosed cases. Therefore, DIF examination made a difference in only 3% of cases. Routine DIF examination does not seem to be cost effective. In specific instances, DIF examination may be helpful, especially in determining whether the alopecia may be caused by LE.

J. C. Maize, MD

Placebo-controlled Oral Pulse Prednisolone Therapy in Alopecia Areata

Kar BR, Handa S, Dogra S, et al (Postgraduate Inst of Med Education and Research, Chandigarh, India)
J Am Acad Dermatol 52:287-290, 2005   7–19

Background.—Systemic corticosteroids administered as pulse therapy have been found helpful in a wide array of diseases including alopecia areata (AA). None of the studies published so far regarding their use in AA have been randomized or placebo-controlled.

Objective.—We sought to compare the efficacy of weekly oral prednisolone pulse therapy in a placebo-controlled trial for patients with extensive AA.

Methods.—A total of 43 patients were randomly divided into two groups. Patients in group A (23 patients) were treated with oral prednisolone (200 mg once weekly, 5 40-mg tablets) and patients in group B (20 patients) were given placebo tablets on an identical schedule. The total study period was 6 months, consisting of 3 months of active therapy followed by another 3 months of observation.

Results.—Significant hair regrowth was obtained in 8 patients in the prednisolone-treated group. Two of the responders experienced a relapse during the observation period of 3 months. In the placebo group, none of the patients had significant hair regrowth at the end of the study.

Conclusion.—Oral prednisolone pulse therapy is useful in AA. Placebo-controlled studies with varying dosage schedules are required to standardize the dose of prednisolone used in pulse therapy, optimize the therapeutic efficacy, and minimize side effects.

▶ Other than demonstrating the well-known fact that systemic steroids are beneficial in AA, the significance of this study is uncertain. The usual prognostic factors for a favorable response were noted (first episode of the disease and disease of less than 2 years' duration) as were the indicators of a poor response (atopy, nail involvement, multiple episodes, and prolonged duration of disease). Common steroid-related side effects were seen in more than half the patients in the group treated with systemic steroids.

B. H. Thiers, MD

Modern External Beam Radiation Therapy for Refractory Dissecting Cellulitis of the Scalp

Chinnaiyan P, Tena LB, Brenner MJ, et al (Univ of Wisconsin, Madison; New York Med College; Sinai Hosp, Baltimore, Md)
Br J Dermatol 152:777-779, 2005   7–20

Background.—Dissecting cellulitis of the scalp can be an extremely painful and disfiguring dermatological condition. The associated pain can be severe enough in some cases to require opioid analgesics, and this pain in conjunction with the disfigurement can induce significant emotional distress.

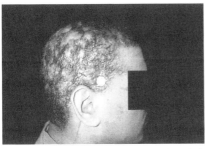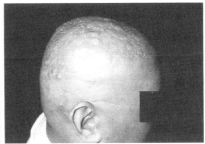

FIGURE 1.—Photographs showing scalp (**a**) before and (**b**) 3 months after treatment. After treatment, nodules diminished in size, and seropurulent discharge entirely ceased. The use of opioid analgesics (oxycodone 10 mg/acetaminophen 1000 mg tablets every 4 hours) was discontinued posttherapy. During radiotherapy, the patient experienced a slight increase in seropurulent discharge, mild erythema, and xeroderma. No long-term sequelae have developed. (Courtesy of Chinnaiyan P, Tena LB, Brenner MJ, et al: Modern external beam radiation therapy for refractory dissecting cellulites of the scalp. *Br J Dermatol* 152:777-779, 2005. Reprinted by permission of Blackwell Publishing.)

Conservative treatments often fail to provide relief. Radiation therapy has been successfully used in the past but with outdated equipment and techniques.

Objectives.—To evaluate the efficacy and toxicity of modern external beam radiation therapy techniques for the treatment of dissecting cellulitis of the scalp.

Methods.—Four patients with intractable dissecting cellulitis of the scalp were treated with electrons or a combination of electrons and photons to the entire scalp. Daily fraction sizes were 2.5 or 3 Gy and initially prescribed to 15-21 Gy. Patients were re-evaluated 3-4 weeks after completion of therapy. Any residual hair growth was treated with additional radiation treatments to ensure full epilation, up to a maximum dose of 35 Gy.

Results.—Rapid resolution of pain was seen in all patients with pain. Regression of nodules and decreased discharge was seen in all patients following treatment and cosmesis was subjectively improved. No long-term toxicity has been observed.

Conclusions.—Using modern techniques and equipment, radiation therapy appears to be a reasonable option for patients with severe/refractory dissecting cellulitis of the scalp. Acute effects are mild and well tolerated. Aside from alopecia, which was present to some extent in all patients before treatment, no long-term complications have been observed (Fig 1; see color plate X).

▶ Dissecting cellulitis of the scalp can be a disabling, life-altering condition. Although some degree of alopecia can be expected (either from the condition or its treatment), radiotherapy appears to be a reasonable option for patients with otherwise unresponsive conditions.

B. H. Thiers, MD

8 Pigmentary Disorders

Increased Prevalence of Chronic Autoimmune (Hashimoto's) Thyroiditis in Children and Adolescents With Vitiligo
Kakourou T, Kanaka-Gantenbein C, Papadopoulou A, et al (Athens Univ, Greece)
J Am Acad Dermatol 53:220-223, 2005   8–1

Background.—An increased prevalence of autoimmune (Hashimoto's) thyroiditis in adult patients with vitiligo has been described. This association has scarcely been studied in children.

Objective.—We sought to assess children and adolescents with vitiligo for autoimmune thyroid disorder and to identify any predisposing factors of this association.

Methods.—In all, 54 children and adolescents (23 boys, 31 girls; mean age 11.4 years) with known vitiligo were studied by physical examination and laboratory studies.

Results.—Four patients with vitiligo were already known to have Hashimoto's thyroiditis. In 9 of the remaining 50 patients, autoimmune thyroiditis was revealed at the time of the investigation. Of the 54 patients with vitiligo, 13 (24.1%) had autoimmune thyroiditis as compared with 9.6% of school-aged children from an iodine-replete area of Greece ($P = .002$). There was no association between thyroiditis and clinical type of vitiligo, age at onset, mean duration of vitiligo, or sex.

Conclusions.—Hashimoto's thyroiditis is 2.5 times more frequent among children and adolescents with vitiligo than in a healthy age- and sex-matched population. It usually follows the onset of vitiligo. We propose that children and adolescents with vitiligo should be screened annually for thyroid dysfunction, particularly autoimmune thyroiditis.

▶ In this study from an iodine-replete area of Greece, the authors noted a 2.5 times increase in the incidence of Hashimoto's thyroiditis among children and adolescents with vitiligo as compared with controls. Since the thyroiditis usually appeared after the vitiligo, monitoring thyroid function on an annual basis, as suggested by these authors, seems quite reasonable.

S. Raimer, MD

Useful Treatment of Vitiligo in 10 Children With UV-B Narrowband (311 nm)

Brazzelli V, Prestinari F, Castello M, et al (Univ of Pavia, Italy)
Pediatr Dermatol 22:257-261, 2005

8–2

Introduction.—We report our experience with UV-B narrowband (UV-B–NB) therapy in children affected by vitiligo. We studied 10 Caucasian Italian children (six boys, four girls, mean age 9.7 years ± 2.67). Treatment mean term was 5.6 months; frequency was three times a week on nonconsecutive days or only twice a week, because of school or family duties. The percentage of repigmentation was evaluated by comparing photographs taken before, during, and after the treatment, and showed a repigmentation level higher than 75% in five patients (5/10, 50%) and between 26% and 75% in three patients (3/10, 30%). Of our patients, 80% had a satisfactory response to phototherapy. Adverse events were limited and transient. No significant relationships between repigmentation grades and variables such as skin type, positive family history, and disease extension were observed. Some areas responded better than others; the best results were shown on the face and neck. Perhaps we studied too few patients to be conclusive, but the results obtained so far seem to indicate that children affected by recent vitiligo have a better response to the therapy. We feel that UV-B–NB therapy is a valuable and safe option for the treatment of pediatric vitiligo, and should be started as soon as possible.

▶ Although this is a very small study, it does suggest that UV-B–NB therapy is an effective treatment modality for children with vitiligo who are capable of standing still in a light box. The face and neck, areas that are generally the most cosmetically important for patients, respond best. Application of a midstrength topical corticosteroid to the vitiliginous skin might further potentiate the beneficial effects of UV-B–NB therapy.

S. Raimer, MD

9 Collagen Vascular and Related Disorders

Combined Oral Contraceptives in Women With Systemic Lupus Erythematosus

Petri M, for the OC-SELENA Trial (Johns Hopkins Univ, Baltimore, Md; et al)

N Engl J Med 353:2550-2558, 2005   9–1

Background.—Oral contraceptives are rarely prescribed for women with systemic lupus erythematosus, because of concern about potential negative side effects. In this double-blind, randomized, noninferiority trial, we prospectively evaluated the effect of oral contraceptives on lupus activity in premenopausal women with systemic lupus erythematosus.

Methods.—A total of 183 women with inactive (76 percent) or stable active (24 percent) systemic lupus erythematosus at 15 U.S. sites were randomly assigned to receive either oral contraceptives (triphasic ethinyl estradiol at a dose of 35 μg plus norethindrone at a dose of 0.5 to 1 mg for 12 cycles of 28 days each; 91 women) or placebo (92 women) and were evaluated at months 1, 2, 3, 6, 9, and 12. Subjects were excluded if they had moderate or high levels of anticardiolipin antibodies, lupus anticoagulant, or a history of thrombosis.

Results.—The primary end point, a severe lupus flare, occurred in 7 of 91 subjects receiving oral contraceptives (7.7 percent) as compared with 7 of 92 subjects receiving placebo (7.6 percent). The 12-month rates of severe flare were similar: 0.084 for the group receiving oral contraceptives and 0.087 for the placebo group ($P=0.95$; upper limit of the one-sided 95 percent confidence interval for this difference, 0.069, which is within the prespecified 9 percent margin for noninferiority). Rates of mild or moderate flares were 1.40 flares per person-year for subjects receiving oral contraceptives and 1.44 flares per person-year for subjects receiving placebo (relative risk, 0.98; $P=0.86$). In the group that was randomized to receive oral contraceptives, there was one deep venous thrombosis and one clotted graft; in the placebo group, there was one deep venous thrombosis, one ocular thrombosis, one superficial thrombophlebitis, and one death (after cessation of the trial).

Conclusions.—Our study indicates that oral contraceptives do not increase the risk of flare among women with systemic lupus erythematosus whose disease is stable.

A Trial of Contraceptive Methods in Women With Systemic Lupus Erythematosus

Sánchez-Guerrero J, Uribe AG, Jiménez-Santana L, et al (Instituto Nacional de Ciencias Médicas y Nutrición Salvador Zubirán, Mexico City; World Health Organization, Geneva)

N Engl J Med 353:2539-2549, 2005   9–2

Background.—The effects of estrogen-containing contraceptives on disease activity in women with systemic lupus erythematosus have not been determined.

Methods.—We conducted a single-blind clinical trial involving 162 women with systemic lupus erythematosus who were randomly assigned to combined oral contraceptives, a progestin-only pill, or a copper intrauterine device (IUD). Disease activity was assessed at 0, 1, 2, 3, 6, 9, and 12 months according to the Systemic Lupus Erythematosus Disease Activity Index (SLEDAI). The primary outcome was global disease activity, which we estimated by measuring the area under the SLEDAI curve. Secondary outcomes included the maximum SLEDAI score, change in SLEDAI score, incidence of lupus flares, median time to first flare, systemic lupus erythematosus treatment, and adverse events. The results were analyzed by the intention-to-treat method.

Results.—At baseline, all demographic features and disease characteristics were similar in the three groups. The mean (±SD) SLEDAI score was 6.1±5.6 in the group assigned to combined oral contraceptives, 6.4±4.6 in the group assigned to the progestin-only pill, and 5.0±5.3 in the group assigned to the IUD (54 patients in each group) (P−0.36). Disease activity remained mild and stable in all groups throughout the trial. There were no significant differences among the groups during the trial in global or maximum disease activity, incidence or probability of flares, or medication use. The median time to the first flare was three months in all groups. Thromboses occurred in four patients (two in each of the two groups receiving hormones), and severe infections were more frequent in the IUD group. One patient receiving combined oral contraceptives died from amoxicillin-related severe neutropenia.

Conclusions.—Global disease activity, maximum SLEDAI score, incidence of flares, time to first flare, and incidence of adverse events were similar among women with systemic lupus erythematosus, irrespective of the type of contraceptive they were using.

▶ Circumstantial data suggest a role for estrogen in the pathogenesis of systemic lupus erythematosus. This includes the high prevalence of the disease (9:1) in women of childbearing age compared with men, presentation of the disease after menarche and before menopause, reported flares of the disease in women receiving exogenous hormone therapy, and exacerbation of lupus in mice by the administration of estrogen. For these and other reasons, many clinicians are reluctant to prescribe oral contraceptives to women with systemic lupus erythematosus. The articles by Petri et al (Abstract 9–1) and Sánchez-

Guerrero et al (Abstract 9–2) provide data to support the use of oral contraceptives in patients with the disease, although neither report addresses their use in women with severe active lupus erythematosus. Thus, it remains uncertain whether combined oral contraceptives can be used safely in this subgroup of the disease. In addition, thrombotic events were noted in both trials, suggesting that patients with lupus should be tested for the presence of antiphospholipid antibodies before oral contraceptives are started, and that these agents should probably be avoided among those who are positive or who manifest other hypercoagulable states.[1]

B. H. Thiers, MD

Reference

1. Bermas BL: Oral contraceptives in systemic lupus erythematosus: A tough pill to swallow? *N Engl J Med* 353:2602-2604, 2005.

The Effect of Combined Estrogen and Progesterone Hormone Replacement Therapy on Disease Activity in Systemic Lupus Erythematosus: A Randomized Trial

Buyon JP, Petri MA, Kim MY, et al (New York Univ; Johns Hopkins Univ, Baltimore, Md)
Ann Intern Med 142:953-962, 2005
9–3

Background.—There is concern that exogenous female hormones may worsen disease activity in women with systemic lupus erythematosus (SLE).

Objective.—To evaluate the effect of hormone replacement therapy (HRT) on disease activity in postmenopausal women with SLE.

Design.—Randomized, double-blind, placebo-controlled noninferiority trial conducted from March 1996 to June 2002.

Setting.—16 university-affiliated rheumatology clinics or practices in 11 U.S. states.

Patients.—351 menopausal patients (mean age, 50 years) with inactive (81.5%) or stable-active (18.5%) SLE.

Interventions.—12 months of treatment with active drug (0.625 mg of conjugated estrogen daily, plus 5 mg of medroxyprogesterone for 12 days per month) or placebo. The 12-month follow-up rate was 82% for the HRT group and 87% for the placebo group.

Measurements.—The primary end point was occurrence of a severe flare as defined by Safety of Estrogens in Lupus Erythematosus, National Assessment-Systemic Lupus Erythematosus Disease Activity Index composite.

Results.—Severe flare was rare in both treatment groups: The 12-month severe flare rate was 0.081 for the HRT group and 0.049 for the placebo group, yielding an estimated difference of 0.033 ($P = 0.23$). The upper limit of the 1-sided 95% CI for the treatment difference was 0.078, within the pre-specified margin of 9% for noninferiority. Mild to moderate flares were significantly increased in the HRT group: 1.14 flares/person-year for HRT and

0.86 flare/person-year for placebo (relative risk, 1.34; $P = 0.01$). The probability of any type of flare by 12 months was 0.64 for the HRT group and 0.51 for the placebo group ($P = 0.01$). In the HRT group, there were 1 death, 1 stroke, 2 cases of deep venous thrombosis, and 1 case of thrombosis in an arteriovenous graft; in the placebo group, 1 patient developed deep venous thrombosis.

Limitations.—Findings are not generalizable to women with high-titer anticardiolipin antibodies, lupus anticoagulant, or previous thrombosis.

Conclusions.—Adding a short course of HRT is associated with a small risk for increasing the natural flare rate of lupus. Most of these flares are mild to moderate. The benefits of HRT can be balanced against the risk for flare because HRT did not significantly increase the risk for severe flare compared with placebo.

▶ The authors provide valuable information to help menopausal women balance the risks versus the benefits of HRT. Despite the overall favorable findings, certain women with special disease characteristics might well avoid HRT. For example, patients with active SLE and those with renal disease had a greater chance of a flare than those with inactive disease. Thus, the risk-to-benefit ratio of HRT appears to vary with the severity and the activity of the underlying lupus.[1]

B. H. Thiers, MD

Reference

1. Hess EV: Help for menopausal patients with lupus? *Ann Intern Med* 142:1014-1015, 2005.

Ultraviolet Radiation–Induced Injury, Chemokines, and Leukocyte Recruitment: An Amplification Cycle Triggering Cutaneous Lupus Erythematosus
Meller S, Winterberg F, Gilliet M, et al (Heinrich-Heine Univ, Dusseldorf, Germany; Univ of Zurich, Switzerland; Dynavax Technologies, Berkeley, Calif; et al)
Arthritis Rheum 52:1504-1516, 2005   9–4

Objective.—To investigate the activation and recruitment pathways of relevant leukocyte subsets during the initiation and amplification of cutaneous lupus erythematosus (LE).

Methods.—Quantitative real-time polymerase chain reaction was used to perform a comprehensive analysis of all known chemokines and their receptors in cutaneous LE lesions, and the cellular origin of these chemokines and receptors was determined using immunohistochemistry. Furthermore, cytokine- and ultraviolet (UV) light-mediated activation pathways of relevant chemokines were investigated in vitro and in vivo.

Results.—In the present study, we identified the CXCR3 ligands CXCL9 (interferon-γ [IFNγ]-induced monokine), CXCL10 (IFNγ-inducible protein

10), and CXCL11 (IFN-inducible T cell α chemoattractant) as being the most abundantly expressed chemokine family members in cutaneous LE. Expression of these ligands corresponded with the presence of a marked inflammatory infiltrate consisting of mainly CXCR3-expressing cells, including skin-homing lymphocytes and blood dendritic cell antigen 2-positive plasmacytoid dendritic cells (PDCs). Within cutaneous LE lesions, PDCs accumulated within the dermis and were activated to produce type I IFN, as detected by the expression of the IFNα-inducible genes IRF7 and MxA. IFNα, in turn, was a potent and rapid inducer of CXCR3 ligands in cellular constituents of the skin. Furthermore, we demonstrated that the inflammatory CXCR3 ligands cooperate with the homeostatic chemokine CXCL12 (stromal cell-derived factor 1) during the recruitment of pathogenically relevant leukocyte subsets. Moreover, we showed that UVB irradiation induces the release of CCL27 (cutaneous T cell-attracting chemokine) from epidermal compartments into dermal compartments and up-regulates the expression of a distinct set of chemokines in keratinocytes.

Conclusion.—Taken together, our data suggest an amplification cycle in which UV light-induced injury induces apoptosis, necrosis, and chemokine production. These mechanisms, in turn, mediate the recruitment and activation of autoimmune T cells and IFNα-producing PDCs, which subsequently release more effector cytokines, thus amplifying chemokine production and leukocyte recruitment, finally leading to the development of a cutaneous LE phenotype.

▶ The authors offer a theory to explain the link between UV radiation-induced injury and the development of cutaneous LE. If correct, the immunopathogenic mechanism described offers a series of new molecular targets to treat this condition. For example, a small-molecule antagonist against CXCR3 is currently in the process of clinical development, and other small-molecule antagonists or neutralizing biologicals against chemokines and their receptors will likely follow.

B. H. Thiers, MD

Thalidomide for the Treatment of Resistant Cutaneous Lupus: Efficacy and Safety of Different Therapeutic Regimens
Cuadrado MJ, Karim Y, Sanna G, et al (Rayne Inst, London)
Am J Med 118:246-250, 2005   9–5

Purpose.—Thalidomide is effective for the treatment of severe cutaneous lupus. Our aim was to study the safety and efficacy of different doses of thalidomide in this condition.

Methods.—We studied patients with severe cutaneous lupus that was unresponsive to antimalarials, prednisolone, methotrexate, azathioprine, and cyclosporin A. Starting doses of 100 mg daily (n = 16 patients), 50 mg daily (n = 17), or 50 mg on alternate days (n = 15) were compared. The response to thalidomide was categorized as complete remission, partial remission, or no visible improvement. All patients received a baseline electromyogram (EMG) followed by repeat EMG every 3 to 6 months, or sooner if neuropathic symptoms developed.

Results.—Forty-eight patients (46 female; mean [± SD] age, 44 ± 12 years; range, 22 to 71 years) with discoid lupus (n = 18), subacute cutaneous lupus (n = 6), or systemic lupus erythematosus with skin involvement (n = 24) were included. The response rate was 81%, including 29 patients (60%) in complete remission and 10 (21%) in partial remission. Nine patients (19%) failed to respond. Thirteen patients (27%) developed peripheral neuropathy, which was EMG-proven in 11, including 4 patients in the 50-mg alternate-day group. Other side effects included drowsiness, constipation or abdominal pain, and amenorrhea. The relapse rate after stopping thalidomide was 67% (26/39). There was no association between a positive response to the drug and either starting doses or cumulative dose. Similarly, no association was found between peripheral neuropathy and the starting or cumulative dose.

Conclusion.—Thalidomide is effective for the treatment of severe cutaneous lupus. There were no clear dose-dependent effects. However, the high incidence of neurotoxicity, even at low doses, suggests that it may be most useful as a remission-inducing drug.

▶ Despite its efficacy, the use of thalidomide was associated with a high rate of neurotoxicity and a high incidence of relapse. Thus, it is probably best used to induce remission in treatment-resistant cases with subsequent transition to an alternative maintenance agent.

B. H. Thiers, MD

Mycophenolate Mofetil or Intravenous Cyclophosphamide for Lupus Nephritis

Ginzler EM, Dooley MA, Aranow C, et al (State Univ of New York, Brooklyn; Univ of North Carolina, Chapel Hill; Albert Einstein College of Medicine, Bronx, NY; et al)
N Engl J Med 353:2219-2228, 2005   9–6

Background.—Since anecdotal series and small, prospective, controlled trials suggest that mycophenolate mofetil may be effective for treating lupus nephritis, larger trials are desirable.

Methods.—We conducted a 24-week randomized, open-label, noninferiority trial comparing oral mycophenolate mofetil (initial dose, 1000 mg per day, increased to 3000 mg per day) with monthly intravenous cyclophosphamide (0.5 g per square meter of body-surface area, increased to 1.0 g per square meter) as induction therapy for active lupus nephritis. A change to the alternative regimen was allowed at 12 weeks in patients who did not have an early response. The study protocol specified adjunctive care and the use and tapering of corticosteroids. The primary end point was complete remission at 24 weeks (normalization of abnormal renal measurements and maintenance of baseline normal measurements). A secondary end point was partial remission at 24 weeks.

Results.—Of 140 patients recruited, 71 were randomly assigned to receive mycophenolate mofetil and 69 were randomly assigned to receive cyclophosphamide. At 12 weeks, 56 patients receiving mycophenolate mofetil and 42 receiving cyclophosphamide had satisfactory early responses. In the intention-to-treat analysis, 16 of the 71 patients (22.5 percent) receiving mycophenolate mofetil and 4 of the 69 patients receiving cyclophosphamide (5.8 percent) had complete remission, for an absolute difference of 16.7 percentage points (95 percent confidence interval, 5.6 to 27.9 percentage points; P=0.005), meeting the prespecified criteria for noninferiority and demonstrating the superiority of mycophenolate mofetil to cyclophosphamide. Partial remission occurred in 21 of the 71 patients (29.6 percent) and 17 of the 69 patients (24.6 percent), respectively (P=0.51). Three patients assigned to cyclophosphamide died, two during protocol therapy. Fewer severe infections and hospitalizations but more diarrhea occurred among those receiving mycophenolate.

Conclusions.—In this 24-week trial, mycophenolate mofetil was more effective than intravenous cyclophosphamide in inducing remission of lupus nephritis and had a more favorable safety profile.

▶ In this study, significantly more complete remissions occurred in the mycophenolate mofetil group than in patients treated with IV cyclophosphamide. However, more than half of the patients either did not complete the study or did not achieve remission, according to the rigorous criteria used by the authors. Nevertheless, the reduced toxicity profile of mycophenolate mofetil compared with cyclophosphamide makes it a welcome treatment option for patients with lupus nephritis.[1]

B. H. Thiers, MD

Reference

1. McCune WJ: Mycophenolate mofetil for lupus nephritis. *N Engl J Med* 353:2282-2284, 2005.

Improvement in Digital Flexibility and Dexterity Following Ingestion of Sildenafil Citrate (Viagra) in Limited Systemic Sclerosis

Yung A, Reay N, Goodfield MD (Leeds Gen Infirmary, England)
Arch Dermatol 141:831-833, 2005   9–7

Background.—Systemic sclerosis (scleroderma) can be of the limited or diffuse cutaneous type. Some differences are notable between these types, but in both varieties Raynaud phenomenon is present, along with involvement of peripheral skin areas. Slowly progressive sclerodactyly occurs, and the skin over the fingers thickens. The fingers eventually lose dexterity, and fixed flexion deformities develop. The "prayer sign" is seen when both hands are held in opposition. A case of sclerodactyly of all the digits was reported that showed some response to sildenafil citrate, a guanosine monophosphate–specific phosphodiesterase type 5 inhibitor developed to treat erectile dysfunction.

> *Case Report.*—Man, 66, had limited systemic sclerosis and discoid lupus erythematosus–induced scarring alpecia over a period of 20 years. In addition, he reported erectile dysfunction lasting a comparable length of time. When he held his palms against one another with maximum extension of the small hand joints, he exhibited a prayer sign. He had sclerodactyly of all his fingers, with fixed flexion deformities of the small hand joints. He could not clench his fist tightly enough to eliminate all spaces between the fingers. He also had a limited mouth opening distance. He was taking hydroxychloroquine 200 mg daily, omeprazole 20 mg daily, 2% ketoconazole shampoo, clobetasol propionate as needed, and 2 annual prostacycline infusions during the winter. The erectile dysfunction had responded to the intermittent use of sildenafil citrate over a period of 5 years. In addition to the expected adverse effects of sildenafil of flushing and headache, the patient reported less frequent Raynaud phenomenon and improved finger function and flexibility beginning about 2 hours after taking the drug. The effects lasted for up to 3 days after each dose of sildenafil. This relationship was evaluated by giving him 50 mg of sildenafil citrate, then examining him 12 hours later. He was able to clench his fist without spaces between the fingers, and his mouth opening distance increased. These effects disappeared after 3 days.

Conclusions.—Further studies are needed to confirm the possible role of 5-phosphodiesterase inhibitors in treating Raynaud phenomenon and improving digital dexterity for patients with sclerodactyly. Women would not have the side effect of penile erection and may benefit particularly from this treatment. The dose-response relationship between these agents and improved function was not addressed, and the effects lasted only 3 days.

Sildenafil in the Treatment of Raynaud's Phenomenon Resistant to Vasodilatory Therapy

Fries R, Shariat K, von Wilmowsky H, et al (Universitätsklinikum des Saarlandes, Homburg/Saar, Germany; Knappschaftskrankenhaus, Püttlingen, Germany)
Circulation 112:2980-2985, 2005   9–8

Background.—Vasodilatory therapy of Raynaud's phenomenon represents a difficult clinical problem because treatment often remains inefficient and may be not tolerated because of side effects.

Method and Results.—To investigate the effects of sildenafil on symptoms and capillary perfusion in patients with Raynaud's phenomenon, we performed a double-blinded, placebo-controlled, fixed-dose, crossover study in 16 patients with symptomatic secondary Raynaud's phenomenon resistant to vasodilatory therapy. Patients were treated with 50 mg sildenafil or placebo twice daily for 4 weeks. Symptoms were assessed by diary cards including a 10-point Raynaud's Condition Score. Capillary flow velocity was measured in digital nailfold capillaries by means of a laser Doppler anemometer. While taking sildenafil, the mean frequency of Raynaud attacks was significantly lower (35 ± 14 versus 52 ± 18, $P=0.0064$), the cumulative attack duration was significantly shorter (581 ± 133 versus 1046 ± 245 minutes, $P=0.0038$), and the mean Raynaud's Condition Score was significantly lower (2.2 ± 0.4 versus 3.0 ± 0.5, $P=0.0386$). Capillary blood flow velocity increased in each individual patient, and the mean capillary flow velocity of all patients more than quadrupled after treatment with sildenafil (0.53 ± 0.09 versus 0.13 ± 0.02 mm/s, $P=0.0004$). Two patients reported side effects leading to discontinuation of the study drug.

Conclusions.—Sildenafil is an effective and well-tolerated treatment in patients with Raynaud's phenomenon.

▶ In patients with secondary Raynaud's phenomenon resistant to vasodilator therapy, sildenafil may be a reasonable therapeutic option. Clearly, the drug is not FDA-approved for that indication.

B. H. Thiers, MD

Pulsed High-Dose Corticosteroids Combined With Low-Dose Methotrexate in Severe Localized Scleroderma

Kreuter A, Gambichler T, Breuckmann F, et al (Ruhr-Univ Bochum, Germany)
Arch Dermatol 141:847-852, 2005   9–9

Objective.—To evaluate the efficacy of pulsed high-dose corticosteroids combined with orally administered low-dose methotrexate therapy in patients with severe localized scleroderma (LS).

Design.—A prospective, nonrandomized, open pilot study.

Setting.—Dermatology department at a university hospital in Bochum, Germany.

Patients.—Fifteen patients with histologically confirmed severe LS.

Interventions.—Oral methotrexate (15 mg/wk) combined with pulsed intravenous methylprednisolone (1000 mg for 3 days monthly) for at least 6 months.

Main Outcome Measures.—Treatment outcome was evaluated by means of a clinical score, 20-MHz ultrasonography, and histopathologic analysis. Safety assessment included the monitoring of adverse effects and clinical laboratory parameters.

Results.—One patient discontinued therapy. In most of the remaining 14 patients, significant elimination of all signs of active disease (inflammation) and remarkable softening of formerly affected sclerotic skin that resulted in a decrease of the mean ± SD clinical score from 10.9 ± 5.3 at the beginning to

5.5 ± 2.5 at the end of therapy was observed ($P < .001$). Clinical improvement was confirmed by histologic and ultrasonographic assessments. No serious adverse effects were noted.

Conclusions.—These data suggest that pulsed high-dose corticosteroids combined with orally administered low-dose methotrexate therapy is beneficial and safe in the treatment of patients with LS. This treatment regimen should especially be considered for severe forms of LS in which conventional treatments have failed.

Combination Antimalarials in the Treatment of Cutaneous Dermatomyositis: A Retrospective Study

Ang GC, Werth VP (Univ of Pennsylvania, Philadelphia)
Arch Dermatol 141:855-859, 2005   9–10

Objective.—To observe whether the use of antimalarials in combination resulted in significant improvement in the cutaneous signs and symptoms of patients with dermatomyositis who did not otherwise respond to the use of single-agent antimalarial therapy.

Design.—Retrospective case series of 17 patients treated between January 1, 1991, and December 31, 2002.

Setting.—An ambulatory medical dermatology clinic in an academic center.

Patients.—Patients had adult-onset dermatomyositis with predominantly cutaneous symptoms and a follow-up period at our clinic of at least 6 months. Cases in which it was not possible to assess the effect of treatment on cutaneous symptoms were not included.

Intervention.—Treatment regimens varied and included the use of antimalarials, prednisone, methotrexate, and other medications.

Main Outcome Measures.—Physician-observed and patient-reported improvement based on erythema, pruritus, and extent of affected skin.

Results.—Seven of 17 patients experienced at least near clearance in cutaneous symptoms with the use of antimalarial therapy alone: 4 of these patients required combination therapy (hydroxychloroquine sulfate-quinacrine hydrochloride or chloroquine phosphate-quinacrine), while 3 of them responded well to antimalarial monotherapy. The median time required to reach the response milestones on the final working therapeutic regimen was 3 months (mean, 4.8 months; range, 2-14 months). Six patients did not respond significantly to any type of therapy, including nonantimalarials.

Conclusion.—Our experience suggests that a significant subgroup of patients whose skin lesions have been unresponsive to a single antimalarial benefit from combination therapy with hydroxychloroquine and quinacrine or chloroquine and quinacrine, but controlled clinical trials are warranted to assess the extent of benefit.

▶ These 2 articles (Abstracts 9–9 and 9–10) detail innovative approaches to difficult therapeutic problems encountered in patients with connective tissue diseases. It would be helpful to have larger randomized, controlled, blinded trials with standardized measures to assess therapeutic response. However, given the rarity of the diseases, this ideal might be difficult to achieve.

B. H. Thiers, MD

Mortality in Systemic Sclerosis: An International Meta-analysis of Individual Patient Data
Ioannidis JPA, Vlachoyiannopoulos PG, Haidich A-B, et al (Univ of Ioannina, Greece; Found for Research and Technology—Hellas, Ioannina, Greece; Tufts Univ, Boston; et al)
Am J Med 118:2-10, 2005   9–11

Purpose.—Studies on mortality associated with systemic sclerosis have been limited by small sample sizes. We aimed to obtain large-scale evidence on survival outcomes and predictors for this disease.

Methods.—We performed a meta-analysis of individual patient data from cohorts recruited from seven medical centers in the United States, Europe, and Japan, using standardized definitions for disease subtype and organ system involvement. The primary outcome was all-cause mortality. Standardized mortality ratios and predictors of mortality were estimated. The main analysis was based only on patients enrolled at each center within 6 months of diagnosis (incident cases).

Results.—Among 1645 incident cases, 578 deaths occurred over 11,521 person-years of follow-up. Standardized mortality ratios varied by cohort (1.5 to 7.2). In multivariate analyses that adjusted for age and sex, renal (hazard ratio [HR] = 1.9; 95% confidence interval [CI]: 1.4 to 2.5), cardiac (HR = 2.8; 95% CI: 2.1 to 3.8), and pulmonary (HR = 1.6; 95% CI: 1.3 to 2.2) involvement, and anti-topoisomerase I antibodies (HR = 1.3; 95% CI: 1.0 to 1.6), increased mortality risk. Renal, cardiac, and pulmonary involvement tended to occur together (*P* <0.001). For patients without adverse predictors for 3 years after enrollment, the subsequent risk of death was not significantly different from that for the general population in three cohorts, but was significantly increased in three cohorts that comprised mostly referred patients. Analyses that included all cases in each center (n = 3311; total follow-up: 19,990 person-years) yielded largely similar results.

Conclusion.—Systemic sclerosis confers a high mortality risk, but there is considerable heterogeneity across settings. Internal organ involvement and anti-topoisomerase I antibodies are important determinants of mortality.

▶ This heroic effort demonstrates that for clinically important but relatively uncommon diseases such as systemic sclerosis, it is possible to accumulate large-scale evidence by collating standardized information from diverse sources. The presence of anti-topoisomerase I antibodies as well as renal, cardiac, and pulmonary involvement (but not esophageal involvement) independently increased the risk of death after adjusting for age, sex, and year of enrollment. Patients who had 1 major organ involved were more likely to have another involved as well. Anticentromere antibodies, anti-U3RNP antibodies, and esophageal involvement did not adversely effect patient survival.

B. H. Thiers, MD

History of Infection Before the Onset of Juvenile Dermatomyositis: Results From the National Institute of Arthritis and Musculoskeletal and Skin Diseases Research Registry

Pachman LM, Lipton R, Ramsey-Goldman R, et al (Northwestern Univ, Chicago; Univ of Chicago; Children's Hosp of Orange County, Orange, Calif; et al)
Arthritis Rheum 53:166-172, 2005   9–12

Objective.—To obtain data concerning a history of infection occurring in the 3 months before recognition of the typical weakness and rash associated with juvenile dermatomyositis (JDM).

Methods.—Parents or caretakers of children within 6 months of JDM diagnosis were interviewed by the registry study nurse concerning their child's symptoms, environment, family background, and illness history. Physician medical records were reviewed, confirming the JDM diagnosis.

Results.—Children for which both a parent interview and physician medical records at diagnosis were available (n = 286) were included. Diagnoses were as follows: definite/probable JDM (n = 234, 82%), possible JDM (n = 43, 15%), or rash only (n = 9, 3%). The group was predominantly white (71%) and had a girl:boy ratio of 2:1. Although the mean age at onset was 6.7 years for girls and 7.3 years for boys, 25% of the children were ≤4 years old at disease onset. In the 3 months before onset, 57% of the children had respiratory complaints, 30% had gastrointestinal symptoms, and 63% of children with these symptoms of infection were given antibiotics.

Conclusion.—This study provides evidence that JDM affects young children. The symptoms of the typical rash and weakness often follow a history of respiratory or gastrointestinal complaints. These data suggest that the response to an infectious process may be implicated in JDM disease pathogenesis.

▶ It is difficult to accept the authors' conclusions without data from a comparable control group without newly diagnosed dermatomyositis.

B. H. Thiers, MD

Rituximab in the Treatment of Refractory Dermatomyositis

Chiappetta N, Steier J, Gruber B (Stony Brook Univ, New York)
J Clin Rheumatol 11:264-266, 2005   9–13

Background.—Increasingly, B cells are being identified as the cause of autoimmune disorders. B-cell–depleting therapy with rituximab has been used for various diseases, such as rheumatoid arthritis. In a case report, rituximab appeared to have usefulness for a patient with dermatomyositis.

> *Case Report.*—Man, 56, had diffuse myalgias, arthralgias, and progressive proximal muscle weakness of 3 weeks' duration. It was hard for him to raise his arms and legs or get out of bed. He also had paresthesias of both legs. The man had undergone L4-L5 laminectomy 1 month before admission. An erythematous rash was noted in a V-neck distribution on the chest and neck, and he reported fatigue. Laboratory tests showed mild normocytic anemia, creatinine kinase level of 11,321 IU/L, and transaminase levels of about 300 U/L. Erythrocyte sedimentation rate was 32 mm/h. Pulmonary function tests did not indicate pulmonary involvement, and no malignancies were detected. Muscle tests revealed an inflammatory myopathy and possible myophagocytosis.
>
> Solumedrol induced little improvement, so IV immunoglobulin was added. The patient had significant muscle weakness even when methotrexate therapy was begun. Hydroxychloroquine, azathioprine, and oral cyclophosphamide were added over the ensuing year, but his weakness progressed and creatine kinase levels increased. Infliximab was begun, but the patient developed right middle lobe pneumonia 2 weeks after receiving his third infusion, requiring 14 days of antibiotics for resolution. He was taken off all immunosuppressive agents except prednisone. Within 1 month, his creatine kinase level reached 15,084 U/L and he was confined to a wheelchair. Rituximab was then begun, with 6 weekly infusions of 210 mg, then maintenance doses of 210 mg/m² every 3 months. Flow cytometry performed 3 weeks after completing the 6 weekly infusions revealed an absolute B-lymphocyte count of 0. At this point, the patient showed increased muscle strength, resolution of the rash, ability to walk without assistance, and a creatine kinase level of 1413 U/L. After 20 months, the patient is taking 7.5 mg of prednisone daily, 25 mg of azathioprine daily, 20 mg of methotrexate weekly, and 210 mg of rituximab every 3 months. His creatine kinase level has declined to 64 U/L, and he has regained full strength in all proximal muscles except the left lower extremity.

Conclusions.—B-cell depletion therapy with rituximab was able to restore the patient's muscle strength, resolve his rash, permit unassisted ambulation, and lower his creatine kinase level. More long-term results may require the addition of a plasma cell depletion agent. Patients with autoimmune diseases that have not responded to current therapies may be managed with rituximab or other B-cell depletion therapies.

▶ This report provides circumstantial evidence that B-cell activation plays a role in the pathogenesis of dermatomyositis.

B. H. Thiers, MD

Opportunistic Infections in Polymyositis and Dermatomyositis

Marie I, Hachulla E, Chérin P, et al (Centre Hospitalier Universitaire de Rouen-Boisguillaume, France; Centre Hospitalier Universitaire de Lille, France; Groupe Hospitalier Pitié-Salpêtrière, Paris)

Arthritis Rheum 53:155-165, 2005   9–14

Objective.—To assess prevalence and characteristics of opportunistic infections in patients with polymyositis/dermatomyositis (PM/DM). To determine the predictive values for opportunistic infections on clinical presentation, biochemical findings, and paraclinical features of PM/DM to detect patients at risk of opportunistic infections.

Methods.—The medical records of 156 consecutive PM/DM patients in 3 medical centers were reviewed.

Results.—Eighteen PM/DM patients (11.5%) developed opportunistic infections. The majority of patients exhibited an opportunistic infection after the onset of PM/DM (89% of cases). Opportunistic infections occurred most frequently during the first year following PM/DM diagnosis (62.5%). The pathogen microorganisms responsible for opportunistic infections were various, i.e., *Candida albicans, Pneumocystis carinii, Aspergillus fumigatus, Geotrichum capitatum, Mycobacterium avium-intracellulare* complex, *M. xenopi, M. marinum, M. tuberculosis, Helicobacter heilmanii,* cytomegalovirus, and herpes simplex virus. Mortality rates were as high as 27.7% in these PM/DM patients. Higher mean daily doses of steroids, lymphopenia, and lower serum total protein levels were significantly more frequent in the group of PM/DM patients with opportunistic infections.

Conclusion.—Our study underscores the high frequency of opportunistic infections in PM/DM, resulting in an increased mortality rate. It also indicates that a great variety of microorganisms are responsible for opportunistic infections, although they were more often due to fungi (>50% of cases). Our series highlights a predominance of both lung and digestive opportunistic infections (89% of cases). In addition, our results suggest that PM/DM patients presenting with factors predictive of opportunistic infection may require closer monitoring.

▶ One of the more vivid memories of my dermatology residency was a young girl with juvenile DM who died of *P carinii* pneumonia, a new and presumed to be untreatable condition at the time. Clearly, opportunistic infections in patients with PM/DM are still a problem and are an expected consequence of immunosuppressive therapy. The lung and digestive system appear to be the most common targets.

B. H. Thiers, MD

Leflunomide or Methotrexate for Juvenile Rheumatoid Arthritis

Silverman E, for the Leflunomide in Juvenile Rheumatoid Arthritis (JRA) Investigator Group (Univ of Toronto; et al)

N Engl J Med 352:1655-1666, 2005

9–15

Background.—We compared the safety and efficacy of leflunomide with that of methotrexate in the treatment of polyarticular juvenile rheumatoid arthritis in a multinational, randomized, controlled trial.

Methods.—Patients 3 to 17 years of age received leflunomide or methotrexate for 16 weeks in a double-dummy, blinded fashion, followed by a 32-week blinded extension. The rates of American College of Rheumatology Pediatric 30 percent responses (ACR Pedi 30) and the Percent Improvement Index were assessed at baseline and every 4 weeks for 16 weeks and every 8 weeks during the 32-week extension study.

Results.—Of 94 patients randomized, 86 completed 16 weeks of treatment, 70 of whom entered the extension study. At week 16, more patients in the methotrexate group than in the leflunomide group had an ACR Pedi 30 response (89 percent vs. 68 percent, P=0.02), whereas the values for the Percent Improvement Index did not differ significantly (-52.87 percent vs. -44.41 percent, P=0.18). In both groups, the improvements achieved at week 16 were maintained at week 48. The most common adverse events in both groups included gastrointestinal symptoms, headache, and nasopharyngeal symptoms. Aminotransferase elevations were more frequent with methotrexate than with leflunomide during the initial study and the extension study.

Conclusions.—In patients with polyarticular juvenile rheumatoid arthritis, methotrexate and leflunomide both resulted in high rates of clinical improvement, but the rate was slightly greater for methotrexate. At the doses used in this study, methotrexate was more effective than leflunomide.

▶ Leflunomide is an orally administered inhibitor of pyrimidine synthesis that appears to be safe and effective long-term therapy for adults with rheumatoid arthritis. The current study in patients with juvenile rheumatoid arthritis showed it to be not quite as effective as methotrexate in this group of individuals. As we have seen time and again, what is new and expensive is not always better than what is old and inexpensive.

B. H. Thiers, MD

Abatacept for Rheumatoid Arthritis Refractory to Tumor Necrosis Factor α Inhibition

Genovese MC, Becker J-C, Schiff M, et al (Stanford Univ, Calif; Bristol-Myers Squibb, Priceton, NJ; Denver Arthritis Clinic, Denver; et al)

N Engl J Med 353:1114-1123, 2005

9–16

Background.—A substantial number of patients with rheumatoid arthritis have an inadequate or unsustained response to tumor necrosis factor α

(TNF-α) inhibitors. We conducted a randomized, double-blind, phase 3 trial to evaluate the efficacy and safety of abatacept, a selective costimulation modulator, in patients with active rheumatoid arthritis and an inadequate response to at least three months of anti-TNF-α therapy.

Methods.—Patients with active rheumatoid arthritis and an inadequate response to anti-TNF-α therapy were randomly assigned in a 2:1 ratio to receive abatacept or placebo on days 1, 15, and 29 and every 28 days thereafter for 6 months, in addition to at least one disease-modifying antirheumatic drug. Patients discontinued anti-TNF-α therapy before randomization. The rates of American College of Rheumatology (ACR) 20 responses (indicating a clinical improvement of 20 percent or greater) and improvement in functional disability, as reflected by scores for the Health Assessment Questionnaire (HAQ) disability index, were assessed.

Results.—After six months, the rates of ACR 20 responses were 50.4 percent in the abatacept group and 19.5 percent in the placebo group (P<0.001); the respective rates of ACR 50 and ACR 70 responses were also significantly higher in the abatacept group than in the placebo group (20.3 percent vs. 3.8 percent, P<0.001; and 10.2 percent vs. 1.5 percent, P=0.003). At six months, significantly more patients in the abatacept group than in the placebo group had a clinically meaningful improvement in physical function, as reflected by an improvement from baseline of at least 0.3 in the HAQ disability index (47.3 percent vs. 23.3 percent, P<0.001). The incidence of adverse events and peri-infusional adverse events was 79.5 percent and 5.0 percent, respectively, in the abatacept group and 71.4 percent and 3.0 percent, respectively, in the placebo group. The incidence of serious infections was 2.3 percent in each group.

Conclusions.—Abatacept produced significant clinical and functional benefits in patients who had had an inadequate response to anti-TNF-α therapy.

▶ These results are particularly impressive in that the patients selected for this study had previously responded poorly to TNF-α inhibition. Abatacept is the first in a new class of drugs that selectively modulate the CD80 or CD86-CD28 costimulatory signal required for full T-cell activation. Preclinical studies have suggested a potential therapeutic role for this immunomodulatory approach in psoriasis; however, clinical data are lacking.[1,2]

B. H. Thiers, MD

References

1. Abrams JR, Lebwohl MG, Guzzo CA, et al: CTLA4Ig-mediated blockade of T-cell costimulation in patients with psoriasis vulgaris. *J Clin Invest* 103:1243-1252, 1999.
2. Abrams JR, Kelley SL, Hayes E, et al: Blockade of T lymphocyte costimulation with cytotoxic T lymphocyte-associated antigen 4-immunoglobulin (CTLA4Ig) reverses the cellular pathology of psoriatic plaques, including the activation of keratinocytes, dendritic cells, and endothelial cells. *J Exp Med* 192:681-694, 2000.

No Evidence for Increased Risk of Cutaneous Squamous Cell Carcinoma in Patients With Rheumatoid Arthritis Receiving Etanercept for Up to 5 Years

Lebwohl M, Blum R, Berkowitz E, et al (Mount Sinai School of Medicine, New York)
Arch Dermatol 141:861-864, 2005   9–17

Objective.—To determine the incidence of cutaneous squamous cell carcinoma (SCC) in patients with rheumatoid arthritis receiving etanercept, a tumor necrosis factor antagonist, for up to 5 years.

Design.—An etanercept clinical trials' database and an etanercept postmarketing surveillance database were retrospectively analyzed for the incidence of SCC.

Setting.—Patients enrolled in clinical trials of etanercept were from private and institutional practices. The postmarketing database comprised reports from postmarketing trials and solicited and spontaneous reports.

Patients.—A total of 1442 patients with rheumatoid arthritis with 4257 patient-years of etanercept exposure (median exposure, 3.7 years) are included in the clinical trials' database. More than 125 000 patients with more than 250 000 patient-years of etanercept exposure are included in the etanercept postmarketing database.

Interventions.—Most patients enrolled in clinical trials of etanercept received a dosage of 25 mg of etanercept subcutaneously twice weekly for most of the time they received etanercept therapy.

Results.—Only 4 cases of SCC were observed in the etanercept clinical trials' database, an incidence that compares favorably with the expected incidences based on general population data from Arizona (13.1) and Minnesota (5.9). Similarly, few cases of SCC (1 per 10,000 patient-years) have been reported during postmarketing surveillance of etanercept therapy.

Conclusion.—In patients with rheumatoid arthritis, etanercept use of up to 5 years does not seem to be associated with an increase in the incidence of cutaneous SCC.

▶ The results are reassuring, given the known association of SCC with therapeutic immunosuppression.

B. H. Thiers, MD

A Randomized Clinical Trial of Acupuncture Compared With Sham Acupuncture in Fibromyalgia

Assefi NP, Sherman KJ, Jacobsen C, et al (Univ of Washington, Seattle)
Ann Intern Med 143:10-19, 2005   9–18

Background.—Fibromyalgia is a common chronic pain condition for which patients frequently use acupuncture.

Objective.—To determine whether acupuncture relieves pain in fibromyalgia.

Design.—Randomized, sham-controlled trial in which participants, data collection staff, and data analysts were blinded to treatment group.

Setting.—Private acupuncture offices in the greater Seattle, Washington, metropolitan area.

Patients.—100 adults with fibromyalgia.

Intervention.—Twice-weekly treatment for 12 weeks with an acupuncture program that was specifically designed to treat fibromyalgia, or 1 of 3 sham acupuncture treatments: acupuncture for an unrelated condition, needle insertion at nonacupoint locations, or noninsertive simulated acupuncture.

Measurements.—The primary outcome was subjective pain as measured by a 10-cm visual analogue scale ranging from 0 (no pain) to 10 (worst pain ever). Measurements were obtained at baseline; 1, 4, 8, and 12 weeks of treatment; and 3 and 6 months after completion of treatment. Participant blinding and adverse effects were ascertained by self-report. The primary outcomes were evaluated by pooling the 3 sham-control groups and comparing them with the group that received acupuncture to treat fibromyalgia.

Results.—The mean subjective pain rating among patients who received acupuncture for fibromyalgia did not differ from that in the pooled sham acupuncture group (mean between-group difference, 0.5 cm [95% CI, −0.3 cm to 1.2 cm]). Participant blinding was adequate throughout the trial, and no serious adverse effects were noted.

Limitations.—A prescription of acupuncture at fixed points may differ from acupuncture administered in clinical settings, in which therapy is individualized and often combined with herbal supplementation and other adjunctive measures. A usual-care comparison group was not studied.

Conclusion.—Acupuncture was no better than sham acupuncture at relieving pain in fibromyalgia.

Reporting of Harm in Randomized, Controlled Trials of Nonpharmacologic Treatment for Rheumatic Disease

Ethgen M, Boutron I, Baron G, et al (Centre Hospitalier Universitaire de Hautepierre, Strasbourgh, France: Hôpital Bretonneau, Tours, France; Université Paris VII)
Ann Intern Med 143:20-25, 2005   9–19

Background.—Reports of clinical trials usually emphasize benefits and give less attention to harms.

Purpose.—To compare the reporting of harm in trials of pharmacologic and nonpharmacologic treatment.

Data Sources. MEDLINE and the Cochrane Central Register of Controlled Trials.

Study Selection.—Reports of randomized, controlled trials assessing treatment of rheumatic disease that were published between January 1999 and January 2005.

Data Extraction.—A standardized abstraction form was used to extract data.

Data Synthesis.—193 articles were analyzed. After adjustment for medical area, sample size, funding source, and multicenter trials, data on harm were more often described in pharmacologic treatment reports than in nonpharmacologic treatment reports in reporting adverse events (odds ratio, 5.2 [95% CI, 2.1 to 12.9]), reporting withdrawals due to adverse events (odds ratio, 4.6 [CI, 2.0 to 10.9]), reporting severity (odds ratio, 3.7 [CI, 1.5 to 9.1]), and allocating space for describing harm (odds ratio, 1.6 [CI, 1.2 to 2.3]).

Limitations.—Extrapolating results to trials in areas other than rheumatic disease is questionable.

Conclusions.—The lack of reporting harm in trials assessing nonpharmacologic treatment in rheumatic disease is an important barrier to evaluating the benefit-harm balance of nonpharmacologic treatments.

▶ Randomized controlled trials assessing pharmacologic treatments generally include detailed adverse event reporting. Ethgen et al (Abstract 9–18) demonstrate that such disclosure is rarely found in reports of randomized controlled trials assessing nonpharmacologic treatments, such as surgery, arthroscopy, joint lavage, exercise, physiotherapy, orthosis, spa therapy, acupuncture, and education (Abstract 9–19). Adverse event reporting is necessary for both pharmacologic and nonpharmacologic treatments so that clinicians and patients can make informed decisions about the benefits and risks of these approaches.

B. H. Thiers, MD

10 Blistering Disorders

Genetic and Functional Characterization of Human Pemphigus Vulgaris Monoclonal Autoantibodies Isolated by Phage Display
Payne AS, Ishii K, Kacir S, et al (Univ of Pennsylvania, Philadelphia; Keio Univ, Tokyo)
J Clin Invest 115:888-899, 2005   10–1

Introduction.—Pemphigus is a life-threatening blistering disorder of the skin and mucous membranes caused by pathogenic autoantibodies to desmosomal adhesion proteins desmoglein 3 (Dsg3) and Dsg1. Mechanisms of antibody pathogenicity are difficult to characterize using polyclonal patient sera. Using antibody phage display, we have isolated repertoires of human anti-Dsg mAbs as single-chain variable-region fragments (scFvs) from a patient with active mucocutaneous pemphigus vulgaris. ScFv mAbs demonstrated binding to Dsg3 or Dsg1 alone, or both Dsg3 and Dsg1. Inhibition ELISA showed that the epitopes defined by these scFvs are blocked by autoantibodies from multiple pemphigus patients. Injection of scFvs into neonatal mice identified 2 pathogenic scFvs that caused blisters histologically similar to those observed in pemphigus patients. Similarly, these 2 scFvs, but not others, induced cell sheet dissociation of cultured human keratinocytes, indicating that both pathogenic and nonpathogenic antibodies were isolated. Genetic analysis of these mAbs showed restricted patterns of heavy and light chain gene usage, which were distinct for scFvs with different desmoglein-binding specificities. Detailed characterization of these pemphigus mAbs should lead to a better understanding of the immunopathogenesis of disease and to more specifically targeted therapeutic approaches.

▶ The authors have cloned and characterized pathogenic human monoclonal pemphigus vulgaris autoantibodies that reproduce disease in both animal and human keratinocyte models. This represents a major step in better understanding the pathophysiology of this autoimmune blistering disease and may help in the design of innovative therapeutic strategies.

B. H. Thiers, MD

Detection of Laminin 5-Specific Auto-antibodies in Mucous Membrane and Bullous Pemphigoid Sera by ELISA

Bekou V, Thoma-Uszynski S, Wendler O, et al (Friedrich Alexander Univ Erlangen-Nürnberg, Germany; Univ Hosp, Bern, Switzerland; Charité Univ Medicine, Berlin; et al)
J Invest Dermatol 124:732-740, 2005   10–2

Introduction.—Mucous membrane pemphigoid (MMP) is an autoimmune bullous disease that primarily affects mucous membranes leading to a scarring phenotype. MMP patients produce auto-antibodies (auto-ab) that preferentially recognize two components of the dermoepidermal basement membrane zone (BMZ): bullous pemphigoid (BP)180 and laminin 5 (LN5). Since detection of disease-specific auto-ab may be critical for diagnosis of MMP, we developed an ELISA with affinity-purified native human LN5. A total of 24 MMP, 72 BP, and 51 control sera were analyzed for LN5-specific auto-ab: 18/24 (75.0%) MMP and 29/72 (40.3%) BP sera were LN5 reactive. Sensitivity and specificity of the LN5 ELISA for MMP were 75% and 84.3%, respectively, and 40.3% and 88.2% for BP, respectively. The LN5 ELISA was more sensitive than a dot blot assay with native LN5, which detected LN5-reactive IgG in 14/24 (58.3%) MMP and 16/72 (22.2%) BP sera. In MMP, but not BP, levels of LN5-reactive IgG correlated with disease severity. Furthermore, IgG reactivity to LN5 of the MMP and BP sera was not significantly associated with IgG reactivity against other autoantigens of the BMZ, such as BP180 or BP230. Thus, the established LN5 ELISA holds great promise as a novel diagnostic and prognostic parameter for MMP.

▶ The authors developed a native LN5 ELISA that is sensitive and specific in detecting LN5-reactive IgG in MMP and a subgroup of patients with BP. It appears, therefore, that LN5 is a major autoantigen in MMP, and that antibodies against LN5 play an important role in its pathogenesis. Widespread use of this assay might allow earlier recognition and aggressive treatment of the disease, which often is associated with significant morbidity secondary to mucosal scarring.

B. H. Thiers, MD

Evidence That Anti-Type VII Collagen Antibodies Are Pathogenic and Responsible for the Clinical, Histological, and Immunological Features of Epidermolysis Bullosa Acquisita

Woodley DT, Chang C, Saadat P, et al (Univ of Southern California, Los Angeles; Univ of North Carolina, Chapel Hill)
J Invest Dermatol 124:958-964, 2005   10–3

Introduction.—Epidermolysis bullosa acquisita (EBA) is an autoimmune blistering disease characterized by autoantibodies to type VII (anchoring fibril) collagen. Therefore, it is a prototypic autoimmune disease defined by a well-known autoantigen and autoantibody. In this study, we injected hairless immune competent mice with purified immunoglobulin G (IgG) fraction of serum from rabbits immunized with the non-collagenous amino-terminal domain (NC1) of human type VII collagen, the domain known to contain immunodominant epitopes. As a control, identical mice were injected with the IgG fraction of serum from non-immunized rabbits. Mice injected with immune IgG developed subepidermal skin blisters and erosions, IgG deposits at the epidermal–dermal junction of their skin, and circulating anti-NC1 antibodies in their serum—all features reminiscent of patients with EBA. Similar concentrations of control IgG purified from normal rabbits did not induce disease in the mice. These findings strongly suggest that autoantibodies that recognize human type VII collagen in EBA are pathogenic. This murine model, with features similar to the clinical, histological, and immunological features of EBA, will be useful for the fine dissection of immunopathogenic mechanisms in EBA and for the development of new therapeutic interventions.

▶ The authors used a murine model to demonstrate the pathogenetic properties of anti-type VII collagen antibodies, which are found in patients with EBA. The use of this murine model may help to better define the immunopathogenesis of this condition and may lead to better treatments for it.

B. H. Thiers, MD

Lymphoma in Patients With Dermatitis Herpetiformis and Their First-Degree Relatives

Hervonen K, Vornanen M, Kautiainen H, et al (Tampere Univ, Finland; Rheumatism Found Hosp, Heinola, Finland)
Br J Dermatol 152:82-86, 2005   10–4

Background.—The risk for lymphoma is increased in both dermatitis herpetiformis (DH) and in coeliac disease. The lymphoma most associated with coeliac disease is enteropathy-associated T-cell lymphoma.

Objectives.—To study the occurrence and type of lymphoma in a large series of patients with DH and their first-degree relatives.

Methods.—The occurrence of lymphoma was studied in 1104 patients consecutively diagnosed with DH in two university hospitals during 1969-2001. A questionnaire was sent to 341 patients to examine the occurrence of lymphoma in their 1825 first-degree relatives. To analyse whether the DH patients with lymphoma had adhered to a gluten-free diet similarly to the patients without lymphoma, two age- and sex-matched patients with DH served as controls for each index case. Data on the gluten-free diet were collected from prospectively completed dietary forms and also from medical records.

Results.—Eleven (1%) patients contracted lymphoma 2-31 years after the diagnosis of DH. Eight had B-cell-type lymphoma, two enteropathy-associated T-cell lymphoma and one remained unclassified due to missing material. Three (0.2%) of the first-degree relatives contracted lymphoma, all

B-cell type. The 11 DH patients with lymphoma had adhered to a gluten-free diet significantly less strictly than the DH controls without lymphoma.

Conclusions.—The present study documents that patients with DH can have both B- and T-cell lymphoma. The DH patients with lymphoma had not adhered as strictly to the gluten-free diet as the control patients without lymphoma. The occurrence of lymphoma in the first-degree relatives was lower than in the patients with DH.

▶ The data presented here confirm the association of DH with lymphoma and suggest that the risk of lymphoma is higher in patients who do not adhere to a strict gluten-free diet.

B. H. Thiers, MD

11 Genodermatoses

Mutations in Lipid Transporter ABCA12 in Harlequin Ichthyosis and Functional Recovery by Corrective Gene Transfer
Akiyama M, Sugiyama-Nakagiri Y, Sakai K, et al (Hokkaido Univ, Sapporo, Japan; Japanese Red Cross Sendai Hosp, Yagiyama, Tashiro, Sendai, Japan; Natl Ctr for Child Health and Development, Okura, Setagaya, Tokyo)
J Clin Invest 115:1777-1784, 2005   11–1

Introduction.—Harlequin ichthyosis (HI) is a devastating skin disorder with an unknown underlying cause (Fig 1; see color plate XI). Abnormal ke-

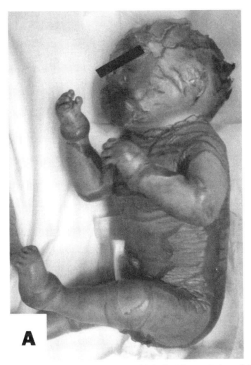

A

FIGURE 1.—Clinical features of HI patients. (Republished with permission of the *Journal of Clinical Investigation* from Akiyama M, Sugiyama-Nakagiri Y, Sakai K, et al: Mutations in Lipid Transporter ABCA12 in Harlequin Ichthyosis and Functional Recovery by Corrective Gene Transfer. *J Clin Invest* 115:1777-1784, 2005. Reproduced by permission of the publisher via Copyright Clearance Center, Inc.)

ratinocyte lamellar granules (LGs) are a hallmark of HI skin. ABCA12 is a member of the ATP-binding cassette transporter family, and members of the ABCA subfamily are known to have closely related functions as lipid transporters. ABCA3 is involved in lipid secretion via LGs from alveolar type II cells, and missense mutations in *ABCA12* have been reported to cause lamellar ichthyosis type 2, a milder form of ichthyosis. Therefore, we hypothesized that HI might be caused by mutations that lead to serious ABCA12 defects. We identify 5 distinct *ABCA12* mutations, either in a compound heterozygous or homozygous state, in patients from 4 HI families. All the mutations resulted in truncation or deletion of highly conserved regions of ABCA12. Immunoelectron microscopy revealed that ABCA12 localized to LGs in normal epidermal keratinocytes. We confirmed that ABCA12 defects cause congested lipid secretion in cultured HI keratinocytes and succeeded in obtaining the recovery of LG lipid secretion after corrective gene transfer of *ABCA12*. We concluded that ABCA12 works as an epidermal keratinocyte lipid transporter and that defective ABCA12 results in a loss of the skin lipid barrier, leading to HI. Our findings not only allow DNA-based early prenatal diagnosis but also suggest the possibility of gene therapy for HI.

▶ HI is a severe congenital disease resulting in abnormal skin keratinization. Mutations in the gene coding for *ABCA12,* a lipid transporter, have been shown to be associated with a mild form of ichthyosis (lamellar ichthyosis type 2). In this elegant study, Akiyama et al performed mutation analysis and expression studies of the *ABCA12* gene in 4 families with HI. They demonstrated 5 different mutations in patients of all the families, and defective protein expression in those patients was studied. Further studies revealed disturbed lipid secretion by lamellar granules of patient epidermal keratinocytes. Furthermore, glucosylceramide, which is a component of lamellar granules that plays a major role in maintenance of the epidermal barrier, was found throughout the epidermis of patients; this lipid is normally restricted to the stratum corneum. A most exciting aspect of this study was the in vitro transfer of the normal *ABCA12* gene into patient keratinocytes that resulted in the correction of protein expression and a normal distribution of glucosylceramide. These findings suggest that gene therapy may become a viable therapeutic option for patients with this grave disease.

G. M. P. Galbraith, MD

Pregnancy and Obstetrical Outcomes in Pseudoxanthoma Elasticum
Bercovitch L, Leroux T, Terry S, et al (Brown Med School, Providence, RI; PXE Internatl, Inc, Washington, DC)
Br J Dermatol 151:1011-1018, 2004   11–2

Background.—Pseudoxanthoma elasticum (PXE) is a genetic multisystem disorder characterized by calcified dystrophic elastic fibres in skin, retina and arteries. Much of the earlier literature on pregnancy in PXE contained reports of severe complications, leading some healthcare providers to advise women with PXE against becoming pregnant and some women with PXE to avoid pregnancy.

Objectives.—To evaluate the obstetrical outcomes and the incidence of pregnancy complications in women with PXE and to determine if pregnancy is associated with an adverse effect on the course of the disease.

Methods.—Women with PXE (n = 407) answered detailed questionnaires regarding reproductive history and pregnancy as well as the course of their disease. The frequency of reported pregnancy outcomes and complications was determined. Severity indices for the major clinical manifestations of PXE were developed and correlated with gravidity of affected women aged 40 years or over.

Results.—Among the 306 respondents with PXE who had ever been pregnant, there were 795 pregnancies. Of these, 83% ended in live births and 1% in stillbirth. The median birth weight was within the normal range and the incidence of low birth weight for gestation was low. Hypertension occurred in 10% of pregnancies, gastric bleeding and retinal complications in < 1%, and 12% of pregnancies were associated with worsening of skin manifestations. There was no effect of gravidity and clinical severity on cutaneous ($P = 0.07$), ocular ($P = 0.59$) or cardiac ($P = 0.42$) manifestations of PXE in women aged 40+ years, nor did ever having been pregnant adversely affect these clinical severity indices. Of the 101 women who had never been pregnant, 17% made the decision because they were advised against becoming pregnant by a healthcare professional and 11% did not become pregnant because they feared an adverse outcome either in their pregnancy or disease.

Conclusions.—PXE is not associated with markedly increased fetal loss or adverse reproductive outcomes. The incidence of gastric bleeding, although probably higher than in the unaffected population, is much lower than previously reported, and retinal complications are uncommon. Although a few pregnancies were associated with worsening of skin manifestations, there was no correlation of either gravidity or ever having been pregnant with ultimate severity of skin, ocular or cardiovascular manifestations. There is no basis for advising women with PXE to avoid becoming pregnant, and most pregnancies in PXE are uncomplicated.

▶ This article attempts to counter the common belief that women with PXE should not become pregnant. Bercovitch et al analyzed questionnaires from 407 women with this condition and found that the vast majority had successful pregnancies with a live birth and minimal complications.

B. H. Thiers, MD

Evolution of Skin Lesions in Proteus Syndrome

Twede JV, Turner JT, Biesecker LG, et al (Uniformed Services Univ of the Health Sciences, Bethesda, Md; NIH, Bethesda, Md)
J Am Acad Dermatol 52:834-838, 2005   11–3

Background.—Proteus syndrome is a rare overgrowth disorder that is generally progressive, but the natural history of the skin lesions is not known.

Objective.—Our purpose was to document the evolution of 4 common skin lesions in 16 patients with Proteus syndrome.

Results.—Most epidermal nevi and vascular malformations were reported to appear in the first month of life and had little tendency for expan-

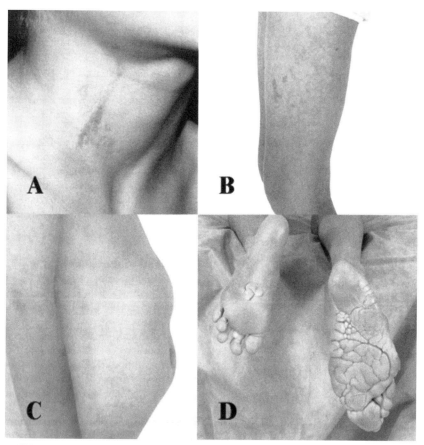

FIGURE 1.—Representative examples of 4 skin lesions in patients with Proteus syndrome. **A,** Linear, brown epidermal nevus on neck of affected patient. **B,** Red capillary malformations and ectatic veins on leg of patient. **C,** Three subcutaneous lipomas on abdomen of patient. **D,** Cerebriform connective tissue nevi on feet of patient with Proteus syndrome who also has overgrowth of the right foot. (Reprinted by permission of the publisher from Twede JV, Turner JT, Biesecker LG, et al: Evolution of skin lesions in Proteus syndrome. *J Am Acad Dermatol* 52:834-838, 2005. Copyright 2005 by Elsevier.)

sion or development of additional lesions. Subcutaneous lipomas and cerebriform connective tissue nevi were commonly noted in the first year of life, but not in the first month. Most patients reported that subcutaneous lipomas and cerebriform connective tissue nevi progressively increased in size, and in most patients additional lesions developed at new locations. Of the 4 types of skin lesions, plantar cerebriform connective tissue nevi were most frequently cited as a source of symptoms.

Conclusion.—Skin lesions of Proteus syndrome may not appear until later infancy or early childhood, making it difficult to diagnose in young children (Fig 1; see color plate XII).

▶ Sixteen patients with Proteus syndrome evaluated at the National Institutes of Health or by their caregivers completed a lengthy questionnaire regarding the age of onset and progression of skin lesions associated with the syndrome. Skin lesions fell into 2 groups. Group I lesions, consisting of epidermal nevi and vascular malformations, tended to be present at birth or developed in the neonatal period, and the area of involvement remained stable. These lesions likely result from mosaicism. Group II lesions, including lipomas and cerebriform connective tissue nevi, appeared postnatally and were progressive. Their delayed onset and tendency to progress suggests that the growth of group II lesions may require additional, as yet unknown genetic events or other stimuli.

S. Raimer, MD

Prevalence of Fabry Disease in Patients With Cryptogenic Stroke: A Prospective Study

Rolfs A, Böttcher T, Zschiesche M, et al (Univ of Rostock, Germany; Univ of Tübingen, Germany; Univ College London; et al)
Lancet 366:1794-1796, 2005   11–4

Background.—Strokes are an important cause of morbidity and mortality in young adults. However, in most cases the cause of the stroke remains unclear. Anderson-Fabry disease is an X-linked recessive lysosomal storage disease resulting from deficient α-galactosidase and causes an endothelial vasculopathy followed by cerebral ischaemia. To determine the importance of Fabry disease in young people with stroke, we measured the frequency of unrecognised Fabry disease in a cohort of acute stroke patients.

Methods.—Between February, 2001, and December, 2004, 721 German adults aged 18 to 55 years suffering from acute cryptogenic stroke were screened for Fabry disease. The plasma α-galactosidase activity in men was measured followed by sequencing of the entire α-*GAL* gene in those with low enzyme activity. By contrast, the entire α-*GAL* gene was genetically screened for mutations in women even if enzyme activity was normal.

Findings.—21 of 432 (4.9%) male stroke patients and seven of 289 (2.4%) women had a biologically significant mutation within the α-*GAL* gene. The mean age at onset of symptomatic cerebrovascular disease was

38.4 years (SD 13.0) in the male stroke patients and 40.3 years (13.1) in the female group. The higher frequency of infarctions in the vertebrobasilar area correlated with more pronounced changes in the vertebrobasilar vessels like dolichoectatic pathology (42.9% *vs* 6.8%).

Interpretation.—We have shown a high frequency of Fabry disease in a cohort of patients with cryptogenic stroke, which corresponds to about 1.2% in young stroke patients. Fabry disease must be considered in all cases of unexplained stroke in young patients, especially in those with the combination of infarction in the vertebrobasilar artery system and proteinuria.

▶ The authors found that some cases of cryptogenic stroke (ie, a cerebrovascular event for which no specific cause can be identified) may be associated with Fabry disease. As cutaneous manifestations (eg, angiokeratomas, hypohidrosis) can occur in these patients, the dermatologist can aid in providing an accurate diagnosis. Enzyme replacement therapy is available for patients with Fabry disease, although there is no clear evidence of its benefit in patients with cerebrovascular events. Nevertheless, such treatment does appear to have an effect on resting cerebral blood flow abnormalities.[1]

B. H. Thiers, MD

Reference

1. Moore DF, Scott LTC, Gladwin MT, et al: Regional cerebral hyperperfusion and nitric oxide pathway dysregulation in Fabry disease. Reversal by enzyme replacement therapy. *Circulation* 104:1506-1512, 2001.

Glycogen Storage Diseases Presenting as Hypertrophic Cardiomyopathy
Arad M, Maron BJ, Gorham JM, et al (Harvard Med School, Boston; Minneapolis Heart Inst Found; Univ of Alabama at Birmingham; et al)
N Engl J Med 352:362-372, 2005   11–5

Background.—Unexplained left ventricular hypertrophy often prompts the diagnosis of hypertrophic cardiomyopathy, a sarcomere-protein gene disorder. Because mutations in the gene for AMP-activated protein kinase γ_2 (PRKAG2) cause an accumulation of cardiac glycogen and left ventricular hypertrophy that mimics hypertrophic cardiomyopathy, we hypothesized that hypertrophic cardiomyopathy might also be clinically misdiagnosed in patients with other mutations in genes regulating glycogen metabolism.

Methods.—Genetic analyses performed in 75 consecutive unrelated patients with hypertrophic cardiomyopathy detected 40 sarcomere-protein mutations. In the remaining 35 patients, PRKAG2, lysosome-associated membrane protein 2 (LAMP2), α-galactosidase (GLA), and acid α-1,4-glucosidase (GAA) genes were studied.

Results.—Gene defects causing Fabry's disease (GLA) and Pompe's disease (GAA) were not found, but two LAMP2 and one PRKAG2 mutations were identified in probands with prominent hypertrophy and electrophysiological abnormalities. These results prompted the study of two additional, independent series of patients. Genetic analyses of 20 subjects with massive hypertrophy (left ventricular wall thickness, ≤30 mm) but without electrophysiological abnormalities revealed mutations in neither LAMP2 nor PRKAG2. Genetic analyses of 24 subjects with increased left ventricular wall thickness and electrocardiograms suggesting ventricular preexcitation revealed four LAMP2 and seven PRKAG2 mutations. Clinical features associated with defects in LAMP2 included male sex, severe hypertrophy, early onset (at 8 to 17 years of age), ventricular preexcitation, and asymptomatic elevations of two serum proteins.

Conclusions.—LAMP2 mutations typically cause multisystem glycogen-storage disease (Danon's disease) but can also present as a primary cardiomyopathy. The glycogen-storage cardiomyopathy produced by LAMP2 or PRKAG2 mutations resembles hypertrophic cardiomyopathy but is distinguished by electrophysiological abnormalities, particularly ventricular preexcitation.

▶ Most dermatologists are quite familiar with Fabry disease, a glycogen-storage disease that can be associated with hypertrophic cardiomyopathy and other systemic abnormalities. The authors performed genetic analyses in 75 consecutive unrelated patients presenting with hypertrophic cardiomyopathy and found none with Fabry disease. However, 2 had a genetic defect (LAMP2 mutation) previously associated with another multisystem glycogen-storage disorder (Danon disease). The other patient had a PRKAG2 mutation.

B. H. Thiers, MD

12 Drug Actions, Reactions, and Interactions

Risk of Stevens-Johnson Syndrome and Toxic Epidermal Necrolysis in New Users of Antiepileptics
Mockenhaupt M, Messenheimer J, Tennis P, et al (Univ of Freiburg, Germany; GlaxoSmithKline, Research Triangle Park, NC, RTI Health Solutions, Research Triangle Park, NC)
Neurology 64:1134-1138, 2005
12–1

Background.—Estimates of risk of Stevens-Johnson syndrome (SJS) and toxic epidermal necrolysis (TEN) associated with some antiepileptic drugs (AEDs) have used denominators based on the number of prescriptions or daily doses. Because the risk of SJS is highest in new users of drugs, the use of denominators reflective of all users can lead to low estimates of risk associated with drugs. In this study, risk in new users is assessed.

Methods.—Data on all hospitalized patients with SJS and TEN with use of carbamazepine (CBZ), lamotrigine (LTG), phenobarbital (PHB), phenytoin (PHT), or valproic acid (VPA) were obtained from the German Registry for Serious Cutaneous Reactions. For 1998-2001, the numbers of new users were estimated from number of dispensed prescriptions in Germany, the average prescribed doses, and the duration of use in the Mediplus database (IMS Health) Germany, and assumptions that relate new use to growth in national dispensings. To minimize the probability of underestimating risk in new users, conservative estimates of new use that were somewhat lower than predicted from national prescription data were used.

Results.—More than 90% of SJS and TEN cases occurred in the first 63 days of AED use. Over the 4 years, increases in dispensing were 5% for CBZ, 65% for LTG, 6% for PHB, -16% for PHT, and 26% for VPA. Across a range of assumptions about frequency of incident use, the risk estimates vary between 1 and 10 per 10,000 new users for CBZ, LTG, PHT, and PHY and were consistently lower for VPA.

Conclusion.—Across a range of assumptions used, the risk of hospitalization for Stevens-Johnson syndrome or toxic epidermal necrolysis in new users is low for carbamazepine, lamotrigine, phenytoin, phenobarbital, and valproic acid. Because conservative incidence use fractions were used, it is likely that some risks were overestimated.

▶ Although rare, reactions to antiepileptic drugs can be quite serious and even life threatening. They generally occur during the first 2 months of therapy, and thus a high index of suspicion is warranted when evaluating patients during this time window.

B. H. Thiers, MD

HLA-B*5801 Allele as a Genetic Marker for Severe Cutaneous Adverse Reactions Caused by Allopurinol

Hung-S-I, Chung W-H, Liou L-B, et al (Inst of Biomedical Sciences, Taipei, Taiwan; Chang Gung Mem Hosp, Taipei, Taiwan; Mackay Mem Hosp, Taipei, Taiwan; et al)
Proc Natl Acad Sci U S A 102:4134-4139, 2005   12–2

Introduction.—Allopurinol, a commonly prescribed medication for gout and hyperuricemia, is a frequent cause of severe cutaneous adverse reactions (SCAR), which include the drug hypersensitivity syndrome, Stevens-Johnson syndrome, and toxic epidermal necrolysis. The adverse events are unpredictable and carry significant morbidity and mortality. To identify genetic markers for allopurinol-SCAR, we carried out a case-control association study. We enrolled 51 patients with allopurinol-SCAR and 228 control individuals (135 allopurinol-tolerant subjects and 93 healthy subjects from the general population), and genotyped for 823 SNPs in genes related to drug metabolism and immune response. The initial screen revealed strong association between allopurinol-SCAR and SNPs in the MHC region, including *BAT3* (encoding HLA-B associated transcript 3), *MSH5* (mutS homolog 5), and *MICB* (MHC class I polypeptide-related sequence B) ($P < 10^{-7}$). We then determined the alleles of HLA loci A, B, C, and DRB1. The HLA-B*5801 allele was present in all (100%) 51 patients with allopurinol-SCAR, but only in 20 (15%) of 135 tolerant patients [odds ratio 580.3 (95% confidence interval, 34.4-9780.9); corrected P value = 4.7×10^{-24}] and in 19 (20%) of 93 of healthy subjects [393.51 (23.23-6665.26); corrected P value = 8.1×10^{-18}]. HLA alleles A*3303, Cw*0302, and DRB1*0301 were in linkage disequilibrium and formed an extended haplotype with HLA-B*5801. Our results indicated that allopurinol-SCAR is strongly associated with a genetic predisposition in Han Chinese. In particular, HLA-B*5801 allele is an important genetic risk factor for this life-threatening condition.

Medical Genetics: A Marker for Stevens-Johnson Syndrome

Chung W-H, Hung S-I, Hong H-S, et al (Chang Gung Mem Hosp, Taipei, Taiwan; Inst of Biomedical Sciences, Taipei, Taiwan)

Nature 428:486, 2004   12–3

Background.—Stevens-Johnson syndrome (SJS) and toxic epidermal necrosis are life-threatening skin reactions to particular medications. In this study, it was demonstrated that a strong association exists between a genetic marker, *HLA-B*1502*, and SJS induced by carbamazepine (CBZ-SJS), which is commonly prescribed for the treatment of seizures. Whether it is possible to utilize this association as a marker for predicting severe adverse reactions was determined.

Methods.—A group of 44 Taiwanese (Han Chinese) patients with CBZ-SJS were studied. Included in this group were 5 patients with overlapping toxic epidermal necrolysis, in whom the clinical morphology met Roujeau's diagnostic criteria. These patients had widespread skin rashes with blisters, skin detachment, and mucosa involvement. Also included was a control group of 101 patients who had been receiving carbamazepine for at least 3 months with no adverse reactions (CBZ-tolerant patients) and 93 normal subjects. Because genetic factors that influence drug metabolism and the immune response, including *HLA* genotype, might have a role in drug hypersensitivity, genotyping was done for 157 cytochrome-P450 single-nucleotide polymorphisms by using high-throughput MALDI-TOF mass spectrometry. In addition, all *HLA-B, -C, -A,* and *-DRBI* alleles were genotyped by sequence-specific oligonucleotide reverse lineblot and sequence-based typing.

Results.—When the CPZ-tolerant group is used as the control, the presence of *B*1502* has a 93.6% positive predictive value for CBZ-SJS, while its negative predictive value is 100%. Thus, the *HLA-B*1502* allele should have 100% sensitivity and 97% specificity in a test for CBZ-SJS.

Conclusions.—The incidence of SJS in Han Chinese is significantly higher than in white persons, and carbamazepine is the drug most commonly associated with this syndrome in Asian patients. A strong association was found between *HLA-B*1502* and CBZ-SJS. While these findings could affect more than 1 billion Chinese throughout the world, their application to other populations is unknown. It has yet to be determined whether genes in the vicinity of the *HLA-B* locus, if not *B*1502* itself, are involved in the pathogenesis of CBZ-SJS.

▶ The specifics of these studies (Abstracts 12–2 and 12–3) are less important than the concepts they demonstrate. Why do certain patients respond to a given drug whereas other patients with clinically similar disease do not? Why do certain patients have a severe adverse reaction to a given drug while others do not? Quite likely, genetic factors affecting drug metabolism underlie these phenomena. Better understanding of these factors will eventually lead to more effective and specific therapies for individual patients.[1]

B. H. Thiers, MD

Reference

1. Wilkinson GR: Drug metabolism and variability among patients in drug response. *N Engl J Med* 352:2211-2221, 2005.

Pruritus After Intrathecal Baclofen Withdrawal: A Retrospective Study
Smail DB, Hugeron C, Denys P, et al (Hôpıtal Raymond Poincaré, Garches, France)
Arch Phys Med Rehabil 86:494-497, 2005   12–4

Objectives.—To determine the frequency of pruritus after intrathecal baclofen (ITB) withdrawal and to study the pathophysiology of this symptom.

Design.—Retrospective cohort study.

Setting.—Rehabilitation department of a general hospital.

Participants.—Patients (N=102) implanted with an ITB pump who had been followed up since 1988.

Interventions.—Not applicable.

Main Outcome Measures.—Incidence of pruritus after withdrawal. We studied the relation between pruritus and daily dose, concentration and mode of infusion of baclofen, and cause of the central nervous system lesion inducing spasticity.

Results.—Pruritus was observed in 10 of 23 cases of ITB withdrawal. It never occurred during the first 3 months after pump implantation. It seems likely that the segmental spinal action of baclofen is responsible for pruritus. There was no statistically significant difference between patients with ITB deprivation who did and did not experience pruritus in their daily infused dosage or in concentration and mode of infusion. Surprisingly, no pruritus was observed in patients with multiple sclerosis.

Conclusions.—Pruritus is a frequent symptom after ITB withdrawal. Its occurrence is probably subsequent to chronic blocking of the liberation of substance P by baclofen at the spinal level. This symptom is a good clinical predictor of baclofen withdrawal, in contrast to an isolated increase of spasticity that may be due to drug tolerance or irritant factors. Pruritus requires investigation of a possible dysfunction of the infusion system.

▶ Abrupt withdrawal of ITB can lead to serious consequences, including death; thus, although pruritus is an inconsistent symptom, it can be an early indicator of pump malfunction. It is postulated that ITB inhibits substance P release by acting at primary afferent terminals. Abrupt withdrawal is associated with release of substance P, which interacts with hypersensitive postsynaptic substance P receptors to activate sensory pathways that induce itching.

B. H. Thiers, MD

Tissue Eosinophils and the Perils of Using Skin Biopsy Specimens to Distinguish Between Drug Hypersensitivity and Cutaneous Graft-Versus-Host Disease

Marra DE, McKee PH, Nghiem P, et al (Harvard Med School, Boston; Dana-Farber Cancer Inst, Boston)
J Am Acad Dermatol 51:543-546, 2004   12–5

Introduction.—Graft-versus-host disease (GvHD) is a frequent and serious complication of bone-marrow transplantation (BMT), and carries a high morbidity and mortality if not promptly recognized and treated. The rash of acute GvHD is often difficult to distinguish clinically from a drug eruption, and skin biopsies are often performed in an attempt to render a diagnosis. Histologically, eosinophils are classically associated with hypersensitivity reactions, and their presence in inflamed tissue is considered suggestive of a drug-induced dermatitis. We present 3 cases of acute exanthema in BMT recipients in whom the presence of eosinophils on skin biopsy specimen led to an initial diagnosis of drug eruption over GvHD. As a result, these patients experienced delays in the institution of definitive immunosuppressive therapy for GvHD. We review the growing literature suggesting that no single or combined histologic feature, including tissue eosinophils, is useful in differentiating GvHD from drug eruptions in BMT recipients. Indeed, in most cases, the cause of a new-onset blanchable erythematous rash in a BMT recipient is most accurately determined by close examination and follow-up of the clinical features without a skin biopsy.

▶ When eosinophils are detected in the inflammatory infiltrate of a skin biopsy, it is often a knee-jerk reflex for the observer to conclude that an allergic reaction is involved. The extrapolation of this is that eosinophils have been gauged to be a marker for drug reactions in the clinical setting of a macular and papular exanthem. This study clearly indicates that eosinophils cannot discriminate between the exanthem of GvHD and the exanthem of drug hypersensitivity. Physicians should always remember that clinicopathologic correlation is of the utmost importance in the interpretation of histopathologic findings in skin biopsy specimens.

J. C. Maize, MD

13 Drug Development and Promotion

Payment to Healthcare Professionals for Patient Recruitment to Trials: A Systematic Review
Bryant J, Powell J (Univ of Southampton, England; Univ of Warwick, England)
BMJ 331:1377-1378, 2005   13–1

Background.—Randomized controlled trials (RCTs) are vital to the establishment of the clinical effectiveness and cost-effectiveness of interventions in health care. One important element in determining the quality of RCTs is the recruitment of enough participants in the study to test a priori hypotheses with statistical confidence and to minimize bias. One strategy for increasing the number of participants in RCTs is to provide financial incentives either by paying the study participants outright or by reimbursing the excess costs incurred. Such arrangements are common in studies conducted by pharmaceutical companies but are not common practice in publicly funded research programs. Demonstrating that payments are worthwhile is necessary if such an approach is to be adopted by publicly funded programs. In the present study, the evidence on the effectiveness of payment to health care professionals for patient recruitment to trials was synthesized.

Methods.—Electronic databases were searched from inception to July 2004 for published English-language studies that paid or reimbursed health care professionals for recruiting patients to trials with reported recruitment rates. Bibliographies and gray literature were also searched.

Results.—Only a few studies were identified, and the quality of the studies was inconclusive. No controlled trials comparing recruitment rates achieved with and without financial incentives were identified. One primary care study reported no relationship between incentive-driven motivation and the number of patients recruited. A second primary care study did not report a correlation between financial reimbursement and recruitment rates but concluded from multivariate analysis that patient recruitment by general practitioners may be assisted by several strategies, including financial incentives.

Conclusions.—Evidence is insufficient on the effectiveness of payment to health care professionals for recruiting patients to RCTs. Rigorous evidence from well-conducted studies is needed to guide recruitment strategies before publicly funded research programs can consider the use of financial incentives.

▶ Clinical trials require a certain number of patients to generate valid findings. Thus, sponsors often provide financial incentives to increase patient recruitment. Bryant and Powell found no evidence that payment to health care professionals is an effective strategy for recruiting patients to trials.

B. H. Thiers, MD

Contradicted and Initially Stronger Effects in Highly Cited Clinical Research

Ioannidis JPA (Univ of Ioannina, Greece; Tufts-New England Med Ctr, Boston)
JAMA 294:218-228, 2005   13–2

Context.—Controversy and uncertainty ensue when the results of clinical research on the effectiveness of interventions are subsequently contradicted. Controversies are most prominent when high-impact research is involved.

Objectives.—To understand how frequently highly cited studies are contradicted or find effects that are stronger than in other similar studies and to discern whether specific characteristics are associated with such refutation over time.

Design.—All original clinical research studies published in 3 major general clinical journals or high-impact-factor specialty journals in 1990-2003 and cited more than 1000 times in the literature were examined.

Main Outcome Measure.—The results of highly cited articles were compared against subsequent studies of comparable or larger sample size and similar or better controlled designs. The same analysis was also performed comparatively for matched studies that were not so highly cited.

Results.—Of 49 highly cited original clinical research studies, 45 claimed that the intervention was effective. Of these, 7 (16%) were contradicted by subsequent studies, 7 others (16%) had found effects that were stronger than those of subsequent studies, 20 (44%) were replicated, and 11 (24%) remained largely unchallenged. Five of 6 highly-cited nonrandomized studies had been contradicted or had found stronger effects vs 9 of 39 randomized controlled trials ($P = .008$). Among randomized trials, studies with contradicted or stronger effects were smaller ($P = .009$) than replicated or unchallenged studies although there was no statistically significant difference in their early or overall citation impact. Matched control studies did not have a significantly different share of refuted results than highly cited studies, but they included more studies with "negative" results.

Conclusions.—Contradiction and initially stronger effects are not unusual in highly cited research of clinical interventions and their outcomes. The extent to which high citations may provoke contradictions and vice versa needs more study. Controversies are most common with highly cited nonrandomized studies, but even the most highly cited randomized trials may be challenged and refuted over time, especially small ones.

▶ As my mother always said, "Don't believe everything you read!" Ioannidis shows that contradicted and potentially exaggerated findings are common in the most influential and visible clinical research; indeed, 16% of the top-cited clinical research articles on medical therapies published in the past 15 years were contradicted by subsequent studies, and another 16% were found to report initially stronger effects than subsequent research could confirm. Contradictions were most common with nonrandomized trials but even randomized trials did not escape controversy. Overall, approximately one third of the top-cited randomized trials published from 1990 through 1995 have been challenged.

B. H. Thiers, MD

Extent and Impact of Industry Sponsorship Conflicts of Interest in Dermatology Research

Perlis CS, Harwood M, Perlis RH (Brown Med School, Boston; Harvard Med School, Boston)
J Am Acad Dermatol 52:967-971, 2005   13–3

Background.—Many published clinical trials are authored by investigators with financial conflicts of interest. The general medical literature documents the pervasive extent and sometimes problematic impact of these conflicts. Accordingly, there is renewed discussion about author disclosure and clinical trial registry to minimize publication bias from financial conflicts of interest. Despite this evolving discussion in the general medical literature, little is known about the extent or role of financial conflicts of interest in dermatology research.

Objective.—Our purpose was to determine the extent and impact of industry sponsorship conflicts of interest in dermatology research.

Methods.—We recorded potential financial conflicts of interest, study design, and study outcome in 179 clinical trials published between Oct 1, 2000 and Oct 1, 2003 in four leading dermatology journals.

Results.—Forty-three percent of analyzed studies included at least one author with a reported conflict of interest. These studies were more likely to report a positive result, demonstrate higher methodological quality, and include a larger sample size.

Conclusions.—Conflict of interest in clinical investigations in dermatology appears to be prevalent and associated with potentially significant differences in study methodology and reporting.

▶ A recently published study[1] (which was reviewed in the 2003 YEAR BOOK OF DERMATOLOGY AND DERMATOLOGIC SURGERY) found that readers are more suspect of the results of studies performed by conflicted investigators compared with those in which the investigators report no industry affiliations. Many articles reviewed in past YEAR BOOKS have addressed the sometimes uneasy relationship between physicians and pharmaceutical companies.

B. H. Thiers, MD

Reference

1. Chaudhry S, Schroter S, Smith R, et al: Does declaration of competing interests affect readers' perceptions? A randomized trial. *BMJ* 325:1391-1392, 2002.

Academic Medical Centers' Standards for Clinical-Trial Agreements With Industry

Mello MM, Clarridge BR, Studdert DM (Harvard School of Public Health, Boston; Univ of Massachusetts, Boston)
N Engl J Med 352:2202-2210, 2005   13–4

Background.—Although industry sponsors provide approximately 70 percent of the funding for clinical drug trials in the United States, little is known about the legal agreements that exist between industry sponsors and academic investigators. We studied institutional standards regarding contractual provisions that restrict investigators' control over trials.

Methods.—We used a structured, cross-sectional mail survey of medical-school research administrators responsible for negotiating clinical-trial agreements with industry sponsors.

Results.—Of 122 institutions approached, 107 participated. There was a high degree of consensus among administrators about the acceptability of several contractual provisions relating to publications. For example, more than 85 percent reported that their office would not approve provisions giving industry sponsors the authority to revise manuscripts or decide whether results should be published. There was considerable disagreement about the acceptability of provisions allowing the sponsor to insert its own statistical analyses in manuscripts (24 percent allowed them, 47 percent disallowed them, and 29 percent were not sure whether they should allow them), draft the manuscript (50 percent allowed it, 40 percent disallowed it, and 11 percent were not sure whether they should allow it), and prohibit investigators from sharing data with third parties after the trial is over (41 percent allowed it, 34 percent disallowed it, and 24 percent were not sure whether they should allow it). Disputes were common after the agreements had been signed and most frequently centered on payment (75 percent of administrators reported at least one such dispute in the previous year), intellectual property (30 percent), and control of or access to data (17 percent).

Conclusions.—Standards for certain restrictive provisions in clinical-trial agreements with industry sponsors vary considerably among academic medical centers. Greater sharing of information about legal relationships with industry sponsors is desirable in order to build consensus about appropriate standards.

▶ As noted by Steinbrook[1] in an accompanying editorial, clinical trial agreements often contain gag clauses that prevent investigators from independently evaluating the data or submitting a manuscript for publication without the express consent of the sponsor. This can result in suppression of unfavorable efficacy or safety data.[1] One particular egregious example was that of a Toronto hematologist who was sued by a pharmaceutical company when she tried to publish unfavorable findings about a drug she was contracted to investigate; this incident was related in a series of articles in the *New England Journal of Medicine*.[2-4] Academic institutions need to adhere to strict policies about access to data and publication rights so that sponsors will be unable to seek more favorable terms from one institution than from another.

B. H. Thiers, MD

References

1. Steinbrook R: Gag clauses in clinical-trial agreements (editorial). *N Engl J Med* 352:2160-2162, 2005.
2. Drazen JM: Institutions, contracts, and academic freedom. *N Engl J Med* 347:1362-1363, 2002.
3. Nathan DG, Weatherall DJ: Academic freedom in clinical research. *N Engl J Med* 347:1368-1371, 2002.
4. Moses H III, Braunwald E, Martin JB, et al: Collaborating with industry: Choices for the academic medical center. *N Engl J Med* 347:1371-1375, 2002.

Health Industry Practices That Create Conflicts of Interest: A Policy Proposal for Academic Medical Centers
Brennan TA, Rothman DJ, Blank L, et al (Harvard Med School, Boston; Columbia Univ, New York; Assoc of American Med Colleges, Washington, DC; et al)
JAMA 295:429-433, 2006   13–5

Introduction.—Conflicts of interest between physicians' commitment to patient care and the desire of pharmaceutical companies and their representatives to sell their products pose challenges to the principles of medical professionalism. These conflicts occur when physicians have motives or are in situations for which reasonable observers could conclude that the moral requirements of the physician's roles are or will be compromised. Although physician groups, the manufacturers, and the federal government have instituted self-regulation of marketing, research in the psychology and social science of gift receipt and giving indicates that current controls will not satisfactorily protect the interests of patients. More stringent regulation is necessary, including the elimination or modification of common practices related to small gifts, pharmaceutical samples, continuing medical education, funds for physician travel, speakers bureaus, ghostwriting, and consulting and research contracts. We propose a policy under which academic medical centers would take the lead in eliminating the conflicts of interest that still characterize the relationship between physicians and the health care industry.

▶ This article generated a great deal of controversy when it was published early in 2006. The authors believe that the implementation of their proposals would substantially reduce the need for external regulation to safeguard the public against market-driven conflicts of interest and would allow the medical profession to reaffirm its commitment to put the interests of patients first.

B. H. Thiers, MD

Do Drug Samples Influence Resident Prescribing Behavior? A Randomized Trial
Adair RF, Holmgren LR (Univ of Minnesota, Minneapolis; Abbott Northwestern Hosp, Minneapolis)
Am J Med 118:881-884, 2005   13–6

Purpose.—The purpose of the study was to determine whether access to drug samples influences resident prescribing decisions.

Subjects and Methods.—The authors observed 390 decisions to initiate drug therapy by 29 internal medicine residents over a 6-month period in an inner-city primary care clinic. By random selection, half of the residents agreed not to use available free drug samples. Five drug class pairs were chosen for study prospectively. Highly advertised drugs were matched with drugs commonly used for the same indication that were less expensive, available over-the-counter, or available in generic formulation.

Results.—Resident physicians with access to drug samples were less likely to choose unadvertised drugs (131/202 decisions) than residents who did not have access to samples (138/188 decisions; $P = .04$) and less likely to choose over-the-counter drugs (51/202, 73/188; $P = .003$). There was a trend toward less use of inexpensive drugs.

Conclusion.—Access to drug samples in clinic influences resident prescribing decisions. This could affect resident education and increase drug costs for patients.

▶ Adair and Holmgren found that access to drug samples influences the prescribing decisions of resident physicians. Who would have thought otherwise? The results appear to contradict 2 widespread beliefs: (1) drug samples are inherently different from other forms of marketing, and (2) samples help manage drug costs in the long term. The latter concept seems invalid because drug samples are generally available only for high-priced, brand-name drugs. When accompanied by a prescription for the same product (as samples often are), the savings conferred by the samples do little to offset the high price of the prescription.

B. H. Thiers, MD

Differences in Antibiotic Prescribing Among Physicians, Residents, and Nonphysician Clinicians

Roumie CL, Halasa NB, Edwards KM, et al (Vanderbilt Univ, Nashville, Tenn)
Am J Med 118:641-648, 2005   13–7

Purpose.—State legislatures have increased the prescribing capabilities of nurse practitioners and physician assistants and broadened the scope of their practice roles. To determine the impact of these changes, we compared outpatient antibiotic prescribing by practicing physicians, nonphysician clinicians, and resident physicians.

Methods.—Using the National Ambulatory Medical Care Survey (NAMCS) and the National Hospital Ambulatory Medical Care Survey (NHAMCS), we conducted a cross-sectional study of patients ≥18 years of age receiving care in 3 outpatient settings: office practices, hospital practices, and emergency departments, 1995-2000. We measured the proportion of all visits and visits for respiratory diagnoses where antibiotics are rarely indicated in which an antibiotic was prescribed by practitioner type.

Results.—For all patient visits, nonphysician clinicians were more likely to prescribe antibiotics than practicing physicians for visits in office practices (26.3% vs 16.2%), emergency departments (23.8% vs 18.2%), and hospital clinics (25.2% vs 14.6%). Similarly, for the subset of visits for respiratory conditions where antibiotics are rarely indicated, nonphysician clinicians prescribed antibiotics more often than practicing physicians in office practices (odds ratio [OR] 1.86, 95% confidence intervals [CI]: 1.05 to 3.29), and in hospital practices (OR 1.55, 95% CI: 1.12 to 2.15). In hospital practices, resident physicians had lower prescribing rates than practicing physicians for all visits as well as visits for respiratory conditions where antibiotics are rarely indicated (OR 0.56, 95% CI: 0.36 to 0.86).

Conclusion.—Nonphysician clinicians were more likely to prescribe antibiotics than practicing physicians in outpatient settings, and resident physicians were less likely to prescribe antibiotics. These differences suggest that general educational campaigns to reduce antibiotic prescribing have not reached all providers.

▶ The use of physician extenders is increasing.[1] Thus, the relatively high rate of antibiotic use among these practitioners is a concern and indicates that strategies to decrease the inappropriate use of these drugs should extend beyond physicians. Interestingly, Roumie et al found lower prescribing rates among house officers than among practicing physicians.

B. H. Thiers, MD

Reference

1. Druss GB, Marcus SC, Olfson M, et al: Trends in care by nonphysician clinicians in the United States. *N Engl J Med* 348:130-137, 2003.

"Breakthrough" Drugs and Growth in Expenditure on Prescription Drugs in Canada

Morgan SG, Bassett KL, Wright JM, et al (Univ of British Columbia, Vancouver, Canada)
BMJ 331:815-816, 2005   13–8

Background.—Spending on prescription drugs in Canada has doubled between 1996 and 2003. This dramatic increase in spending has been driven by the increased use of prescription drugs and by a shift from old to new pharmaceuticals. In an effort to determine which drugs account for this growth in expenditures, the Canadian Patented Medicine Prices Review Board appraises the therapeutic novelty of every patented medicine in Canada. The goal of this review is to distinguish "breakthrough" drugs from other medicines. In the present study, the review board's classification for breakthrough drugs was applied to total expenditures on and use of prescription drugs in British Columbia.

Methods.—From 1990 to 2003, the board appraised 1147 newly patented drugs, including derivatives of existing medicines. Of these new drugs, 68 (5.9%) met the criterion of being breakthrough drugs. The term *breakthrough drug* was defined as "the first drug to treat effectively a particular illness or which provides a substantial improvement over existing drug products." The remaining 1005 drugs were not determined to meet the breakthrough criteria and were designated as "me-too" drugs. Drugs marketed before 1990 were classified as either "vintage brand" or "vintage generic" drugs.

Results.—From 1996 to 2003, the per capita expenditure on prescription drugs rose from $141 to $316, and the per capita days of treatment increased from 194 to 301 days. The cost per day supplied rose from $0.73 to $1.05. The use of breakthrough drugs accounted for 6% of expenditure and 1% of use in 1996 and 10% of expenditure and 2% of use in 2003. The use of vintage brand and vintage generic drugs combined accounted for 75% of the total use in 1996 and 54% of the total use in 2003 but only 53% and 27% of the total annual expenditure for those 2 years, respectively. In contrast, the use of me-too drugs accounted for 44% of use and 63% of expenditure by 2003. The average cost per day of treatment for me-too drugs was twice that of vintage brand drugs and 4 times that of vintage generic drugs.

Conclusions.—In British Columbia, 80% of the increase in spending on prescription drugs from 1996 to 2003 was attributable to the use of new, patented pharmaceutical products that did not offer substantial improvements on less-expensive alternatives available before 1990. The rising cost of using these me-too drugs at prices far in excess of those of time-tested competitors should be carefully examined. It is likely that me-too drugs dominate spending trends in most of the developed world.

▶ New drugs are more expensive and more heavily promoted than their predecessors, but are they better? This is a question physicians need to ask, especially in the context of this study, which showed that 80% of expenditure growth in the authors' province was attributable to new drugs launched in established chemical subclasses.

B. H. Thiers, MD

14 Practice Management and Managed Care

Patients' Attitudes Toward Resident Participation in Dermatology Outpatient Clinics

Crawford GH, Gutman A, Kantor J, et al (Univ of Pennsylvania, Philadelphia)

J Am Acad Dermatol 53:710-712, 2005   14–1

Introduction.—The attitudes of patients toward resident participation in a university-based dermatology outpatient clinic were evaluated. Of 206 patients asked to participate, 191 patients completed the self-administered questionnaire (92.7%). The overwhelming majority of patients (99.5%) were satisfied (81.8% "very satisfied" and 17.7% "satisfied") with the resident's participation in their care. Many more patients expressed a willingness to allow residents to take histories (93.6%), perform physical examinations (87.2%), and counsel on preventive measures (74.5%), than to allow surgical excisions of skin cancers (19.7%), perform skin biopsies (43.6%), or prescribe medications (44.7%). Of respondents to the questionnaire, 83.2% self-reported an understanding of the difference between "resident" and "attending" physicians. However, only 31.3% (95% confidence interval 24.5-38.1) were able to broadly categorize the amount of training completed by dermatology residents. Dermatology resident participation in outpatient clinics is essential to quality dermatologic education. Consistent with the results of prior studies in other medical disciplines, our study demonstrated an overwhelming patient satisfaction with the participation of dermatology residents in their care.

▶ The time a patient spends with a resident physician is often of longer duration than the time spent with the attending physician. I believe patients enjoy this attention and that the resident physician is a valuable asset in the academic medical setting.

B. H. Thiers, MD

Disciplinary Action by Medical Boards and Prior Behavior in Medical School

Papadakis MA, Teherani A, Banach MA, et al (Univ of California, San Francisco; Federation of State Med Boards, Dallas; Thomas Jefferson Univ, Philadelphia; et al)

N Engl J Med 353:2673-2682, 2005   14–2

Background.—Evidence supporting professionalism as a critical measure of competence in medical education is limited. In this case–control study, we investigated the association of disciplinary action against practicing physicians with prior unprofessional behavior in medical school. We also examined the specific types of behavior that are most predictive of disciplinary action against practicing physicians with unprofessional behavior in medical school.

Methods.—The study included 235 graduates of three medical schools who were disciplined by one of 40 state medical boards between 1990 and 2003 (case physicians). The 469 control physicians were matched with the case physicians according to medical school and graduation year. Predictor variables from medical school included the presence or absence of narratives describing unprofessional behavior, grades, standardized-test scores, and demographic characteristics. Narratives were assigned an overall rating for unprofessional behavior. Those that met the threshold for unprofessional behavior were further classified among eight types of behavior and assigned a severity rating (moderate to severe).

Results.—Disciplinary action by a medical board was strongly associated with prior unprofessional behavior in medical school (odds ratio, 3.0; 95 percent confidence interval, 1.9 to 4.8), for a population attributable risk of disciplinary action of 26 percent. The types of unprofessional behavior most strongly linked with disciplinary action were severe irresponsibility (odds ratio, 8.5; 95 percent confidence interval, 1.8 to 40.1) and severely diminished capacity for self-improvement (odds ratio, 3.1; 95 percent confidence interval, 1.2 to 8.2). Disciplinary action by a medical board was also associated with low scores on the Medical College Admission Test and poor grades in the first two years of medical school (1 percent and 7 percent population attributable risk, respectively), but the association with these variables was less strong than that with unprofessional behavior.

Conclusions.—In this case–control study, disciplinary action among practicing physicians by medical boards was strongly associated with unprofessional behavior in medical school. Students with the strongest association were those who were described as irresponsible or as having diminished ability to improve their behavior. Professionalism should have a central role in medical academics and throughout one's medical career.

▶ This study demonstrates that among some individuals, unprofessional behavior is sustained over decades. It extends the finding of another recent report that showed that medical students who lack thoroughness are unable to perceive their weaknesses the first 2 years of medical school and are more likely than those who do not have these deficiencies to be identified as unprofessional in the clinical years.[1]

B. H. Thiers, MD

Reference

1. Stern DT, Frohna AZ, Gruppen LD: The predication of professional behaviour. *Med Educ* 39:75-82, 2005.

What to Wear Today? Effect of Doctor's Attire on the Trust and Confidence of Patients

Rehman SU, Nietert PJ, Cope DW, et al (Med Univ of South Carolina, Charleston; Univ of California at Los Angeles)
Am J Med 118:1279-1286, 2005   14–3

Purpose.—There are very few studies about the impact of physicians' attire on patients' confidence and trust. The objective of this study was to determine whether the way a doctor dresses is an important factor in the degree of trust and confidence among respondents.

Methods.—A cross-sectional descriptive study using survey methodology was conducted of patients and visitors in the waiting room of an internal medicine outpatient clinic. Respondents completed a written survey after reviewing pictures of physicians in four different dress styles. Respondents were asked questions related to their preference for physician dress as well as their trust and willingness to discuss sensitive issues.

Results.—Four hundred respondents with a mean age of 52.4 years were enrolled; 54% were men, 58% were white, 38% were African-American, and 43% had greater than a high school diploma. On all questions regarding physician dress style preferences, respondents significantly favored the professional attire with white coat (76.3%, $P <.0001$), followed by surgical scrubs (10.2%), business dress (8.8%), and casual dress (4.7%). Their trust and confidence was significantly associated with their preference for professional dress ($P <.0001$). Respondents also reported that they were significantly more willing to share their social, sexual, and psychological problems with the physician who is professionally dressed ($P <.0001$). The importance of physician's appearance was ranked similarly between male and female respondents ($P=.54$); however, female physicians' dress appeared to be significantly more important to respondents than male physicians' dress ($P <.001$).

Conclusion.—Respondents overwhelmingly favor physicians in professional attire with a white coat. Wearing professional dress (ie, a white coat with more formal attire) while providing patient care by physicians may favorably influence trust and confidence-building in the medical encounter.

▶ The message is quite clear: appearance does make a difference. Further studies should address whether the increased confidence that may be shown in appropriately dressed physicians is associated with better patient compliance with their recommendations.

B. H. Thiers, MD

The Relation of Patient Satisfaction With Complaints Against Physicians and Malpractice Lawsuits

Stelfox HT, Ghandi TK, Orav EJ, et al (Massachusetts Gen Hosp, Boston; Brigham and Women's Hosp, Boston)
Am J Med 118:1126-1133, 2005   14–4

Purpose.—A small number of physicians generate a disproportionate share of complaints from patients and of malpractice lawsuits. If these grievances relate to patients' dissatisfaction with care, it might be possible to use commonly distributed patient satisfaction surveys to identify physicians at high risk of complaints from patients and of malpractice lawsuits. We sought to examine associations among patients' satisfaction survey ratings of physicians' performance and complaints from patients, risk management episodes, and rates of malpractice lawsuits.

Subjects and Methods.—We examined 353 physicians at a large US teaching hospital whose inpatient performance was rated by 10 or more patients between January 1, 2001, and March 31, 2003. Physicians were divided into 3 tertiles according to satisfaction on a commercial survey instrument administered to recently discharged patients. Records of unsolicited complaints from patients (January 1, 2000, to March 31, 2003) and risk management episodes (January 1, 1983, to March 31, 2003) were analyzed after adjusting for the physician's specialty and panel characteristics of the physician's patients.

Results.—Decreases in physicians' patient satisfaction survey scores from the highest to the lowest tertile were associated with increased rates of unsolicited complaints from patients (200 vs 243 vs 492 complaints per 100,000 patient discharges; $P < 0.0001$) and risk management episodes (29 vs 43 vs 56 risk management episodes per 100,000 patient discharges; $P = 0.007$). Compared with physicians with the top satisfaction survey ratings, physicians in the middle tertile had malpractice lawsuit rates that were 26% higher (rate ratio [RR] = 1.26; 95% confidence interval [CI]: 0.72 to 2.18; $P = 0.41$), and physicians in the bottom tertile had malpractice lawsuit rates that were 110% higher (RR = 2.10; 95% CI: 1.13 to 3.90; $P = 0.019$).

Conclusion.—Patient satisfaction survey ratings of inpatient physicians' performance are associated with complaints from patients and with risk management episodes. Commonly distributed patient satisfaction surveys may be useful quality improvement tools, but identifying physicians at high risk of complaints from patients and of malpractice lawsuits remains challenging.

▶ This study found that a small number of physicians generate a disproportionate share of complaints from patients and malpractice law suits. The authors demonstrate that physicians who receive low patient satisfaction ratings are more likely to have complaints from patients and malpractice lawsuits than are those who receive high ratings. Malpractice risks could be differentiated based on patient satisfaction measures even after controlling for physician specialty and characteristics of the patient panel. This study emphasizes the importance of soliciting feedback from patients.

B. H. Thiers, MD

Evaluation of a General Practitioner With Special Interest Service for Dermatology: Randomised Controlled Trial
Salisbury C, Noble A, Horrocks S, et al (Univ of Bristol, England; Univ of West of England, Glenside Campus; Univ of Southampton, Lymington, England; et al)
BMJ 331:1441-1446, 2005   14–5

Objective.—To assess the effectiveness, accessibility, and acceptability of a general practitioner with special interest service for skin problems compared with a hospital dermatology clinic.

Design.—Randomised controlled trial.

Setting.—General practitioner with special interest dermatology service and hospital dermatology clinic.

Participants.—Adults referred to a hospital dermatology clinic and assessed by a consultant or the general practitioner with special interest service. Suitable patients had non-urgent skin problems and had been identified from the referral letter as suitable for management by a general practitioner with special interest.

Interventions.—Participants were randomised in 2:1 ratio to receive management by a general practitioner with special interest or usual hospital outpatient care.

Main Outcome Measures.—Primary outcomes were disease related quality of life (dermatology life quality index) and improvement in patients' perception of access to services, assessed nine months after randomisation. Secondary outcomes were patient satisfaction, preference for site of care, proportion of failed appointments, and waiting times to first appointment.

Results.—49% of the participants were judged suitable for care by the general practitioner with special interest service. Of 768 patients eligible, 556 (72.4%) were randomised (354 to general practitioner with special interest, 202 to hospital outpatient care). After nine months, 422 (76%) were followed up. No noticeable differences were found between the groups in clinical outcome (median dermatology life quality index score = 1 both arms, ratio of geometric means 0.99, 95% confidence interval 0.85 to 1.15). The general practitioner with special interest service was more accessible (difference between means on access scale 14, 11 to 19) and waited a mean of 40 (35 to 46) days less. Patients expressed slightly greater satisfaction with consultations with a general practitioner with special interest (difference in mean satisfaction score 4, 1 to 7), and at baseline and after nine months 61% said they preferred care at the service.

Conclusions.—The general practitioner with special interest service for dermatology was more accessible and preferred by patients than hospital outpatient care, achieving similar clinical outcomes. Trial registration ISRCTN31962758.

Economic Evaluation of a General Practitioner With Special Interests Led Dermatology Service in Primary Care
Coast J, Noble S, Noble A, et al (Univ of Bristol, England; Univ of West of England, Bristol; Univ of Oxford, England)
BMJ 331:1444-1449, 2005   14–6

Objective.—To carry out an economic evaluation of a general practitioner with special interest service for non-urgent skin problems compared with hospital outpatient care.

Design.—Cost effectiveness analysis and cost consequences analysis alongside a randomised controlled trial.

Setting.—General practitioner with special interest dermatology service covering 29 general practices in Bristol.

Participants.—Adults referred to a hospital dermatology clinic who were potentially suitable for management by a general practitioner with special interest.

Interventions.—Participants were randomised 2:1 to receive either care by general practitioner with special interest service or usual hospital outpatient care.

Main Outcome Measures.—Costs to NHS, patients, and companions, and costs of lost production. Cost effectiveness, using the two primary outcomes of dermatology life quality index scores and improved patient perceived access, was assessed by incremental cost effectiveness ratios and cost effectiveness acceptability curves. Cost consequences are presented in relation to all costs and both primary and secondary outcomes from the trial.

Results.—Costs to the NHS for patients attending the general practitioner with special interest service were 208 pounds sterling (361 dollars; 308 euro) compared with 118 pounds sterling for hospital outpatient care. Based on analysis with imputation of missing data, costs to patients and companions were 48 pounds sterling and 51 pounds sterling, respectively; costs of lost production were 27 pounds sterling and 34 pounds sterling, respectively. The incremental cost effectiveness ratios for general practitioner with special interest care over outpatient care were 540 pounds sterling per one point gain in the dermatology life quality index and 66 pounds sterling per 10 point change in the access scale.

Conclusions.—The general practitioner with special interest service for dermatology is more costly than hospital outpatient care, but this additional cost needs to be weighed against improved access and broadly similar health outcomes.

▶ The concept of a general practitioner with a special area of interest was promoted in the British National Health Service Plan made public several years ago,[1] and data published since then have demonstrated that more general practitioners claim dermatology as a special interest than any other clinical specialty, with the exception of diabetes care.[2] This approach has been used by selected managed care organizations in the United States as well, where general practitioners have been urged to refer patients with skin problems to their colleagues who claim special expertise in dermatology rather than utilizing the services of a board-certified specialist. There is no evidence that this type of service provides good clinical outcomes, improves accessibility, or is acceptable to patients. Salisbury et al (Abstract 14–5) found no evidence that British patients with nonurgent skin problems treated by a general practitioner with a special interest in dermatology had outcomes different than those patients who received routine nonspecialist care. However, these patients were seen more quickly, found the services to be more accessible than hospital outpatient care, and were somewhat more satisfied. Coast et al (Abstract 14–6) studied the economics of such special interest schemes in terms of their relative cost-effectiveness compared with routine outpatient hospital care. They found that the general practitioner with a special interest is more expensive than routine nonspecialist outpatient care while providing little difference in clinical outcome. They note that this higher cost must be offset against improved accessibility. Neither study addresses outcomes, accessibility, or costs when utilizing a consultant (ie, specialist), compared with the nonspecialist approaches used to generate these data. In an accompanying editorial, Roland[3] asserts that general practitioners with special interests need to work in close collaboration with local specialists to obtain ongoing training and education and to maximize effectiveness and safety. Unfortunately, in the United Kingdom, as in the United States, many general practitioners with special interests are not receiving nationally standardized levels of training.[4]

B. H. Thiers, MD

References

1. Department of Health: *The NHS Plan. A Plan for Investment. A Plan for Reform.* London, DoH, 2000.
2. Jones R, Bartholomew J: General practitioners with special clinical interests: A cross-sectional survey. *Br J Gen Pract* 52:833-834, 2002.
3. Roland M: General practitioners with special interests: Not a cheap option (commentary). *BMJ* 331:1448-1449, 2005.
4. Schofield JK, Irvine A, Jackson S, et al: General practitioners with a special interest in dermatology: Results of an audit against Department of Health (DH) guidance. *Br J Dermatol* 153:O-1, 2005.

Quality of Care in For-Profit and Not-For-Profit Health Plans Enrolling Medicare Beneficiaries

Schneider EC, Zaslavsky AM, Epstein AM (Harvard School of Public Health, Boston; Harvard Med School, Boston)
Am J Med 118:1392-1400, 2005   14–7

Background.— For profit health plans now enroll the majority of Medicare beneficiaries who select managed care. Prior research has produced conflicting results about whether for-profit health plans provide lower quality of care.

Objective.—The objective was to compare the quality of care delivered by for-profit and not-for-profit health plans using Medicare Health Plan Employer Data and Information Set (HEDIS) clinical measures.

Research Design.—This was an observational study comparing HEDIS scores in for-profit and not-for-profit health plans that enrolled Medicare beneficiaries in the United States during 1997.

Outcome Measures.—Outcome measures included health plan quality scores on each of 4 clinical services assessed by HEDIS: breast cancer screening, diabetic eye examination, beta-blocker medication after myocardial infarction, and follow-up after hospitalization for mental illness.

Results.—The quality of care was lower in for-profit health plans than not-for-profit health plans on all 4 of the HEDIS measures we studied (67.5% vs 74.8% for breast cancer screening, 43.7% vs 57.7% for diabetic eye examination, 63.1% vs 75.2% for beta-blocker medication after myocardial infarction, and 42.1% vs 60.4% for follow-up after hospitalization for mental illness). Adjustment for sociodemographic case-mix and health plan characteristics reduced but did not eliminate the differences, which remained statistically significant for 3 of the 4 measures (not beta-blocker medication after myocardial infarction). Different geographic locations of for-profit and not-for-profit health plans did not explain these differences.

Conclusion.—By using standardized performance measures applied in a mandatory measurement program, we found that for-profit health plans provide lower quality of care than not-for-profit health plans. Special efforts to monitor and improve the quality of for-profit health plans may be warranted.

▶ The authors found that the quality of care delivered to Medicare beneficiaries was substantially higher in not-for-profit health plans than in for-profit health plans. This is particularly disturbing in light of the prominent role of for-profit health plans in Medicare and the payment changes designed to accelerate enrollment in these plans. It appears that the financial incentives of for-profit plans lead to less aggressive efforts to manage the quality of care, which suggests that strict monitoring of these plans is mandatory. The variability of performance within both not-for-profit and for-profit plans indicates that a blanket indictment of the latter may be premature.

B. H. Thiers, MD

Potential Savings From Substituting Generic Drugs for Brand-Name Drugs: Medical Expenditure Panel Survey, 1997-2000

Haas JS, Phillips KA, Gerstenberger EP, et al (Brigham and Women's Hosp, Boston; Univ of California, San Francisco)
Ann Intern Med 142:891-897, 2005   14–8

Background.—Generic substitution is one mechanism of curtailing prescription drug expenditures. Limited information is available about the potential savings associated with generic substitution.

Objective.—To estimate the potential savings associated with broad substitution of generic drugs.

Design.—Cross-sectional, nationally representative survey of noninstitutionalized adults.

Setting.—United States.

Participants.—Adults included in the Medical Expenditure Panel Survey Household Component, 1997–2000.

Measurements.—Use of a multisource drug (that is, a drug available in a brand-name and ≥ 1 generic formulation) or a generic drug and the potential cost savings associated with broad generic substitution for all multisource products.

Results.—Fifty-six percent of all outpatient drugs were multisource products, accounting for 41% of total outpatient drug expenditures. Of these multisource drugs, 61% were dispensed as a generic. If a generic had been substituted for all corresponding brand-name outpatient drugs in 2000, the median annual savings in drug expenditures per person would have been $45.89 (interquartile range, $10.35 to $158.06) for adults younger than 65 years of age and $78.05 (interquartile range, $19.94 to $241.72) for adults at least 65 years of age. In these age groups, the national savings would have been $5.9 billion (95% CI, $5.5 billion to $6.2 billion) and $2.9 billion (CI, $2.6 billion to $3.1 billion), respectively, representing approximately 11% of drug expenditures.

Limitations.—Specific information about an individual's formulary was not available, so the authors could not estimate how much of the potential savings would benefit an individual or his or her health plan.

Conclusion.—Although broad substitution of generic drugs would affect only a modest percentage of drug expenditures, it could result in substantial absolute savings.

▶ Clearly, substitution of cheaper generic drugs for the more expensive brand-name counterparts might reduce prescription costs. Haas et al estimated that substitution of a generic for brand-name drugs when available would save $46 to $78 per person annually, depending on the patient's age. This translates into considerable savings nationwide, which the authors approximate to be $3 billion to $6 billion.

B. H. Thiers, MD

15 Miscellaneous Topics in Clinical Dermatology

Are the Clinical Effects of Homoeopathy Placebo Effects? Comparative Study of Placebo-controlled Trials of Homoeopathy and Allopathy
Shang A, Huwiler-Müntener K, Nartey L, et al (Univ of Berne, Switzerland; Univ of Bristol, England; Univ of Zürich, Switzerland; et al)
Lancet 366:726-732, 2005   15–1

Background.—Homoeopathy is widely used, but specific effects of homoeopathic remedies seem implausible. Bias in the conduct and reporting of trials is a possible explanation for positive findings of trials of both homoeopathy and conventional medicine. We analysed trials of homoeopathy and conventional medicine and estimated treatment effects in trials least likely to be affected by bias.

Methods.—Placebo-controlled trials of homoeopathy were identified by a comprehensive literature search, which covered 19 electronic databases, reference lists of relevant papers, and contacts with experts. Trials in conventional medicine matched to homoeopathy trials for disorder and type of outcome were randomly selected from the Cochrane Controlled Trials Register (issue 1, 2003). Data were extracted in duplicate and outcomes coded so that odds ratios below 1 indicated benefit. Trials described as double-blind, with adequate randomisation, were assumed to be of higher methodological quality. Bias effects were examined in funnel plots and meta-regression models.

Findings.—110 homoeopathy trials and 110 matched conventional-medicine trials were analysed. The median study size was 65 participants (range ten to 1573). 21 homoeopathy trials (19%) and nine (8%) conventional-medicine trials were of higher quality. In both groups, smaller trials and those of lower quality showed more beneficial treatment effects than larger and higher-quality trials. When the analysis was restricted to large trials of higher quality, the odds ratio was 0.88 (95% CI 0.65-1.19) for homoeopathy (eight trials) and 0.58 (0.39-0.85) for conventional medicine (six trials).

Interpretation.—Biases are present in placebo-controlled trials of both homoeopathy and conventional medicine. When account was taken for these biases in the analysis, there was weak evidence for a specific effect of homoeopathic remedies, but strong evidence for specific effects of conventional interventions. This finding is compatible with the notion that the clinical effects of homoeopathy are placebo effects.

▶ Shang et al illustrate the interplay and cumulative effect of different sources of bias. Although they acknowledge that to prove a negative is impossible, they do show that the effects seen in placebo-controlled trials of homeopathy are compatible with the placebo hypothesis. In contrast, using identical methods, they found that the benefits of conventional medicine are unlikely to be explained by nonspecific effects. They compared homeopathy and allopathy in a meta-analysis of 2 sets of 110 placebo-controlled trials. Although initially both seemed effective, a meta-regression and a subgroup of trials of higher quality showed higher sensitivity to potential bias for homeopathic than for allopathic trials. A philosophical approach to the evaluation of homeopathic remedies is presented in a comment[1] that accompanied this study.

B. H. Thiers, MD

Reference

1. Vandenbroucke J: Homoeopathy and "the growth of truth." *Lancet* 366:691-692, 2005.

Neuropathic Scrotal Pruritus: Anogenital Pruritus Is a Symptom of Lumbosacral Radiculopathy

Cohen AD, Vander T, Medvendovsky E, et al (Ben-Gurion Univ, Negev)
J Am Acad Dermatol 52:61-66, 2005   15–2

Background.—Anogenital pruritus is defined as an itch localized to the anus, perianal, and genital skin. Anogenital pruritus is usually a symptom of an underlying disorder of the skin or mucosa or a consequence of anorectal pathology. When no demonstrable cause is found, anogenital pruritus is often described as "idiopathic".

Objective.—To investigate the role of lumbosacral radiculopathy in the pathogenesis of anogenital pruritus.

Methods.—Included in the study were consecutive patients with anogenital pruritus. Radiographs and nerved conduction studies were performed in all patients. Needle electromyography studies and computerized tomography were performed when necessary. Nerve conduction studies included measurement of distal sensory and motor latency, conduction velocity, and F-responses of the peroneal and tibial nerves. Patients with confirmed radiculopathy were treated with paravertebral injection of a mixture of triamcinolone acetonide and lidocaine. Response to the injections was assessed using visual analogue scales by the patients. Mean scores before and after treatment were compared using paired t tests.

Results.—Included in the study were 20 patients with anogenital pruritus. There were 18 men (90%) and 2 (10%) women. The mean age was 52.7 years (standard deviation [SD] 11.7 years). In 16 patients (80%), radiographs demonstrated degenerative changes of the lower spine. In 16 patients (80%) the presence of lumbosacral radiculopathy was confirmed by nerve conduction studies. Fifteen patients (75%) were treated with paravertebral injections, with significant decrease in mean pruritus score as assessed by the patients (6.3 [±2.8]; 4.5 [±2.7], before and after treatment, respectively, $P =$ .033).

Conclusion.—"Idiopathic" anogenital pruritus may be attributable to lumbosacral radiculopathy. Paravertebral blockade may be used for alleviation of symptoms in patients with anogenital pruritus.

▶ This report is reminiscent of previous studies suggesting an association of brachioradial pruritus with cervical radiculopathy.[1,2] The authors' conclusions would be strengthened considerably by a prospective study in which an asymptomatic age-matched control group is investigated for degenerative changes in the lumbosacral spine and a group of patients with anogenital pruritus and lumbosacral radiculopathy is treated with placebo paravertebral injections rather than the triamcinolone/lidocaine mixture.

B. H. Thiers, MD

References

1. Goodkin R, Wingard E, Bernhard JD: Brachioradial pruritus: Cervical spine disease and neurogenic/neuropathic [corrected] pruritus. *J Am Acad Dermatol* 48:521-524, 2003.
2. Cohen AD, Masalha R, Medvedovsky E, et al: Brachioradial pruritus: A symptom of neuropathy. *J Am Acad Dermatol* 48:825-828, 2003.

Efficacy of Lidocaine in the Treatment of Pruritus in Patients With Chronic Cholestatic Liver Diseases

Villamil AG, Bandi JC, Galdame OA, et al (Hospital Italiano de Buenos Aires, Argentina)
Am J Med 118:1160-1163, 2005   15–3

Background.—Pruritus is often a complication in patients with chronic cholestatic liver disease. For decades, pruritus has been associated with the effect of bile salts or other poorly defined pruritogenic substances over free unmyelinated type C nerve endings of dermic nociceptors. However, mounting evidence supports the theory that different putative mediators involved in neurotransmission and neuromodulation over opioid and serotoninergic receptors (ie, enkephalins) may be potential mediators of cholestasis-induced itching in the CNS. Lidocaine is a sodium-channel blocker and may inhibit abnormal activity in peripheral nerve endings; thus, it may be effec-

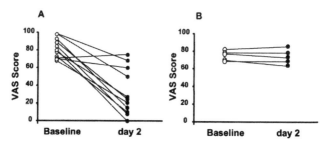

FIGURE 3.—VAS score of pruritus at baseline and at day 2 for each patient treated with (**A**) lidocaine or (**B**) placebo. Data are shown as absolute values. Only 1 patient in the lidocaine group showed no effect over severity of pruritus at day 2 ($P < .05$ vs placebo). *Abbreviation: VAS*, Visual analog scale. (Reprinted from Villamil AG, Bandi JC, Galdame OA, et al: Efficacy of lidocaine in the treatment of pruritus in patients with chronic cholestatic liver diseases. *Am J Med* 118:1160-1163, 2005. Copyright 2005, with permission from Elsevier Science.)

tive in patients who are resistant to conventional antipruritic medications. The efficacy of lidocaine for use in treatment-resistant pruritus was determined in patients with chronic liver disease.

Methods.—The study was conducted from 1999 to 2002 in 18 patients with treatment-resistant pruritus associated with cholestatic liver diseases at a hospital in Buenos Aires, Argentina. The specific liver diseases were primary biliary cirrhosis (13 patients), primary sclerosing cholangitis (4 patients), and drug-induced chronic cholestasis (1 patient). All patients had persistent pruritus in the 3 months preceding enrollment in the study. The patients were randomly assigned to receive 100 mg IV lidocaine over 5 minutes or placebo. They were then asked to record the severity of their pruritus on a visual analog scale at baseline and at every 12 hours for the next 7 days.

Results.—Two patients, one in each group, were excluded from the analysis. No significant changes in the severity of pruritus and fatigue were seen in patients in the placebo group. Lidocaine administration resulted in a significant reduction in the severity of pruritus when compared with placebo administration (Fig 3).

Conclusions.—IV lidocaine may reduce the severity of pruritus in patients with chronic cholestatic liver diseases resistant to conventional antipruritic medications.

▶ The authors present data to support consideration of IV lidocaine as a therapeutic alternative in patients with treatment-resistant pruritus associated with cholestatic liver disease.

B. H. Thiers, MD

Gabapentin for Hot Flashes in 420 Women With Breast Cancer: A Randomised Double-blind Placebo-controlled Trial

Pandya KJ, Morrow GR, Roscoe JA, et al (Univ of Rochester, NY)
Lancet 366:818-824, 2005   15–4

Background.—Most women receiving systemic therapy for breast cancer experience hot flashes. We undertook a randomised, double-blind, placebo-controlled, multi-institutional trial to assess the efficacy of gabapentin in controlling hot flashes in women with breast cancer.

Methods.—420 women with breast cancer who were having two or more hot flashes per day were randomly assigned placebo, gabapentin 300 mg/ day, or gabapentin 900 mg/day by mouth in three divided doses for 8 weeks. Each patient kept a 1-week, self-report diary on the frequency, severity, and duration of hot flashes before the start of the study and during weeks 4 and 8 of treatment. Analyses were by intention to treat.

Findings.—Evaluable data were available on 371 participants at 4 weeks (119 placebo, 123 gabapentin 300 mg, and 129 gabapentin 900 mg) and 347 at 8 weeks (113 placebo, 114 gabapentin 300 mg, and 120 gabapentin 900 mg). The percentage decreases in hot-flash severity score between baseline and weeks 4 and 8, respectively were: 21% (95% CI 12 to 30) and 15% (1 to 29) in the placebo group; 33% (23 to 43) and 31% (16 to 46) in the group assigned gabapentin 300 mg; and 49% (42 to 56) and 46% (34 to 58) in the group assigned gabapentin 900 mg. The differences between the groups were significant ($p=0.0001$ at 4 weeks and $p=0.007$ at 8 weeks by ANCOVA for overall treatment effect, adjusted for baseline values); only the higher dose of gabapentin was associated with significant decreases in hot-flash frequency and severity.

Interpretation.—Gabapentin is effective in the control of hot flashes at a dose of 900 mg/day, but not at a dose of 300 mg/day. This drug should be considered for treatment of hot flashes in women with breast cancer.

Gabapentin Therapy for Pruritus in Haemodialysis Patients: A Randomized, Placebo-controlled, Double-blind Trial

Gunal AI, Ozalp G, Yoldas TK, et al (Firat Univ, Elazig, Turkey)
Nephrol Dial Transplant 19:3137-3139, 2004   15–5

Background.—Uraemic pruritus is a common and distressing symptom in patients on haemodialysis for chronic renal failure. Gabapentin is an anticonvulsant that alleviates neuropathic pain. We conducted a double-blind, placebo-controlled, crossover study to assess its effectiveness against renal itch.

Methods.—We enrolled in the trial 25 adult patients on haemodialysis who were asked to daily record the severity of their pruritus on a visual analogue scale. The patients were randomly assigned to receive gabapentin for 4 weeks followed by placebo for 4 weeks or the reverse sequence. Gabapentin or placebo were administered thrice weekly, at the end of haemodialysis sessions.

Results.—The mean pruritus score of the cohort before the study was 8.4 ± 0.94. After placebo intake, it decreased to 7.6 ± 2.6 ($P = 0.098$). The score of four patients decreased by >50% following placebo. After gabapentin administration, the mean score decreased significantly, to 1.2 ± 1.8 ($P = 0.0001$), although one patient's symptoms did not improve significantly. No patient dropped out of the study due to adverse effects from gabapentin.

Conclusions.—Our study shows that gabapentin is safe and effective for treating uraemic pruritus in haemodialysis patients. Our results also support the neuropathic hypothesis of uraemic pruritus.

▶ Gabapentin is another drug in a long line of treatments that have been proposed for the control of hot flashes in patients with breast cancer and of uremic pruritus in patients on hemodialysis (Abstracts 15–4 and 15–5). Whether it will stand the test of time can only be a matter for speculation. Gabapentin is certainly not a benign drug, and any physician prescribing it should be well versed in its potential side effects.

B. H. Thiers, MD

Deficiency of a Subset of T Cells With Immunoregulatory Properties in Sarcoidosis
Ho L-P, Urban BC, Thickett DR, et al (John Radcliffe Hosp, Oxford, England; Churchill Hosp, Oxford, England; Univ of Birmingham, England)
Lancet 365:1062-1072, 2005   15–6

Background.—Sarcoidosis is a multisystem disorder that predominantly involves the lungs, characterised by a T-helper 1 (Th1) biased CD4-positive T-cell response and granuloma formation, for which the explanation is unknown. A newly identified subset of T-cells with immunoregulatory functions, CD1d-restricted natural-killer T (NKT) cells, has been shown to protect against disorders with increased CD4-positive Th1 responses in animals. We explored whether abnormalities in these cells are implicated in the pathogenesis of sarcoidosis.

Methods.—We generated fluorescence-labelled CD1d-tetrameric complexes and used them, with monoclonal antibodies to Vα24 and Vβ11 T-cell receptor, to assess the frequency of CD1d-restricted NKT cells in the peripheral blood of 60 patients with histologically proven sarcoidosis (16 with Löfgren's syndrome) and 60 healthy controls. Lung lymphocytes were also analysed in 16 of the patients with sarcoidosis.

Findings.—CD1d-restricted NKT cells were absent or greatly reduced in peripheral blood from all patients with sarcoidosis, except those with Löfgren's syndrome (median proportion of lymphocytes 0.01% [IQR 0-0.03] vs 0.06% [0.03-0.12] in controls; p=0.0004). The deficiency was found in both acute and resolved disease and was unrelated to systemic corticosteroid therapy. There was no difference in the proportion of CD1d-restricted NKT cells between peripheral blood and lungs in patients, suggesting that the peripheral-blood deficiency is not due to sequestration of these cells in the lungs. The NKT cells were not observed in mediastinal lymph nodes or granulomatous lesions. CD1d expression on antigen-presenting cells of patients was normal, thus the deficiency of CD1d-restricted NKT cells is not explained by abnormal CD1d expression.

Interpretation.—Loss of immunoregulation by CD1d-restricted NKT cells could explain the amplified and persistent T-cell activity that characterises sarcoidosis.

Relevance to practice.—Our findings give new insight into the pathogenesis of sarcoidosis and draw attention to a potential target for therapeutic modulation in sarcoidosis.

▶ The authors demonstrate a defect in the frequency of and, at times, a complete loss of a subset of T cells with immunoregulatory functions in patients with sarcoidosis. They suggest that this defect could contribute to the prolonged and amplified immune response that characterizes the disease.

B. H. Thiers, MD

Treatment of Sarcoidosis With Infliximab
Doty JD, Mazur JE, Judson MA (Med Univ of South Carolina, Charleston, SC)
Chest 127:1064-1071, 2005   15–7

Background/Objectives.—Many patients with sarcoidosis are unable to tolerate corticosteroids or alternative therapeutic agents due to side effects or have disease refractory to these agents. We report our experience using infliximab to treat such patients.

Methods.—A group of patients in whom traditional sarcoidosis therapy failed, either due to drug failure or intolerable side effects, were prescribed infliximab. Their charts were retrospectively reviewed.

Results.—Ten patients receiving infliximab were reviewed. Nine of the 10 patients reported a symptomatic improvement with therapy, and all 10 demonstrated objective evidence of improvement. A drug reaction developed in one patient after several months of therapy, oral candidiasis developed in one patient, and angioimmunoblastic lymphoma developed in another patient. The corticosteroid dose was reduced in five of the six patients who were receiving corticosteroids at the time of infliximab therapy.

Conclusion.—Infliximab appears to be an effective, safe treatment for patients with refractory sarcoidosis, including such manifestations as lupus pernio, uveitis, hepatic sarcoidosis, and neurosarcoidosis. Infliximab appears to be steroid sparing. Patients receiving the drug should be screened for latent tuberculosis and lymphoproliferative disorders.

▶ This series adds to a growing body of literature supporting infliximab as an effective agent for sarcoidosis. However, the authors' conclusion that infliximab appears to be safe for this indication may be premature, especially given the side effects outlined in the study. Certainly, a double-blind controlled study with long-term follow-up will be essential to establish the exact role of the drug in the treatment of sarcoidosis.

B. H. Thiers, MD

Etanercept Plus Standard Therapy for Wegener's Granulomatosis
Stone JH, for the Wegener's Granulomatosis Etanercept Trial (WGET) Research Group (Johns Hopkins Vasculitis Ctr, Baltimore, Md)
N Engl J Med 352:351-361, 2005   15–8

Background.—The majority of patients with Wegener's granulomatosis have disease flares after conventional medications are tapered. There is no consistently safe, effective treatment for the maintenance of remission.

Methods.—We conducted a randomized, placebo-controlled trial at eight centers to evaluate etanercept for the maintenance of remission in 180 patients with Wegener's granulomatosis. The primary outcome was sustained remission, defined as a Birmingham Vasculitis Activity Score for Wegener's Granulomatosis of 0 for at least six months (scores can range from 0 to 67, with higher scores indicating more active disease). In addition to etanercept or placebo, patients received standard therapy (glucocorticoids plus cyclophosphamide or methotrexate). After remission, standard medications were tapered according to the protocol.

Results.—The mean follow-up for the overall cohort was 27 months. Of the 174 patients who could be evaluated, 126 (72.4 percent) had a sustained remission, but only 86 (49.4 percent) remained in remission for the remainder of the trial. There were no significant differences between the etanercept and control groups in the rates of sustained remission (69.7 percent vs. 75.3 percent, $P=0.39$), sustained periods of low-level disease activity (86.5 percent vs. 90.6 percent, $P=0.32$), or the time required to achieve those measures. Disease flares were common in both groups, with 118 flares in the etanercept group (23 severe and 95 limited) and 134 in the control group (25 severe and 109 limited). There was no significant difference between the etanercept and control groups in the relative risk of disease flares per 100 person-years of follow-up (0.89, $P=0.54$). During the study, 56.2 percent of patients in the etanercept group and 57.1 percent of those in the control group had at least one severe or life-threatening adverse event or died ($P=0.90$). Solid cancers developed in six patients in the etanercept group, as compared with none in the control group ($P=0.01$).

Conclusions.—Etanercept is not effective for the maintenance of remission in patients with Wegener's granulomatosis. Durable remissions were achieved in only a minority of the patients, and there was a high rate of treatment-related complications.

▶ The results clearly were disappointing. As argued in an accompanying editorial by Bacon, more research into the granulomatous nature of Wegener's granulomatosis is needed to help identify new drug targets that may make long-term maintenance of remission as effective as current regimens for the induction of remission.[1]

B. H. Thiers, MD

Reference

1. Bacon PA: The spectrum of Wegener's granulomatosis and disease relapse. *N Engl J Med* 352:330-332, 2005.

Is Oral Granulomatosis in Children a Feature of Crohn's Disease
Khouri JM, Bohane TD, Day AS (Sydney Children's Hosp)
Acta Paediatr 94:501-504, 2005   15–9

Introduction.—Orofacial granulomatosis is a term generally used to describe lip swelling secondary to an underlying granulomatous inflammatory process. Granulomatous cheilitis is the histopathological description of such inflammation occurring in the lips and surrounding tissues. Melkersson-Rosenthal syndrome (a triad of orofacial swelling, facial paralysis and a fissured tongue) is one manifestation of orofacial granulomatosis, which more commonly presents as granulomatous cheilitis alone. Oral Crohn's disease also belongs to the entity of orofacial granulomatosis. Most reported cases of orofacial granulomatosis have been in adults and some in adolescents. We present six children presenting with orofacial granulomatosis at an early age (range 5-8 y) whose course points towards the development of Crohn's disease. Conclusion: Orofacial granulomatosis in the paediatric population may be an initial manifestation of Crohn's disease and so careful surveillance is recommended.

▶ Orofacial granulomatosis in young children is uncommon but, when present, may be related to Crohn's disease. Initially, only subclinical intestinal pathology may be present. When orofacial granulomatosis is present, a detailed history and growth assessment should be done, and children should be followed up for the development of gastrointestinal symptoms. All of the 6 children in this series had a history of perianal disease, so a specific inquiry regarding this may be helpful.

S. Raimer, MD

Erythema Toxicum Neonatorum Is an Innate Immune Response to Commensal Microbes Penetrated Into the Skin of the Newborn Infant
Marchini G, Nelson A, Edner J, et al (Karolinska Univ Hosp in Solna, Stockholm; Karolinska Univ Hosp in Huddinge, Stockholm)
Pediatr Res 58:613-616, 2005   15–10

Introduction.—Erythema toxicum neonatorum is a common rash of unknown etiology affecting healthy newborn infants. In this study, we postulated that the rash reflects a response to microbial colonization of the skin at birth, and that the hair follicle constitutes an "easily opened door" for microbes into the skin of the newborn. We collected microbial cultures from the skin of 69 healthy, 1-d-old infants with and without erythema toxicum to identify the colonizing flora and correlate culture results with clinical findings. We also analyzed biopsies from lesions of erythema toxicum with scanning and transmission electron microscopy in the search for microbes. Finally, each infant's body temperature was measured as a sign of acute phase response. We found that 84% of 1-d-old healthy infants, with and without erythema toxicum were colonized with coagulase-negative staphylococci. In all lesions of erythema toxicum, TEM identified cocci-like bacteria localized in the hair follicle epithelium and into recruited immune cells surrounding the hair follicle; morphology and dimension supported their identification as belonging to the genus *Staphylococcus*. SEM revealed 10 times more hair structures per skin surface unit in newborns compared with adults. Infants with erythema toxicum also had higher body temperature. In erythema toxicum, commensal microbes gain entry into the skin tissue, most probably through the hair canal. This triggers the local immune system and a systemic acute phase response, including an increase in body temperature. We speculate that early microbial exposure to the newborn may be important for the maturation of the immune system.

▶ Erythema toxicum previously has been postulated to be a response of the innate immune system of the newborn to colonization by bacteria. The authors demonstrate perifollicular inflammation and cocci-like microbes within hair follicle epithelium, which strongly suggests that microbes gain access into the skin through the hair follicle. The fact that erythema toxicum can be found over the entire body except for the palms, soles, and penis, which are all regions lacking hair follicles, supports the concept that hair follicles are involved in the development of lesions. Recent studies[1] have shown that skin appendages, especially the hair follicle, act as immunologic sentinels for the skin. The follicle has a complex immunologic profile, including a complement of perifollicular immunocytes that comprise part of the effector arm of the immune system.

S. Raimer, MD

Reference

1. Christoph T, Muller-Röver S, Audring H, et al: The human hair follicle immune system: Cellular composition and immune privilege. *Br J Dermatol* 142:862-873, 2000.

Epidemiologic Study of the Predisposing Factors in Erythema Toxicum Neonatorum

Liu C, Feng J, Qu R, et al (Xi'an Jiaotong Univ, China; Yunyang Med College, Shiyan, China)
Dermatology 210:269-272, 2005   15–11

Background.—Erythema toxicum neonatorum (ETN) is a very common disease, but its predisposing factors are still unknown.

Objective.—To determine the predisposing factors of ETN.

Methods.—Seven hundred and eighty-three neonates born in the same hospital during the same period were investigated, and the factors predisposing to ETN were evaluated in a case-control study.

Results.—(1) The incidence of ETN is about 43.68%, and it is significantly higher in males than in females ($p < 0.001$). (2) Term birth ($p < 0.05$), first-pregnancy birth ($p < 0.001$), the birth season (summer and autumn, $p < 0.005$), being fed with milk powder substitute or a mixed diet ($p < 0.001$) and vaginal delivery ($p < 0.001$) are the predisposing factors of ETN. (3) The severity of ETN in neonates born by vaginal delivery is significantly correlated with the total length of labor ($p < 0.001$).

Conclusion.—Our findings suggest that environmental factors play an important role in the onset of ETN.

▶ Marchini et al (Abstract 15–10) postulated that ETN is an innate immune response to commensal microbes that gain entry into skin, most probably through the hair canal. In this epidemiologic study of predisposing factors to ETN in infants born in Xi'an and Shiyan, China, at least 2 of the factors associated with an increased incidence of ETN, vaginal delivery and birth in a warm, humid climate, might potentiate the ability of microbes to penetrate the skin.

S. Raimer, MD

Circulating Level of Vascular Endothelial Growth Factor in Differentiating Hemangioma From Vascular Malformation Patients

Zhang L, Lin X, Wang W, et al (Affiliated Hosp of Bengbu Med College, Anhui, China; Shanghai Second Med Univ, China)
Plast Reconstr Surg 116:200-204, 2005   15–12

Background.—The majority of vascular anomalies can be diagnosed accurately based on natural history and physical examination; however, there is no convenient, noninvasive, and objective method to (1) differentiate hemangioma from vascular malformation; (2) determine whether a hemangioma is in the proliferating or involuting phase; (3) tell whether or not corticosteroids or interferon alfa-2a is effective for hemangioma; or (4) follow up hemangioma. Although the differences in endothelial cell, protein, and mRNA expression levels of some positive and negative angiogenic factors in the lesions can help to solve these problems, these methods (pathological section, immunohistochemical analysis, and in situ hybridization techniques) necessitate that a biopsy be performed, and the procedures are complicated. A nonsurgical and convenient method would have significant clinical applications.

Methods.—Fifty-nine patients with proliferating hemangiomas, 38 with involuting hemangiomas, 18 with vascular malformations, and 12 negative control subjects were examined for serum levels of vascular endothelial growth factor using enzyme-linked immunosorbent assays.

Results.—The serum level of vascular endothelial growth factor in proliferating hemangiomas was significantly higher than that in involuting hemangiomas, vascular malformations, and negative controls, while differences among involuting hemangiomas, vascular malformations, and negative controls were not statistically significant. In addition, after systemic steroid therapy, the serum level of vascular endothelial growth factor was significantly reduced compared with pretreatment levels in six patients with proliferating hemangiomas.

Conclusions.—The serum level of vascular endothelial growth factor may be useful in differentiating hemangioma from vascular malformations, staging hemangiomas, judging the efficacy of steroid therapy, and evaluating follow-up criteria for hemangiomas. The results probably shed new light on the pathogenesis of hemangiomas.

▶ In patients with large or enlarging vascular lesions, particularly those involving the lips, it occasionally may be difficult to clinically differentiate between hemangiomas and vascular malformations. Having a relatively simple noninvasive test to distinguish between the 2 entities would be of value. In this study, the presence of elevated levels of circulating vascular endothelial growth factor was indicative of the presence of a proliferating hemangioma. If these findings are confirmed by other studies, circulating levels of vascular endothelial growth factor might also be of benefit in staging hemangiomas and in monitoring the effect of treatment of large lesions.

S. Raimer, MD

GLUT-1: An Extra Diagnostic Tool to Differentiate Between Haemangiomas and Vascular Malformations

Leon-Villapalos J, Wolfe K, Kangesu L (St Andrews Centre for Plastic Surgery and Burns, Chelmsford, England; Southend Gen Hosp, Essex, England)
Br J Plast Surg 58:348-352, 2005   15–13

Introduction.—The differential diagnosis between juvenile haemangiomas, vascular malformations, pyogenic granulomas and normally proliferative endothelium (granulation tissue) on the basis of histology alone is sometimes difficult. This is important because haemangiomas, are self-limiting and vascular malformations are not. We report our experience of using the immunohistochemical marker GLUT-1 to distinguish haemangiomas from vascular malformations following the initial report by North and Colleagues (1998). We studied a total of 50 specimens from patients with vascular anomalies, and found that GLUT-1 reactivity was positive in 18 out of 19 juvenile haemangiomas, negative in two out of two noninvoluting congenital haemangiomas (NICH) and negative in 29 out of 29 vascular malformations, that included capillary malformations, lymphatic malformations, venous malformations and arteriovenous malformations (95% sensitivity, 100% specificity). Pyogenic granulomas ($n = 4$) and granulation tissue samples ($n = 4$) were used as negative controls. Placenta tissue was used as positive control. GLUT-1 accurately distinguishes haemangiomas from vascular malformations, and as a result from this work, we use this technique in routine histopathological differentiation of vascular anomalies.

Expression of Wilms Tumor 1 Gene Distinguishes Vascular Malformations From Proliferative Endothelial Lesions

Lawley LP, Cerimele F, Weiss SW, et al (Emory Univ, Atlanta, Ga; Univ of Arkansas, Little Rock; Harvard Med School, Boston)
Arch Dermatol 141:1297-1300, 2005   15–14

Background.—Vascular malformations and hemangiomas, which are endothelial lesions of childhood, may result in considerable morbidity because they can cause discomfort and functional impairment and have a negative affect on the patient's appearance. Although vascular malformations may initially appear very similar to hemangiomas, they have distinct clinical courses. Infantile hemangiomas progress through 3 stages: proliferative, involuting, and involuted. The proliferative phase is characterized by clinical growth. Once hemangiomas reach their maximum size, they begin to regress or involute. Histologically, this stage is characterized by endothelial apoptosis. Finally, the involuted stage of the hemangioma occurs when the original lesion is replaced by a connective tissue remnant. In contrast to hemangiomas, vascular malformations do not involute but continue to enlarge as the patient grows.

Observations.—The biochemical differences between hemangiomas, which involute, and vascular malformations, which do not involute, are not well understood. We found that the transcription factor encoded by the *Wilms tumor 1* (WT1) gene is expressed in the endothelium of hemangiomas but not in vascular malformations.

Conclusions.—Defects in WT1 signaling may underlie the inability of malformation endothelial cells to undergo physiologic apoptosis and remodeling. The availability of WT1 staining in hospital laboratories may allow the clinician to distinguish hemangiomas from vascular malformations and thus to give appropriate therapy to the patient.

► Hemangiomas most commonly develop at birth or shortly thereafter and may be characterized by a rapid growth phase. Hemangiomas on certain critical body sites warrant therapy to prevent compromised function or serious deformity. Vascular malformations may also be present at birth or may develop later in life; however, vascular malformations do not involute or respond to therapy with systemic corticosteroids or interferon. Therefore, it is important to distinguish hemangiomas from vascular malformations (Abstract 15–13). Histologically, some hemangiomas can be difficult to differentiate from venous or arteriovenous malformations. The absence of diagnostic histopathologic features in some cases may lead to the mismanagement of vascular lesions in childhood. Any histologic markers that could help distinguish between juvenile hemangiomas and vascular malformations would be welcome. GLUT-1 is an erythrocyte-type glucose transporter protein that is highly expressed in the endothelium of juvenile hemangiomas but not in vascular malformations, pyogenic granulomas, granulation tissue, or noninvoluting congenital hemangiomas.

Wilms tumor 1 is a transcription factor that is a candidate-signaling molecule in endothelial tumors. Wilms tumor 1 messenger RNA is expressed in high levels in human endothelium that is stimulated by angiopoietin 2. Lawley et al (Abstract 15–14) performed immunohistochemical analysis of human hemangiomas and vascular malformations and observed strong endothelial staining in hemangiomas but greatly decreased endothelial staining in vascular malformations. Wilms tumor 1 gene product also is detected by immunohistochemical methods in the endothelium of pyogenic granulomas, angiosarcomas, and hemangioendotheliomas. Therefore, Wilms tumor 1 expression does not distinguish between juvenile hemangioma and pyogenic granuloma whereas, GLUT-1 labels juvenile hemangioma but not pyogenic granuloma.

At centers where hemangiomas and vascular malformations are evaluated and treated on a regular basis, it would be useful to have the ability to perform immunohistochemical studies of biopsy specimens of these lesions for expression of GLUT-1 and Wilms tumor 1. This would enable a more precise classification of the lesions that may be difficult to differentiate on the basis of clinical findings and routine histopathology. This analysis would be especially critical in cases where therapy with systemic agents is being considered.

J. C. Maize, MD

Palmar-Plantar Fibromatosis in Children and Preadolescents: A Clinico-pathologic Study of 56 Cases With Newly Recognized Demographics and Extended Follow-up Information
Fetsch JF, Laskin WB, Miettinen M (Armed Forces Inst of Pathology, Washington, DC; Northwestern Univ, Chicago)
Am J Surg Pathol 29:1095-1105, 2005   15–15

Introduction.—Palmar-plantar fibromatosis, the most common type of fibromatosis, is well recognized in the adult population, but many clinicians and pathologists are unfamiliar with the fact that children may also be affected by this process. This report describes the clinicopathologic findings in 56 cases of palmar-plantar fibromatosis in children and preadolescents. Our study group included 19 males and 37 females, ranging from 2 to 12 years of age at the time of their first surgical procedure (median age, 9 years). The patients typically presented with solitary, lobular or multilobular masses in the 0.5- to 2.5-cm size range. The preoperative duration of the lesions ranged from 1 month to 6 years, with 1 patient purportedly having clinical evidence of disease since birth. All but two of the initial lesions occurred on the plantar aspect of the feet, typically in the region of the arch. Only 2 patients presented with palmar disease. The tumors were usually painless, except when pressure was applied. Seven patients had a history of trauma, sometimes involving a foreign body. One patient presented with concurrent disease involving both feet, and 12 additional patients subsequently developed palmar-plantar fibromatosis in another extremity, knuckle pads on the hands, or had other clinical findings linked to this disease. A family history was available for 25 patients, and 11 individuals had relatives with palmar-plantar fibromatosis, and 4 others had relatives with a history that was either suspicious for palmar-plantar disease or positive for other disorders associated with this disease. Histologically, the tumors involved aponeurosis and commonly formed discontinuous, moderately cellular, nodular masses composed of spindled cells with intervening collagen. Mitotic counts for 79 separately submitted tumor specimens ranged from 0 to 31 mitotic figures per 25 wide-field high power fields (mean mitotic count, 3.4 mitotic figures per 25 wide-field high power fields). Eight tumor had ≥ 10 mitoses per 25 wide-field high power fields. All patients were initially managed by local excision, and in most of cases, histologic examination showed tumor extending to the tissue edge. Thirty-two of 38 patients (84.2%) with clinical follow-up, ranging from 4 months to 33 years (mean, 14 years 9 months; median, 16 years 1 month), had one (n = 16) or more (n = 16) local recurrence of their fibromatosis.

▶ This is the largest series to date of palmar-plantar fibromatosis in children. Although rare, in children plantar fibromatosis occurred with much greater frequency than palmar fibromatosis and was more likely to develop after age 5 years. The female/male ratio was 2:1 in children. The authors reaffirm the association between palmar-plantar fibromatosis, knuckle pads, and seizures. Optimal treatment is controversial. Plantar disease is often relatively asymptomatic and not all nodular lesions lead to contractures. Surgical intervention can lead to complications, and there is a high incidence of recurrence, especially when early nodular lesions are removed. Triamcinolone acetonide injections may be helpful. Because numerous mitoses can be seen histologically and the fact that palmar-plantar fibromatosis is not a well-recognized entity in children, it occasionally has been misdiagnosed as fibrosarcoma. Fibrosarcomas are extremely rare on the hands and feet and tend to be more deep seated than palmar-plantar fibromatosis, with exhibit infiltrative growth.

S. Raimer, MD

Childhood Neutrophilic Eccrine Hidradenitis: A Clinicopathologic and Immunohistochemical Study of 10 Patients

Shih I-H, Huang Y-H, Yang C-H, et al (Chang Gung Mem Hosp, Taipei, Taiwan)
J Am Acad Dermatol 52:963-966, 2005   15–16

Background.—Neutrophilic eccrine hidradenitis (NEH) is occasionally reported in patients who have not received chemotherapy.

Objective.—The purpose of this study was to describe the clinicopathologic features of NEH occurring in healthy children and to investigate the interleukin (IL)-8 expression in the cutaneous lesions.

Methods.—Ten children with characteristic histologic features of NEH were collected from the Chang Gung Memorial Hospital. Their formalin-fixed, paraffin-embedded specimens were examined by immunohistochemical staining for IL-8.

Results.—The age of first presentation at our clinic ranged from 6 months to 14 months with a median age of 9.1 months. The onset of the disease clustered in the summertime. The most common clinical appearance was multiple erythematous papules and nodules on the limbs. Two of 7 biopsy specimens grew coagulase-negative *Staphylococcus*. None of patients had underlying systemic disease and all had complete resolution of the lesions within 3 weeks. Immunohistochemical staining for IL-8 was negative in the 10 cases studied.

Conclusion.—Childhood NEH appears as urticaria-like erythematous nodules and plaques on the limbs, trunk, or scalp. This benign and limited disease occurs with a predilection for summer months. In our study, onset

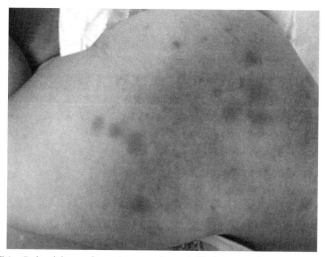

FIGURE 1.—Red nodules, confluent plaques, and pustule-like lesions on the right thigh. (Reprinted by permission of the publisher from Shih I-H, Huang Y-H, Yang C-H, et al: Childhood neutrophilic eccrine hidradenitis: A clinicopathologic and immunohistochemical study of 10 patients. *J Am Acad Dermatol* 52:963-966, 2005. Copyright 2005 by Elsevier.)

was in children less than 15 months of age. IL-8 was not detected in the cutaneous lesions (Fig 1; see color plate XII).

▶ The authors describe a unique presentation of NEH occurring in the summer months in a group of infants 6 to 14 months of age who had not received chemotherapy. The lesions are seen as erythematous nodules or plaques on the extremities and resolve spontaneously without sequelae within 3 weeks.

S. Raimer, MD

Neuro-Sweet Disease: Clinical Manifestations and Criteria for Diagnosis
Hisanaga K, for the Neuro-Sweet Disease Study Group (Miyagi Natl Hosp, Japan; et al)
Neurology 64:1756-1761, 2005   15–17

Background.—Sweet disease, also known as acute febrile neutrophilic dermatosis, is a multisystem inflammatory disorder characterized by painful erythematous plaques and aseptic neutrophilic infiltration of various organs. Skin biopsies typically demonstrate dermal infiltration with neutrophils in the absence of vasculitis. Sweet disease responds to systemic corticosteroids. The CNS can also be involved.

Methods.—The authors performed a survey on neuro-Sweet disease (NSD) in Japan and obtained detailed information about 16 cases. They analyzed 42 cases, including 26 cases documented in the literature, and assessed clinical and laboratory criteria for the diagnosis.

Results.—Thirteen cases also fulfilled the criteria for the diagnosis of Behçet disease. The clinical features of 27 cases, which the authors classified as probable NSD, are as follows: 1) both sexes are almost evenly affected; 2) people of ages 30 to 70 years are affected; 3) encephalitis and meningitis are common neurologic manifestations; 4) any region of the CNS can be involved, resulting in a variety of neurologic symptoms; 5) there is a strong human leukocyte antigen-Cw1 association; 6) systemic corticosteroids are highly effective for most of the neurologic manifestations, although recurrences are not infrequent.

Conclusions.—Neuro-Sweet disease is a distinct entity that may account for some cases of idiopathic encephalomeningitis.

▶ This article reports a systemic variant of Sweet disease that includes encephalitis as a prominent manifestation; the authors have labeled this "neuro-Sweet disease" (NSD). NSD has been observed primarily, but not exclusively, in the Japanese population. A similarity has been recognized with Behçet disease although the genetic associations appear to be different; HLA-B54 has been reported in Japanese patients with Sweet disease in contrast to the high frequency of HLA-B51 and the low frequency of HLA-B54 in Behçet disease. The bottom line is that clinicians must be aware of the possibility of neurologic manifestations when evaluating patients with Sweet disease.

B. H. Thiers, MD

Successful Treatment of Scleromyxedema With Autologous Peripheral Blood Stem Cell Transplantation

Lacy MQ, Hogan WJ, Gertz MA, et al (Mayo Clinic and Found, Rochester, Minn)

Arch Dermatol 141:1277-1282, 2005   15–18

Background.—Scleromyxedema is a rare chronic fibromucinous disorder that can have devastating clinical manifestations, including sclerosis of the skin with progressive pharyngeal and upper airway involvement, resulting in high mortality due to respiratory complications. Herein we describe a novel therapeutic approach. Because autologous hematopoietic stem cell transplantation is effective in other plasma cell proliferative disorders, it may be effective in this setting.

Observations.—We retrospectively evaluated 6 patients who were offered high-dose chemotherapy with stem cell rescue as treatment for scleromyxedema. One heavily pretreated patient was unable to mobilize stem cells. The remaining 5 patients mobilized stem cells and underwent successful transplantation. There was no treatment-related mortality. Hematologic responses were seen in 4 patients, including 2 complete remissions and 2 partial remissions, and all 4 had improvement in extracutaneous manifestations. All 4 patients subsequently had relapse of the monoclonal protein, and 3 developed skin relapses at 14, 37, and 45 months.

Conclusions.—High-dose chemotherapy with stem cell rescue is feasible for patients with scleromyxedema and, although not curative, offers durable remission in most patients. This therapy should be considered before treatment with alkylating agents or other treatments that could adversely affect the ability to collect stem cells.

▶ This is a retrospective report of a small number of patients with scleromyxedema who had a favorable response to autologous hematopoietic progenitor cell transplantation. The large number of treatments that have been described for this condition, including alkylating agents, methotrexate, systemic steroids, isotretinoin, interferon alfa, extracorporeal photochemotherapy, psoralen photochemotherapy, plasmapheresis, thalidomide, and IV IgG suggests that there is no "one size fits all" agent that is appropriate for every patient with this rare condition.

B. H. Thiers, MD

DERMATOLOGIC SURGERY AND CUTANEOUS ONCOLOGY

16 Nonmelanoma Skin Cancer

Ultraviolet Radiation and Skin Cancer: Molecular Mechanisms
Hussein MR (Assuit Univ, Egypt)
J Cutan Pathol 32:191-205, 2005   16–1

Introduction.—Every living organism on the surface of the earth is exposed to the ultraviolet (UV) fraction of the sunlight. This electromagnetic energy has both life-giving and life-endangering effects. UV radiation can damage DNA and thus mutagenize several genes involved in the development of the skin cancer. The presence of typical signature of UV-induced mutations on these genes indicates that the ultraviolet-B part of sunlight is responsible for the evolution of cutaneous carcinogenesis. During this process, variable alterations of the oncogenic, tumor-suppressive, and cell-cycle control signaling pathways occur. These pathways include (a) mutated *PTCH* (in the mitogenic Sonic Hedgehog pathway) and mutated *p53* tumor-suppressor gene in basal cell carcinomas, (b) an activated mitogenic *ras* pathway and mutated *p53* in squamous cell carcinomas, and (c) an activated *ras* pathway, inactive *p16*, and *p53* tumor suppressors in melanomas. This review presents background information about the skin optics, UV radiation, and molecular events involved in photocarcinogenesis.

Somatic Mutations in the *PTCH, SMOH, SUFUH,* and *TP53* Genes in Sporadic Basal Cell Carcinomas
Reifenberger J, Wolter M, Knobbe CB, et al (Heinrich-Heine-Univ, Düsseldorf, Germany)
Br J Dermatol 152:43-51, 2005   16–2

Background.—Basal cell carcinoma (BCC) of the skin is the most common human cancer. The genetic alterations underlying BCC development are only partly understood.

Objectives.—To investigate further the molecular genetics of sporadic BCCs, we performed mutation analyses of 10 skin cancer-associated genes in 42 tumours.

Methods.—Single-strand conformational polymorphism analysis followed by DNA sequencing was used to screen for mutations in the sonic hedgehog pathway genes *PTCH, SMOH, SUFUH* and *GLI1*, in the *TP53* tumour suppressor gene, and in the proto-oncogenes *NRAS, KRAS, HRAS, BRAF* and *CTNNB1*. Microsatellite markers flanking the *PTCH, SUFUH* and *TP53* loci at 9q22, 10q24 and 17p13, respectively, were studied for loss of heterozygosity (LOH).

Results.—*PTCH* mutations were found in 28 of 42 tumours (67%). Microsatellite analysis revealed LOH on 9q22 in 20 of 38 tumours investigated (53%), including 14 tumours with and six tumours without *PTCH* mutations. *SMOH* mutations were identified in four of the 42 BCCs (10%) while two tumours demonstrated mutations in *SUFUH*, including one missense mutation and one silent mutation. None of the BCCs showed LOH at markers flanking the *SUFUH* locus. Seventeen BCCs (40%) carried *TP53* mutations, with only three tumours showing evidence of biallelic *TP53* inactivation. *TP53* mutations were present in BCCs with and without mutations in *PTCH, SMOH* or *SUFUH*. Interestingly, 72% of the *TP53* alterations were presumably ultraviolet (UV)-induced transition mutations. In contrast, only 40% of the *PTCH* and *SMOH* alterations corresponded to UV signature mutations. No mutations were identified in *GLI1, NRAS, KRAS, HRAS, BRAF* or *CTNNB1*.

Conclusions.—Our data confirm the importance of *PTCH, SMOH* and *TP53* mutations in the pathogenesis of sporadic BCCs. *SUFUH* alterations are restricted to individual cases while the other investigated genes do not appear to be important targets for mutations in BCCs.

▶ The authors investigated 10 skin cancer-related genes in an effort to detect genetic alterations in sporadic BCCs. The *PTCH* mutation was most commonly found; interestingly, a drug is currently in development that directly targets this mutation. The different mutations detected support the hypothesis that both UV-dependent and UV-independent mechanisms contribute to the development of BCC (Abstracts 16–1 and 16–2).

B. H. Thiers, MD

In Vitro Sensitivity to Ultraviolet B Light and Skin Cancer Risk: A Case–Control Analysis
Wang L-E, Xiong P, Strom SS, et al (Univ of Texas, Houston; DermSurgery Associates, Houston)
J Natl Cancer Inst 97:1822-1831, 2005   16–3

Background.—Mutagen sensitivity, measured as mutagen-induced chromatid breaks per cell in primary lymphocytes in vitro, has been used to study susceptibility to various epithelial cancers. Patients with xeroderma pigmentosum are highly sensitive to ultraviolet (UV) light due to inherited defects in DNA repair and have a 1000-fold higher risk of UV-induced skin cancer than the general population. However, an association between UV-induced chromosomal aberrations and risk of skin cancer in the general population has not been established.

Methods.—We assessed in vitro UVB-induced chromatid breaks in a hospital-based case–control study. The study included 469 patients with skin cancer (231 with nonmelanoma skin cancer [NMSC] and 238 with cutaneous malignant melanoma [CMM]) and 329 cancer-free control subjects. Multivariable logistic regression was used to calculate odds ratios (ORs) and 95% confidence intervals (CIs). All statistical tests were two-sided.

Results.—Compared with the frequency of UVB-induced chromatid breaks per cell in control subjects (mean = 0.28 breaks per cell, 95% CI = 0.27 to 0.30), that in NMSC patients (basal cell carcinoma [BCC], n = 143, mean = 0.36 breaks per cell, 95% CI = 0.33 to 0.39 and squamous cell carcinoma [SCC], n = 88, mean = 0.35 breaks per cell, 95% CI = 0.32 to 0.38) was higher ($P = .001$ and $P < .001$, respectively), but that in CMM case patients (mean = 0.30 breaks per cell, 95% CI = 0.28 to 0.33) was not ($P = .22$). A frequency of chromatid breaks per cell above the median of control subjects was associated with nearly threefold increased risks for BCC (OR = 2.78, 95% CI = 1.79 to 4.30) and SCC (OR = 2.62, 95% CI = 1.50 to 4.60), but not with an increased risk of CMM. A dose–response relationship was evident between mutagen sensitivity and risk for both BCC ($P_{trend} < .001$) and SCC ($P_{trend} < .001$). Multiplicative interactions between mutagen sensitivity and sun exposure variables on risk, particularly for sunburn in BCC and hair color, tanning ability, and family history of skin cancer in SCC, were seen for NMSC but not CMM.

Conclusions.—UVB-induced mutagen sensitivity may play a role in susceptibility to NMSC but not to CMM.

▶ This in vitro study suggests that UVB-induced skin damage may play a more important role in the pathogenesis of NMSC than for melanoma. The clinical relevance of these findings still needs to be explored.

B. H. Thiers, MD

Prevention of UV Radiation–Induced Immunosuppression by IL-12 Is Dependent on DNA Repair

Schwarz A, Maeda A, Kernebeck K, et al (Univ Münster, Germany; Laboratory of Health Effects Research, Bilthoven, The Netherlands; Univ Kiel, Germany)
J Exp Med 201:173-179, 2005   16–4

Introduction.—The immunostimulatory cytokine IL-12 is able to antagonize immunosuppression induced by solar/ultraviolet (UV) radiation via yet unknown mechanisms. IL-12 was recently found to induce deoxyribonucleic acid (DNA) repair. UV-induced DNA damage is an important molecular trigger for UV-mediated immunosuppression. Thus, we initiated studies into immune restoration by IL-12 to discern whether its effects are linked to DNA repair. IL-12 prevented both UV-induced suppression of the induction of contact hypersensitivity and the depletion of Langerhans cells, the primary APC of the skin, in wild-type but not in DNA repair-deficient mice. IL-12 did not prevent the development of UV-induced regulatory T cells in DNA repair-deficient mice. In contrast, IL-12 was able to break established UV-induced tolerance and inhibited the activity of regulatory T cells independent of DNA repair. These data identify a new mechanism by which IL-12 can restore immune responses and also demonstrate a link between DNA repair and the prevention of UV-induced immunosuppression by IL-12.

▶ Interleukin 12 (IL-12) is a well-characterized immunomodulatory cytokine that has been shown to inhibit immunosuppression induced by UV light and to promote DNA repair after damage by UV light. In this interesting study, the investigators used a murine model to investigate the hypothesis that the latter activity may account for the immunoprotective effect of IL-12. They demonstrated that exposure to UV light prevented sensitization to dinitrofluorobenzene in both wild-type and knockout mice lacking a functional *Xpa* gene that is required for nucleotide excision repair of damaged DNA. In contrast, pretreatment of mice with IL-12 restored the DNFB hypersensitivity response in wild-type but not the *Xpa* knockout mice. Further experiments revealed that IL-12 also prevented both the migration of epidermal Langerhans cells and the DNA damage to such cells induced by UV light in wild-type but not in knockout mice. These findings strongly suggest that the effect of IL-12 in preventing UV-induced cutaneous immunosuppression is mediated by its ability to induce DNA repair. Additional studies will be required to determine the mechanisms underlying this activity.

G. M. P. Galbraith, MD

Predictors of Self-Reported Confidence Ratings for Adult Recall of Early Life Sun Exposure

Relova A-S, Marrett LD, Klar N, et al (Cancer Care Ontario, Toronto; Univ of Toronto; Mount Sinai Hosp, Toronto; et al)
Am J Epidemiol 162:183-192, 2005

16–5

Introduction.—Use of self-reported confidence ratings may be an efficient method for assessing recall bias. In this exploratory application of the method, the authors examined the relation between case-control status and self-reported confidence ratings. In 2002 and 2003, melanoma cases ($n = 141$) and controls ($n = 143$) aged 20–44 years residing in Ontario, Canada, estimated the amounts of time they had spent outdoors in summer activities when they were 6-18 years of age and indicated their confidence in the accuracy of each estimate. The generalized estimating equations extension of logistic regression was used to examine dichotomized confidence ratings (more confident vs. less confident) for activities reported for ages 6–11 years and 12–18 years. Types of activity were associated with more confident reporting for both age strata; as the number of stable outdoor activity periods (total number of similar outdoor periods within each activity) reported by respondents increased, confidence decreased. Cumulative time spent outdoors was also associated with more confidence but reached statistical significance only for the age stratum 12–18 years. There was no statistically significant association between case-control status and self-reported confidence for either age stratum (6–11 years: odds ratio = 0.91; 12–18 years: odds ratio = 1.32), which suggests an absence of recall bias for reported time spent outdoors.

▶ Many studies that examine the epidemiology of skin cancer ask participants to report their prior history of sun exposure. One criticism of such studies is the reliability of such reporting, specifically whether patients with a history of skin cancer may be more cognizant of their past sun exposure. Using self-reported confidence ratings, the authors of this study determined that a prior history of skin cancer did not introduce recall bias.

P. G. Lang, Jr, MD

Randomized Controlled Trial Testing the Impact of High-Protection Sunscreens on Sun-Exposure Behavior
Dupuy A, Dunant A, Grob J-J, et al (Hôpital Saint-Louis, Paris; Institut Gustave Roussy, Villejuif, France; Université de la Méditerranée, Marseille, France)
Arch Dermatol 141:950-956, 2005   16–6

Objective.—High-protection sunscreens have been suspected to prompt people to increase sun exposure, and thus to increase skin cancer risk. We tested the influence of both the actual protection (sun protection factor [SPF]) and the information about protection (label) on sun-exposure behavior.

Design.—Randomized controlled trial.

Setting.—Four French seaside resorts during summer 2001.

Participants.—A total of 367 healthy subjects during their 1-week holiday. Outcome was assessable in 98% of them.

Intervention.—Subjects were offered free sunscreens, with randomization into the following study arms: (1) SPF 40 labeled as "high protection"; (2) SPF 40 labeled as "basic protection"; and (3) SPF 12 labeled as "basic protection." Arm 4, ie, SPF 12 labeled as "high protection," was not implemented for ethical reasons. Subjects were not aware of the real target of the study and were blinded to the SPF value.

Main Outcome Measure.—Duration of sunbathing exposure during 1 week. Secondary outcomes were occurrence of sunburns and amount of sunscreen used. Influences of SPF and label were assessed separately.

Results.—Compared with the low-SPF group, the high-SPF group did not have longer sunbathing exposure (12.9 ± 7.2 h/wk for high SPF vs 14.6 ± 6.7 h/wk for low SPF; $P = .06$), experienced fewer sunburns (14% vs 24%; $P = .049$), and used less sunscreen (median, 30 g vs 109 g; $P<.001$). The label "high protection" or "basic protection" had no influence on these end points.

Conclusions.—In this adult population, higher SPF had no influence on duration of sun exposure and offered better protection against sunburns. Although higher SPF may increase sun exposure duration in specific populations, this effect cannot be viewed as a universal side effect of high-SPF sunscreens.

▶ This study tends to refute the argument that sunscreen use makes people more cavalier about sun exposure and thus actually increases their risk of skin cancer, particularly melanoma.

B. H. Thiers, MD

Incidence of Basal Cell and Squamous Cell Carcinomas in a Population Younger Than 40 Years
Christenson LJ, Borrowman TA, Vachon CM, et al (Mayo Clinic, Rochester, Minn)
JAMA 294:681-690, 2005

16–7

Context.—The incidence of nonmelanoma skin cancer is increasing rapidly among elderly persons, but little is known about its incidence in the population younger than 40 years.

Objectives.—To estimate the sex- and age-specific incidences of basal cell carcinoma and squamous cell carcinoma in persons younger than 40 years in Olmsted County, Minnesota, and to evaluate change in incidence over time; to describe the clinical presentation, rate of recurrence and metastasis, and histologic characteristics of these tumors in this population-based sample.

Design.—Population-based retrospective incidence case review.

Setting.—Residents of Olmsted County, Minnesota, a population with comprehensive medical records captured through the Rochester Epidemiology Project.

Participants.—Patients younger than 40 years with basal cell carcinoma or squamous cell carcinoma diagnosed between 1976 and 2003.

Main Outcome Measures.—Incident basal cell carcinomas and squamous cell carcinomas and change in incidence of these tumors over time.

Results.—During the study period, 451 incident basal cell carcinomas were diagnosed in 417 patients and 70 incident squamous cell carcinomas were diagnosed in 68 patients. Of these tumors, 328 were histologically confirmed basal cell carcinomas and 51 were histologically confirmed squamous cell carcinomas. Overall, the age-adjusted incidence of basal cell carcinoma per 100,000 persons was 25.9 (95% confidence interval [CI], 22.6-29.2) for women and 20.9 (95% CI, 17.8-23.9) for men. The incidence of basal cell carcinoma increased significantly during the study period among women ($P<.001$) but not men ($P=.19$). Nodular basal cell carcinoma was the most common histologic subtype; 43.0% of tumors were solely nodular basal cell carcinoma and 11.0% had a mixed composition, including the nodular subtype. The incidence of squamous cell carcinoma was similar in men and women, with an average age- and sex-adjusted incidence per 100

000 persons of 3.9 (95% CI, 3.0-4.8); the incidence of squamous cell carcinoma increased significantly over the study period among both women ($P=.01$) and men ($P=.04$).

Conclusions.—This population-based study demonstrated an increase in the incidence of nonmelanoma skin cancer among young women and men residing in Olmsted County, Minnesota. There was a disproportionate increase in basal cell carcinoma in young women. This increase may lead to an exponential increase in the overall occurrence of nonmelanoma skin cancers over time as this population ages, which emphasizes the need to focus on skin cancer prevention in young adults.

▶ This study confirms what clinicians have been observing for some time now—we are seeing more young people with basal cell carcinoma and squamous cell carcinoma, especially basal cell carcinoma in young women. As pointed out by the authors, the explanation for this observation may be multifaceted, but in large part is probably related to both indoor and outdoor tanning. The development of basal cell carcinoma is currently thought to be primarily caused by intermittent intense ultraviolet light exposure rather than long-term exposure. The increase in superficial basal cell carcinomas of the trunk reported in this study would support this concept. Educating people at a young age regarding the hazards of tanning and the importance of sunscreen use, along with regulation of the tanning industry, will help reverse this alarming increase in nonmelanoma skin cancer.

P. G. Lang, Jr, MD

Repeated Occurrence of Basal Cell Carcinoma of the Skin and Multifailure Survival Analysis: Follow-up Data From the Nambour Skin Cancer Prevention Trial

Pandeya N, Purdie DM, Green A, et al (Queensland Inst of Med Research, Brisbane, Australia; Univ of Queensland, Brisbane, Australia)
Am J Epidemiol 161:748-754, 2005   16–8

Introduction.—The aim of this study was to apply multifailure survival methods to analyze time to multiple occurrences of basal cell carcinoma (BCC). Data from 4.5 years of follow-up in a randomized controlled trial, the Nambour Skin Cancer Prevention Trial (1992–1996), to evaluate skin cancer prevention were used to assess the influence of sunscreen application on the time to first BCC and the time to subsequent BCCs. Three different approaches of time to ordered multiple events were applied and compared: the Andersen-Gill, Wei-Lin-Weissfeld, and Prentice-Williams-Peterson models. Robust variance estimation approaches were used for all multifailure survival models. Sunscreen treatment was not associated with time to first occurrence of a BCC (hazard ratio = 1.04, 95% confidence interval: 0.79, 1.45). Time to subsequent BCC tumors using the Andersen Gill model resulted in a lower estimated hazard among the daily sunscreen application group, although statistical significance was not reached (hazard ratio = 0.82, 95% confidence interval: 0.59, 1.15). Similarly, both the Wei-Lin-Weissfeld marginal-hazards and the Prentice-Williams-Peterson gap-time models revealed trends toward a lower risk of subsequent BCC tumors among the sunscreen intervention group. These results demonstrate the importance of conducting multiple-event analysis for recurring events, as risk factors for a single event may differ from those where repeated events are considered.

▶ This is yet another study that could be used by critics of sunscreen use to suggest that sunscreen application does not prevent skin cancer. However, there are a number of problems with this study. First, it is not clear whether the subjects had baseline skin examinations. Second, how did the investigators assess compliance with respect to sunscreen use? Also, control patients were allowed to continue their "usual sunscreen use." What does this mean? Finally, we know that the first step in tumorigenesis, initiation, which might be irreversible, has already occurred in these patients. What duration of sunscreen use is required to prevent further initiation and for the clinical benefits of sunscreen use to become apparent? The time period studied might not have been adequate.

P. G. Lang, Jr, MD

Sunscreen Use Before and After Transplantation and Assessment of Risk Factors Associated With Skin Cancer Development in Renal Transplant Recipients

Moloney FJ, Almarzouqui E, O'Kelly P, et al (Beaumont Hosp, Dublin)
Arch Dermatol 141:978-982, 2005

16–9

Objective.—To determine the degree of compliance with sunscreen use among renal transplant recipients before and after transplantation and to determine risk factors associated with skin carcinogenesis.

Design.—Single-observer study with structured interview using a standardized questionnaire. Medical records and histology reports were examined for details of prior skin cancer. Cox proportional hazards regression was used for analysis of risk factors for developing skin cancer after transplantation.

Setting.—Patients attending Beaumont Hospital, the national renal transplantation center in Dublin, Ireland.

Patients.—The study population comprised 270 patients (182 male and 88 female).

Main Outcome Measures.—Patients' use of sunscreens before and after transplantation relative to known skin cancer risk factors and subsequent skin carcinogenesis.

Results.—Prior to transplantation, 68.5% of patients never applied sunscreen on a sunny day compared with 25.9% after transplantation. Patients 50 years or younger were more likely to always apply sunscreen both before and after transplantation ($P = .01$), as were female patients prior to transplantation (*P* = .02). Those patients who participated in an outdoor recreation were more likely to subsequently develop nonmelanoma skin cancer (*P* = .04), as were those older than 50 years (*P*<.001) and those with a history of 2 or more painful sunburns (*P* = .03).

Conclusions.—Transplant recipients are poorly compliant with the use of sunscreens both before and after transplantation. Compliance is poorest in those groups at higher risk of nonmelanoma skin cancer.

▶ Moloney et al show poor compliance with sun protection practices among renal transplant recipients. Motivating people who have significant distractions from other medical concerns to be more compliant with sun protection measures will continue to be a difficult problem. Better patient education might be a small but important step forward.[1]

B. H. Thiers, MD

Reference

1. Cowen EW, Billingsley EM: Awareness of skin cancer by kidney transplant patients. *J Am Acad Dermatol* 40:697-701, 1999.

Skin Cancer in Organ Transplant Recipients: Effect of Pretransplant End-Organ Disease

Otley CC, Cherikh WS, Salasche SJ, et al (Mayo Clinic, Rochester, Minn; United Network for Organ Sharing, Richmond, Va; Univ of Arizona, Tucson; et al)
J Am Acad Dermatol 53:783-790, 2005   16–10

Background.—Solid organ transplant recipients are at increased risk for posttransplant neoplasms.

Objective.—Our purpose was to determine whether various diseases causing end-organ failure are associated with different degrees of risk of skin cancer development after transplantation.

Methods.—The Organ Procurement and Transplantation Network/ United Network for Organ Sharing Transplant Tumor Registry was searched for the incidence of skin cancer among kidney, liver, and heart transplant recipients in the United States between 1996 and 2001. Multivariate analysis was used to determine the association between disease diagnosis and posttransplant skin cancer.

Results.—Transplant recipients with specific pretransplant diseases, such as polycystic kidney disease and cholestatic liver disease, were at increased risk for skin cancer. Patients with diabetes mellitus had a lower incidence of skin cancer after kidney transplantation.

Limitations.—The study had only a brief follow-up period, indirect assessment of photodamage, and possible underreporting.

Conclusion.—Transplant recipients with a history of certain diseases warrant intensive skin cancer surveillance and strict sun-protective practices.

▶ Otley et al present fascinating data to identify which subsets of transplant patients are most likely to develop skin cancer. Nevertheless, all immunosuppressed transplant patients need to practice good sun-protective measures and have regular dermatologic examinations to ensure the prevention and early diagnosis of cutaneous malignancies.

B. H. Thiers, MD

Nonmelanoma Skin Cancer in Relation to Ionizing Radiation Exposure Among US Radiologic Technologists

Yoshinaga S, Hauptmann M, Sigurdson AJ, et al (Natl Cancer Inst, Bethesda, Md; Natl Inst of Radiological Sciences, Chiba, Japan; Univ of Minnesota, Minneapolis)
Int J Cancer 115:828-834, 2005   16–11

Introduction.—Ionizing radiation (IR) is an established cause of nonmelanoma skin cancer, but there is uncertainty about the risk associated with chronic occupational exposure to IR and how it is influenced by ultraviolet radiation (UVR) exposure. We studied 1,355 incident cases with basal cell carcinoma (BCC) and 270 with squamous cell carcinoma (SCC) of the skin in a cohort of 65,304 U.S. white radiologic technologists who responded to the baseline questionnaire survey in 1983–1989 and the follow-up survey in 1994–1998. Cox's proportional-hazards model was used to estimate relative risks of BCC and SCC associated with surrogate measures of occupational exposure to IR and residential UVR exposure during childhood and adulthood, adjusted for potential confounders including pigmentation characteristics. Relative risks of BCC, but not of SCC, were elevated among technologists who first worked during the 1950s (RR = 1.42; 95% CI = 1.12–1.80), 1940s (RR = 2.04; 95% CI = 1.44–2.88) and before 1940 (RR = 2.16; 95% CI = 1.14–4.09), when IR exposures were high, compared to those who first worked after 1960 (p for trend < 0.01). The effect of year first worked on BCC risk was not modified by UVR exposure, but was significantly stronger among individuals with lighter compared to darker eye and hair color (p = 0.013 and 0.027, respectively). This study provides some evidence that chronic occupational exposure to IR at low to moderate levels can increase the risk of BCC, and that this risk may be modified by pigmentation characteristics.

▶ Radiologists whose hands were exposed to IR have been shown to develop squamous cell carcinoma in areas of radiation dermatitis, and individuals treated with low doses of radiation for benign conditions may later develop BCC. Atomic bomb survivors also have developed an increased number of skin cancers, especially BCCs. In this study, the investigators tried to determine if radiologic technologists exposed to low or moderate amounts of radiation are

at increased risk for developing BCC. Although some of the data would support this conclusion, there were some inconsistencies. Moreover, the information gathered for this study was gleaned primarily from questionnaires
(with all their inherent deficiencies), and the amount of UVR exposure was
based on tables of UVR intensity for various areas of the country rather than on
data measuring actual individual UVR exposure. This might influence the findings of the study because the development of BCCs seemed to correlate with
eye and hair color, with them being more common in persons with light hair
and eyes.

P. G. Lang, Jr, MD

**Site-Specific Occurrence of Nonmelanoma Skin Cancers in Patients With
Cutaneous Melanoma**
Neale RE, Forman D, Murphy MFG, et al (Childhood Cancer Research Group,
Oxford, England; Univ of Leeds, England; Royal Brisbane Hosp, Australia)
Br J Cancer 93:597-601, 2005   16–12

Introduction.—In a registry-based case–control study, we compared the
site-specific occurrence of nonmelanoma (keratinocytic) skin cancers
among patients with cutaneous melanoma cases (cases, $n = 3774$) and solid
tumours (controls, $n = 349,923$), respectively. Overall, patients with melanoma were almost five-fold more likely to develop keratinocytic cancers
compared with solid tumour controls (adjusted OR 4.7, 95% CI 4.1–5.3),
but the risks varied depending upon the site of melanoma. Whereas patients
with melanoma of the head and neck had similarly increased risks of
keratinocytic cancers across all body sites, patients with melanoma of the
trunk were significantly more likely to develop keratinocyte cancer diagnosed on the trunk (adjusted OR 12.5, 95% CI 7.2–20.2) than on the head
and neck (adjusted OR 3.0, 95% CI 2.2–4.3). Similar colocalisation of skin
tumours was observed for patients with melanomas of the lower limb. These
findings provide support for the hypothesis that skin cancers at different
anatomical sites may arise through different causal pathways.

▶ The data support the notion that melanoma and basal cell carcinoma share
common causal factors, but that the associations between different types of
skin cancer differ according to the age of the host and to the anatomic site of
the lesion.

B. H. Thiers, MD

Role of Dietary Factors in the Development of Basal Cell Cancer and Squamous Cell Cancer of the Skin

McNaughton SA, Marks GC, Green AC (Univ of Queensland, Herston, Australia)

Cancer Epidemiol Biomarkers Prev 14:1596-1607, 2005   16–13

Introduction.—The role of dietary factors in the development of skin cancer has been investigated for many years; however, the results of epidemiologic studies have not been systematically reviewed. This article reviews human studies of basal cell cancer (BCC) and squamous cell cancer (SCC) and includes all studies identified in the published scientific literature investigating dietary exposure to fats, retinol, carotenoids, vitamin E, vitamin C, and selenium. A total of 26 studies were critically reviewed according to study design and quality of the epidemiologic evidence. Overall, the evidence suggests a positive relationship between fat intake and BCC and SCC, an inconsistent association for retinol, and little relation between β-carotene and BCC or SCC development. There is insufficient evidence on which to make a judgment about an association of other carotenoids with skin cancer. The evidence for associations between vitamin E, vitamin C, and selenium and both BCC and SCC is weak. Many of the existing studies contain limitations, however, and further well-designed and implemented studies are required to clarify the role of diet in skin cancer. Additionally, the role of other dietary factors, such as flavonoids and other polyphenols, which have been implicated in skin cancer development in animal models, needs to be investigated.

▶ Overall, the evidence for a possible relationship between skin cancer and diet is weak. McNaughton et al suggest a possible relationship between fat intake and BCC and SCC. Most studies investigating the role of diet and the pathogenesis of skin cancer have significant limitations, and better studies with adjustment for important confounding factors are needed.

B. H. Thiers, MD

Nonsteroidal Anti-inflammatory Drugs and the Risk of Actinic Keratoses and Squamous Cell Cancers of the Skin

Butler GJ, Neale R, Green AC, et al (Royal Brisbane Hosp, Queensland, Australia)

J Am Acad Dermatol 53:966-972, 2005   16–14

Background.—Although animal studies suggest that nonsteroidal anti-inflammatory drugs (NSAIDs), including aspirin, may protect against cutaneous squamous cell carcinoma (SCC) and actinic keratoses (AKs), possible effects on keratinocytic cancers in humans are unknown.

Objective.—We sought to examine the relationship between ingestion of NSAIDs and the risk of SCC and AKs in humans.

Methods.—We conducted a case-control study nested within a community-based cohort of 1621 people in southern Queensland, Australia. Eighty-six persons with SCC were compared with 187 age- and sex-matched control subjects randomly selected from within the cohort. NSAID use was captured through face-to-face interviews with study participants, supplemented by color photographs of product packaging. We defined regular use of NSAIDs as consumption of at least two tablets per week (low frequency) or at least 8 tablets per week (high frequency) for at least 1 year. AKs were counted on the face, ears, right hand, and right forearm by a single physician.

Results.—Patients with SCC were significantly less likely than control subjects to have used any NSAIDs 8 or more times per week for more than 1 year (multivariate odds ratio [OR] 0.07, 95% confidence interval [CI] 0.01-0.71) and to have used full-dose NSAIDs 2 or more times per week for more than 5 years (OR, 0.20; 95% CI, 0.04-0.96). Among participants without SCC, current regular users of NSAIDs (≥2 times per week) had significantly lower counts of AKs than nonusers (rate ratio [RR], 0.52; 95% CI, 0.30-0.91).

Limitations.—Estimates of NSAID use were based on self-reported data. Statistical power to detect associations was limited by the number of cases with SCC.

Conclusion.—Regular users of NSAIDs appear to have lower risks of SCC and lower counts of AKs than nonusers.

▶ UV light leads to increased cyclo-oxygenase (COX) enzyme expression, which, in turn, leads to increased prostaglandin A synthesis, increased cell proliferation, and, possibly, carcinogenesis. Indeed, this enzyme, especially the COX-2 isoform, is often overexpressed in AKs and some nonmelanoma skin cancers. Inhibition of COX by NSAIDs may explain the lower risk of AKs and SCCs reported in this study. The relevance of these findings is supported by the increased benefits noted with longer duration, higher doses, and more frequent use of these drugs.

B. H. Thiers, MD

Non-Steroidal Anti-inflammatory Drugs and the Risk of Oral Cancer: A Nested Case-Control Study

Sudbø J, Lee JJ, Lippman SM, et al (Norwegian Radium Hosp, Oslo; Univ of Texas, Houston; National Hosp and The Norwegian Cancer Registry, Oslo; et al)
Lancet 366:1359-1366, 2005   16–15

Background.—Non-steroidal anti-inflammatory drugs (NSAIDs) seem to prevent several types of cancer, but could increase the risk of cardiovascular complications. We investigated whether use of NSAIDs was associated with a change in the incidence of oral cancer or overall or cardiovascular mortality.

Methods.—We undertook a nested case-control study to analyse data from a population-based database (Cohort of Norway; CONOR), which consisted of prospectively obtained health data from all regions of Norway. People with oral cancer were identified from the 9241 individuals in CONOR who were at increased risk of oral cancer because of heavy smoking ($\geq$15 pack-years), and matched controls were selected from the remaining heavy smokers (who did not have cancer).

Findings.—We identified and analysed 454 (5%) people with oral cancer (279 men, 175 women, mean [SD] age at diagnosis 63.3 [13.2] years) and 454 matched controls (n=908); 263 (29%) had used NSAIDs, 83 (9%) had used paracetamol (for a minimum of 6 months), and 562 (62%) had used neither drug. NSAID use (but not paracetamol use) was associated with a reduced risk of oral cancer (including in active smokers; hazard ratio 0.47, 95% CI 0.37-0.60, p<0.0001). Smoking cessation also lowered the risk of oral cancer (0.41, 0.32-0.52, p<0.0001). Additionally, long-term use of NSAIDs (but not paracetamol) was associated with an increased risk of cardiovascular-disease-related death (2.06, 1.34-3.18, p=0.001). NSAID use did not significantly reduce overall mortality (p=0.17).

Interpretation.—Long-term use of NSAIDs is associated with a reduced incidence of oral cancer (including in active smokers), but also with an increased risk of death due to cardiovascular disease. These findings highlight the need for a careful risk-benefit analysis when the long-term use of NSAIDs is considered.

▶ The authors demonstrate that long-term use of NSAIDs is associated with about a 50% reduction in the risk of oral cancer in a high risk group of smokers with 15 or more pack-years of smoking history. The magnitude of this protective effect was impressive and was comparable to that observed with smoking cessation. The inverse association between NSAID use and oral cancer risk might be due to inhibition of COX-2 activity.[1] In high-risk patients, such as those with aneuploid oral leukoplakia,[2,3] the possible preventative effects of NSAIDs might outweigh their potential adverse cardiovascular effects.

B. H. Thiers, MD

References

1. Dannenberg AJ, Altorki NK, Boyle JO, et al: Cyclo-oxygenase 2: A pharmacological target for the prevention of cancer. *Lancet Oncol* 2:544-551, 2001.
2. Sudbø J, Kildal W, Risberg B, et al: DNA content as a prognostic marker in patients with oral leukoplakia. *N Engl J Med* 344:1270-1278, 2001.
3. Mao L, Hong WK, Papadimitrakopoulou VA: Focus on head and neck cancer. *Cancer Cell* 5:311-316, 2004.

Human Papillomavirus-DNA Loads in Actinic Keratoses Exceed Those in Non-melanoma Skin Cancers

Weissenborn SJ, Nindl I, Purdie K, et al (Univ of Cologne, Germany; Univ of Berlin; Centre for Cutaneous Research, London; et al)

J Invest Dermatol 125:93-97, 2005   16–16

Introduction.—Recent studies suggest a role of cutaneous human papillomaviruses (HPV) in non-melanoma skin cancer (NMSC) development. In this study viral DNA loads of six frequent HPV types were determined by quantitative, type-specific real-time-PCR (Q-PCR) in actinic keratoses (AK, n=26), NMSC (n=31), perilesional tissue (n=22), and metastases of squamous cell carcinomas (SCC) (n=8) which were previously shown to be positive for HPV5, 8, 15, 20, 24, or 36. HPV-DNA loads in AK, (partially microdissected) NMSC, and perilesional skin ranged between one HPV-DNA copy per 0.02 and 14,200 cell equivalents (median: 1 HPV-DNA copy per 344 cell equivalents; n=48). In 32 of the 79 HPV-positive skin biopsies and in seven of the eight metastases viral loads were even below the detection limit of Q-PCR. Low viral loads in NMSC were confirmed by *in situ*-hybridization showing only a few HPV-DNA-positive nuclei per section. Viral loads in SCC, basal cell carcinomas, and perilesional tissue were similar. But, viral loads found in AK were significantly higher than in SCC (p=0.035). Our data suggest that persistence of HPV is not necessary for the maintenance of the malignant phenotype of individual NMSC cells. Although a passenger state cannot be excluded, the data are compatible with a carcinogenic role of HPV in early steps of tumor development.

▶ A role for HPV in cutaneous carcinogenesis is suggested by a number of factors including (1) the known oncogenic potential of the virus; (2) the increased incidence of NMSC in chronically UV-irradiated skin, which is a relatively immunodeficient site compared with non–UV-irradiated skin; and (3) the increased incidence of NMSC in therapeutically immunosuppressed patients. Weissenborn et al suggest that the virus may be most important in initiating the process of cutaneous carcinogenesis and may not be necessary to maintain it.

B. H. Thiers, MD

Human Papillomavirus Gene Expression in Cutaneous Squamous Cell Carcinomas From Immunosuppressed and Immunocompetent Individuals

Purdie KJ, Surentheran T, Sterling JC, et al (Queen Mary Univ of London; Univ of Cambridge, England)

J Invest Dermatol 125:98-107, 2005   16–17

Introduction.—Epidermodysplasia verruciformis (EV)-type human papillomavirus (HPV) DNA have been detected by PCR in squamous cell carcinomas (SCC) from both organ transplant recipients (OTR) and immunocompetent individuals. Their role in skin cancer remains unclear, and previous studies have not addressed whether the viruses are transcriptionally active. We have used in situ hybridization to investigate the transcriptional activity and DNA localization of HPV. EV-HPV gene transcripts were demonstrated in four of 11 (36%) OTR SCC, one of two (50%) IC SCC, and one of five (20%) OTR warts positive by PCR. Viral DNA co-localized with E2/E4 early region gene transcripts in the middle or upper epidermal layers. Non-EV cutaneous HPV gene transcripts were demonstrated in one of five (20%) OTR SCC and four of 10 (40%) OTR warts. In mixed infections transcripts for both types were detected in two of six (33%) cases. Our results provide evidence of EV-HPV gene expression in SCC; although only a proportion of tumors were positive, the similarly low transcriptional activity in warts suggests this is an underestimate. These observations, together with emerging epidemiological and functional data, provide further reason to focus on the contribution of EV-HPV types to the pathogenesis of cutaneous SCC.

▶ This article presents additional data to support a role for HPV in cutaneous carcinogenesis both in immunocompetent and immunosuppressed patients. In contrast to the findings of Weissenborn et al (Abstract 16–16), the data presented by Purdie et al, demonstrating evidence for HPV gene expression in a proportion of SCC, suggest an active rather than latent role for the virus.[1]

B. H. Thiers, MD

Reference

1. Orth G: Human papillomaviruses associated with epidermodysplasia verruciformis in non-melanoma skin cancers: Guilty or innocent? *J Invest Dermatol* 125:xii, 2005.

Melan-A: Not a Helpful Marker in Distinction Between Melanoma In Situ on Sun-Damaged Skin and Pigmented Actinic Keratosis
Shabrawi-Caelen LE, Kerl H, Cerroni L (Univ of Graz, Austria)
Am J Dermatopathol 26:364-366, 2004   16–18

Introduction.—Pigmented actinic keratosis is one of the simulators of early melanoma in situ from severely sun-damaged skin. Close scrutiny of the hematoxylin and eosin stained section does not always allow an unequivocal diagnosis, because it is sometimes difficult to distinguish pigmented keratinocytes from melanocytes. Immunohistochemical stains, such as S-100 and HMB-45, are used routinely to address this problem. Melan-A, also known as MART-1, is an additional melanocytic marker and has proved to be useful in identifying metastatic tumors of melanocytic origin. The usefulness of this marker to discriminate pigmented actinic keratosis from early melanoma in situ, however, has not yet been a subject of investigation. In this study we evaluated Melan-A expression in ten unequivocal cases of pigmented actinic keratosis and compared the staining pattern with that of S-100, HMB-45, and tyrosinase. In all ten cases the number of cells highlighted with Melan-A was by far larger than those labeled with S-100, HMB-45, and tyrosinase. Four cases showed clusters of Melan-A positive cells being suggestive of melanocytic nests. Even areas of normal skin adjacent to the actinic keratosis featured prominent staining of Melan-A, but only inconsistent labeling of intraepidermal melanocytes with S-100, HMB-45, and tyrosinase. We therefore believe that Melan-A is a more sensitive marker for intraepidermal melanocytes than S-100, HMB-45, and tyrosinase. In addition there may be expression of Melan-A in keratinocytes and nonmelanocytic cells. To avoid an erroneous diagnosis of malignant melanoma one should therefore interpret results obtained from Melan-A stained slides carefully and in the context with other melanocytic markers.

▶ Melan-A (also known as MART-1) is a sensitive marker for normal and neoplastic melanocytes. It has also been shown to be more specific than S-100 protein; however, other cells can mark for Melan-A, including cells in angiomyolipoma and some steroid-producing cells of the adrenal cortex, ovaries, and testes.

This study presents evidence that Melan-A may also label keratinocytes in chronically sun-damaged skin. Melan-A has recently been advocated for use by Mohs surgeons as an aide for determining the margins on melanomas, especially those on chronically sun-damaged skin of the head and neck. The implication of this study is that the use of Melan-A as a sole marker may lead to overaggressive surgery because of the staining of some keratinocytes, as well as melanocytes, in the basal zone of the epidermis. Therefore, it would be prudent to use a battery of melanocyte markers and not rely on only the Melan-A stain, particularly when dealing with melanocytic lesions on sun-damaged skin.

J. C. Maize, MD

Long-term Clinical Outcomes Following Treatment of Actinic Keratosis With Imiquimod 5% Cream

Lee PK, Harwell WB, Loven KH, et al (Univ of Minnesota, Minneapolis; Dermatology Research Associates, Nashville, Tenn; Rivergate Dermatology and Skin Care, Goodlettsville, Tenn; et al)
Dermatol Surg 31:659-663, 2005   16–19

Background.—The results from four phase III, randomized, vehicle-controlled studies showed that imiquimod 5% cream (imiquimod) was safe and effective in the treatment of actinic keratosis (AK). Patients applied imiquimod or vehicle cream to AK lesions on the face or balding scalp, dosing three times per week or two times per week for 16 weeks.

Objective.—To obtain long-term safety follow-up data and estimate AK recurrence in patients who completely cleared their AK lesions in the treatment area at the 8-week post-treatment visit in the phase III studies.

Methods.—One hundred forty-six patients from 30 study centers in the United States were evaluated for clinical evidence of AK, and safety data were collected.

Results.—After a median follow-up period of 16 months, 24.7% (19 of 77) of the patients administered imiquimod three times per week and 42.6% (23 of 54) of the patients administered imiquimod two times per week had a recurrence of AK (the appearance of at least one AK lesion) in the original treatment area. The median number of AK lesions present was one lesion for both patients receiving imiquimod three times and those receiving imiquimod two times per week compared with a median of six lesions at baseline in the combined three times per week and two times per week phase III studies. There were no long-term safety issues, and the skin quality seen in the imiquimod-treated patients at the end of the phase III studies was maintained.

Conclusion.—One and a half years following treatment, imiquimod continued to provide a long-term clinical benefit in a majority of patients who experienced complete clearance of their AK lesions.

▶ This article and a brief report by Stockfleth et al[1] document the long-term beneficial effects of topical imiquimod therapy for AKs. To this reviewer's knowledge, comparative long-term data are not available for other topical treatments of AKs.

B. H. Thiers, MD

Reference

1. Stockfleth E, Christophers E, Benninghoff B, et al: Low incidence of new actinic keratoses after topical 5% imiquimod cream treatment: A long-term follow-up study (letter). *Arch Dermatol* 140:1542, 2004.

Safety and Efficacy of 5% Imiquimod Cream for the Treatment of Skin Dysplasia in High-Risk Renal Transplant Recipients: Randomized, Double-blind, Placebo-controlled Trial
Brown VL, Atkins CL, Ghali L, et al (Univ of London)
Arch Dermatol 141:985-993, 2005   16–20

Objective.—To evaluate the safety and efficacy of 5% imiquimod cream for cutaneous dysplasia in high-risk renal transplant recipients.

Design.—A randomized, blinded, placebo-controlled study comparing treated with control skin.

Setting.—A specialist organ transplant dermatology clinic.

Patients.—Twenty-one high-risk patients with skin cancer with comparable areas of clinically atypical skin on dorsal hands or forearms.

Interventions.—Imiquimod or placebo (randomly assigned) applied 3 times a week for 16 weeks to 1 dorsal hand or forearm, with 8 months of follow-up. At week 16, biopsy samples were collected from pre-assigned sites in the treatment and control areas and were examined for dysplasia.

Main Outcome Measures.—The proportion of patients showing reduced numbers of viral and keratotic lesions and reduced histological severity of dysplasia in the treatment vs control areas at week 16, serum creatinine levels, and tumors developing in the study sites.

Results.—Fourteen patients receiving imiquimod and 6 receiving placebo completed the study. Seven patients using imiquimod (1 taking placebo) had reduced skin atypia, 7 using imiquimod (none taking placebo) had reduced viral warts, and 5 using imiquimod (1 taking placebo) showed less dysplasia histologically. In 1 year, fewer squamous skin tumors arose in imiquimod-treated skin than in control areas. Renal function was not adversely affected.

Conclusions.—Topical 5% imiquimod cream seems to be safe on skin areas up to 60 cm² in renal transplant recipients. It may be effective in reducing cutaneous dysplasia and the frequency of squamous tumors developing in high-risk patients. Larger studies are required to confirm these results.

▶ As noted by the authors, larger studies are needed. Clearly, a 1-year follow-up is inadequate, and study designs should include protocols with periodic (eg, yearly) application. One theoretical hazard of applying an immunostimulatory agent to patients who are therapeutically immunosuppressed, such as renal transplant recipients, is the possibility of enhanced graft rejection. This is another area that will need to be investigated before we can be comfortable using imiquimod in this group of patients.

B. H. Thiers, MD

Topical Photodynamic Therapy Using Intense Pulsed Light for Treatment of Actinic Keratosis: Clinical and Histopathologic Evaluation

Kim HS, Yoo JY, Cho KH, et al (Seoul Natl Univ, Korea)
Dermatol Surg 31:33-37, 2005   16–21

Background.—Photodynamic therapy (PDT) is suitable for the treatment of actinic keratosis, and, recently, topical PDT using intense pulsed light as a light source has been reported. However, evaluations of its therapeutic effects have been clinically based.

Objective.—The objective of this study was to confirm the histopathologic resolution of actinic keratosis treated by topical PDT using intense pulsed light as a light source.

Methods.—Twelve actinic keratosis lesions in seven patients were treated with 5-aminolevulinic acid–PDT using intense pulsed light as a light source. After a single treatment, the clinical response was assessed and histopathologic examinations were performed on clinically resolved lesions.

Results.—Six of 12 (50%) lesions showed clinical clearance after a single treatment, but histologic examinations showed that only 5 of the 12 (42%) lesions had been removed. No complications, such as pigmentary changes or scarring, were observed.

Conclusion.—Intense pulsed light is potentially an effective light source for PDT. However, the determination of complete remission in actinic keratosis requires caution, and long-term follow-up or histologic confirmation may be required.

▶ Topical PDT with aminolevulinic acid (ALA) can be performed with a number of different light sources. Some factors to be considered in carrying out topical PDT are limited penetration of the ALA and limited penetration of the photoactivating irradiation. To circumvent these problems, in some recent studies a deeper penetrating red light has been used in lieu of the traditional blue light, and derivatives of ALA (eg, methyl-ALA) that have enhanced cutaneous penetration have been substituted for ALA. This study addressed the effectiveness of topical ALA in conjunction with intense pulsed light for the treatment of actinic keratoses (AK). Clinically 50% of the lesions cleared with a single treatment, but in one of these cases there was still histologic evidence of persistent AK. When comparing the lesions that did not respond to those that did, the authors found that these lesions often had more atypia, were thicker and more hyperkeratotic, and some had follicular involvement. It should be noted that the patients treated were Koreans with darker skin, which could influence the results because of the broad absorption spectrum of melanin. Also, in prior studies addressing the effectiveness of topical PDT for AKs, multiple treatments have been used. Finally, a very broad-spectrum light source was utilized. Efficacy might be improved if the longer wavelengths were filtered out so that more of the energy delivered was in the 630-nm range (the action spectrum of protoporphyrin IX).

P. G. Lang, Jr, MD

Imiquimod Treatment of Superficial and Nodular Basal Cell Carcinoma: 12-Week Open-Label Trial
Peris K, Campione E, Micantonio T, et al (Univ of L'Aquila, Italy; Univ of Rome)
Dermatol Surg 31:318-323, 2005   16–22

Background.—Imiquimod is an immune response modifier shown to be effective in basal cell carcinoma (BCC).

Objective.—To evaluate the efficacy, tolerability, and response durability of imiquimod 5% cream in selected patients with superficial and/or nodular BCCs.

Methods.—Seventy-five superficial and 19 nodular BCCs in 49 patients were treated with imiquimod once daily three times a week for up to 12 weeks.

Results.—Of the 49 enrolled patients, 1 discontinued the study and 1 was lost to follow-up. After 12 weeks of treatment, a complete response occurred in 70 of 75 (93.3%) superficial BCCs and a partial response in 4 of 75 (5.3%) superficial BCCs. Ten of 19 (52.6%) nodular BCCs cleared after 12 weeks, whereas 7 (36.8%) showed partial remission. Adverse side effects were limited to local skin reactions. Recurrence was observed in 2 of 70 (2.9%) successfully treated superficial BCCs 6 and 8 months after treatment discontinuation. No recurrence was detected in 68 of 70 (97.1%) superficial BCCs and in 10 successfully treated nodular BCCs after 12 to 34 months of follow-up (mean 23 months).

Conclusions.—In our patient population, treatment of superficial BCCs with topical imiquimod for 12 weeks produced an excellent clinical response overall, with complete remission maintained after a mean of 23 months.

▶ Clearly, superficial BCCs respond better than nodular BCCs to treatment with topical imiquimod. The follow-up in this study was too short to come to any definitive conclusions regarding ultimate recurrence rates.

B. H. Thiers, MD

Treatment of Diffuse Basal Cell Carcinomas and Basaloid Follicular Hamartomas in Nevoid Basal Cell Carcinoma Syndrome by Wide-Area 5-Aminolevulinic Acid Photodynamic Therapy
Oseroff AR, Shieh S, Frawley NP, et al (State Univ of New York, Buffalo; Biostatistical Consulting Services, Buffalo, NY; Univ of Tennessee, Memphis)
Arch Dermatol 141:60-67, 2005   16–23

Objective.—To report the use of wide-area 5-aminolevulinic acid photodynamic therapy to treat numerous basal cell carcinomas (BCCs) and basaloid follicular hamartomas (BFHs).

Design.—Report of cases.

Setting.—Roswell Park Cancer Institute.

Patients.—Three children with BCCs and BFHs involving 12% to 25% of their body surface areas.

Interventions.—Twenty percent 5-aminolevulinic acid was applied to up to 22% of the body surface for 24 hours under occlusion. A dye laser and a lamp illuminated fields up to 7 cm and 16 cm in diameter, respectively; up to 36 fields were treated per session.

Main Outcome Measures.—Morbidity, patient response, and light dose–photodynamic therapy response relationship and durability.

Results.—Morbidity was minimal, with selective phototoxicity and rapid healing. After 4 to 7 sessions, with individual areas receiving 1 to 3 treatments, the patients had 85% to 98% overall clearance and excellent cosmetic outcomes without scarring. For laser treatments, a sigmoidal light dose–response relationship predicted more than 85% initial response rates for light doses 150 J/cm^2 or more. Responses were durable up to 6 years.

Conclusion.—5-Aminolevulinic acid photodynamic therapy is safe, well tolerated, and effective for extensive areas of diffuse BCCs and BFHs and appears to be the treatment of choice in children.

▶ The children in this study, who had basal cell nevus syndrome with widespread BCCs and BFHs, had excellent and sustained clearing of lesions with little scarring after 5-aminolevulinic acid photodynamic therapy. This appears to be an excellent treatment option for patients with basal cell nevus syndrome.

S. Raimer, MD

Photodynamic Therapy With Topical Methyl Aminolaevulinate for 'Difficult-to-Treat' Basal Cell Carcinoma

Vinciullo C, Elliott T, Francis D, et al (Dermatology Surgery and Laser Centre, South Perth, Western Australia; Fremantle Hosp, Western Australia; Southeastern Dermatology, Brisbane, Queensland, Australia; et al)
Br J Dermatol 152:765-772, 2005   16–24

Background.—Basal cell carcinoma (BCC) may be difficult to treat by conventional means, particularly if the lesions are large or located in the mid-face (H-zone). Photodynamic therapy (PDT) using topical methyl aminolaevulinate (MAL) may be a good noninvasive option for these patients.

Objectives.—To investigate the efficacy and safety of PDT using MAL for BCCs defined as 'difficult to treat', i.e. large lesions, in the H-zone, or in patients at high risk of surgical complications.

Methods.—This was a prospective, multicentre, noncomparative study. Patients were assessed 3, 12 and 24 months after the last PDT treatment. One hundred and two patients with 'difficult-to-treat' BCC were treated with MAL PDT, using 160 mg g^{-1} cream and 75 J cm^{-2} red light (570–670 nm), after lesion preparation and 3 h of cream exposure. Results Ninety-five patients with 148 lesions were included in the per protocol analysis. The histologically confirmed lesion complete response rate at 3 months was 89%

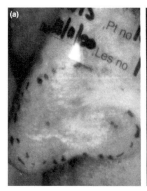 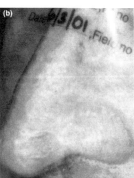 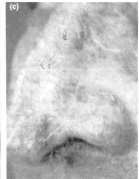

FIGURE 4.—Methyl aminolaevulinate-based photodynamic therapy (MAL PDT) can be used as an alternative therapy when surgery cannot be performed. This patient underwent Mohs' surgery, but because of inadequate local anesthetic effect and excessive bleeding the surgery was abandoned. A full-thickness graft was used to repair the Mohs' surgery defect and the patient was included in the present study 2 months later. The dotted line (a) shows the extent of the lesion prior to MAL PDT. At 3 months after MAL PDT (b), complete response was confirmed by three biopsies. The area remained tumour free at the 3-year follow-up (c). (Courtesy of Vinciullo C, Elliott T, Francis D, et al: Photodynamic therapy with topical methyl aminolaevulinate for 'difficult-to-treat' basal cell carcinoma. *Br J Dermatol* 152:765-772, 2005. Reprinted by permission of Blackwell Publishing.)

(131 of 148). At 12 months, 10 lesions had reappeared, and therefore the cumulative treatment failure rate was 18% (27 of 148). At 24 months, an additional nine lesions had reappeared, resulting in a cumulative treatment failure rate of 24% (36 of 148). The estimated sustained lesion complete response rate (assessed using a time-to-event approach) was 90% at 3 months, 84% at 12 months and 78% at 24 months. Overall cosmetic outcome was judged as excellent or good in 79% and 84% of the patients at 12 and 24 months, respectively (Fig 4; see color plate XIII). Follow-up is continuing for up to 5 years.

Conclusions.—MAL PDT is an attractive option for 'difficult-to-treat' BCC. Because of the excellent cosmetic results, the treatment is particularly well suited for lesions that would otherwise require extensive surgical procedures.

▶ The use of topical PDT to treat BCC, especially invasive lesions, has been problematic because of the limited penetration of delta-aminolevulinic acid. A derivative of this acid, MAL is said to penetrate the skin more readily and thus in theory might be more efficacious in the treatment of BCCs. On the basis of this assumption, the authors of this study looked at the effectiveness of topical PDT by using MAL in the treatment of both superficial and nodular BCCs as well as large BCCs and tumors located in high-risk areas. Although the authors seemed quite excited about their findings, a number of observations need to be made: (1) at 2 years only 82% of superficial BCCs and 67% of nodular BCCs had been cured, and (2) significant scarring can occur. Although PDT continues to evolve, a significant improvement in cure rate needs to be achieved before it can be recommended as a routine treatment modality for BCCs.

P. G. Lang, Jr, MD

Efficacy of Narrow-Margin Excision of Well-Demarcated Primary Facial Basal Cell Carcinomas

Kimyai-Asadi A, Alam M, Goldberg LH, et al (DermSurgery Associates, Houston)
J Am Acad Dermatol 53:464-468, 2005   16–25

Background.—A 4-mm surgical margin of clinically normal skin is the current standard for elliptical excision of basal cell carcinomas (BCCs). However, a 4-mm surgical margin is often not feasible on the face because of cosmetic and functional concerns. As such, facial excisions of BCCs are typically performed with the appropriate margin determined by the surgeon based on clinical features of the tumor.

Objective.—We designed a study to test the efficacy of narrow-margin elliptical excisions for the treatment of small, well-demarcated facial BCCs.

Methods.—A total of 134 primary, small (<1 cm), well-demarcated, facial nodular BCCs were excised as an ellipse with 1-, 2-, or 3-mm margins around the visible border of the tumor. The margin used was decided by the dermatologic surgeon based on cosmetic, anatomic, and functional factors, with the goal of clearing the tumor in a single excision. Using the Mohs technique for elliptical specimens, frozen sections were prepared and examined microscopically to provide complete histologic margin control.

Results.—In all, 134 facial BCCs were included in the study. On average, the tumors measured 0.6×0.5 cm. Of these, 27 (20.1%) had positive margins, requiring additional excision. Excisions with 1-, 2-, and 3-mm margins were associated with positive margins in 16%, 24%, and 13% of tumors, respectively. There was no statistically significant difference in the occurrence of positive margins based on tumor size, anatomic location, or the measured margin used.

Conclusion.—Narrow margins (1-3 mm) are inadequate for the excision of small, well-demarcated, primary nodular BCCs of the face. To avoid repetitive operations and the risk of recurrence in anatomically sensitive areas, these tumors should be treated with standard wide margins (eg, 4 mm), or have Mohs micrographic surgery for histologic margin control.

▶ The surgeon treating BCC of the face must strive to achieve 2 goals—successful tumor extirpation and preservation of function/cosmesis. Even in this series limited to small, well-demarcated facial BCCs, more narrow (<4 mm) surgical margins resulted in a significant number of resection specimens demonstrating positive surgical margins. The resection complicated by involved surgical margins subjects the patient to additional procedural morbidity and expense. Moreover, the resection of skin that is not involved with tumor may complicate reconstructive options, should the need for further surgery arise. For this reason, Mohs surgery remains the gold standard for treating larger, recurrent, or anatomically challenging BCCs of the head and neck.

J. Cook, MD

Accuracy of Serial Transverse Cross-Sections in Detecting Residual Basal Cell Carcinoma at the Surgical Margins of an Elliptical Excision Specimen

Kimyai-Asadi A, Goldberg LH, Jih MH (DermSurgery Associates, Houston)
J Am Acad Dermatol 53:469-474, 2005   16–26

Background.—There has been no published study estimating the proportion of positive surgical margins that is missed when serial transverse cross-sectioning (bread-loafing) is used to histologically evaluate the surgical margins.

Objective.—Our purpose was to estimate the accuracy of serial transverse cross-sectioning (bread-loafing) at 4-mm intervals in detecting the presence of residual tumor at the margins of well-defined facial basal cell carcinomas excised as an ellipse with 2-mm surgical margins.

Methods.—Forty-two small (<1 cm), well-defined, primary, nonmorpheaform facial basal cell carcinomas that had been excised as an ellipse with 2-mm margins and that had positive surgical margins utilizing en-face Mohs sections were included. After longitudinal bisection of each ellipse, frozen sections were prepared encompassing the entire surgical margin.

Transparencies with parallel lines spaced at 4-mm intervals were superimposed on the histologic slides with the lines perpendicular to the epidermal surface. Areas in which the lines intersected tumor at the surgical margin were noted. The percentage of tumors that would be detected by serial cross sections was calculated on the basis of the percentage of these parallel lines that intersected tumor.

Results.—The 42 tumors had a total of 50 positive surgical margins. Overall, the cross-sectional lines intersected tumor 44% of the time (95% confidence interval, 37%-51%). Only 5 (10%) of the residual tumors at the surgical margins exceeded 4 mm in their longitudinal dimension. In the 9 sections containing tumor in the deep margin, tumor intersected the lines 39% of the time.

Conclusion.—Bread-loafing at 4-mm intervals of elliptical excision specimens from facial basal cell carcinomas excised with 2-mm surgical margins is only 44% sensitive in detecting residual tumor at the surgical margins. We recommend complete histologic margin control by using en face tissue orientation (Mohs technique) to identify residual tumor and reduce the risk of tumor recurrence after elliptical excision of facial basal cell carcinomas.

▶ This article simply recapitulates what is widely known; that is, standard pathology bread-loafing of elliptical excision specimens demonstrates low sensitivity in detecting residual tumor at the surgical margins. This underscores the importance of the Mohs technique in more challenging cases.

J. Cook, MD

Basal Cell Carcinoma Treated With Mohs Surgery in Australia. I. Experience Over 10 Years

Leibovitch I, Huilgol SC, Selva D, et al (Univ of Adelaide, Australia; Wakefield Clinic, Adelaide, Australia; Skin & Cancer Found Australia, Sydney)
J Am Acad Dermatol 53:445-451, 2005   16–27

Background.—Only a few prospective studies have been published on surgical treatments for cutaneous basal cell carcinoma (BCC).

Objective.—Our purpose was to report the clinical findings of all patients with BCC treated with Mohs micrographic surgery (MMS) in Australia between 1993 and 2002.

Method.—This prospective, multicenter case series included all patients in Australia treated with MMS for BCC, who were monitored by the Skin and Cancer Foundation between 1993 and 2002. The main outcome measures were patient demographics, reason for referral, duration of tumor, site, preoperative tumor size, recurrences before MMS, histologic classification of malignancy, and postoperative defect size.

Results.—The study included 11,127 patients (47% females and 53% males) with a mean age of 62 years (range, 15-98 years). In 43.8% of cases BCC was a recurrent tumor. Most of the tumors (98.3%) were on the head and neck area, most commonly on the nose (39%), cheek and maxilla

(16.5%), periocular area (12.7%), and auricular region (11.4%). The most common histologic subtypes were infiltrating (30.7%), nodulocystic (24.2%), and superficial (13.6%). Previously recurrent tumors were larger than primary tumors ($P < .001$), had a larger postexcision defect and more subclinical extension, and required more levels of excision ($P < .001$).

Limitations.—Data were missing for some outcome measures.

Conclusion.—This large prospective series of BCC managed by MMS is characterized by a high percentage of high-risk tumors. Most tumors were located in the mid-facial area and the histologic subtype was mainly infiltrating or nodulocystic. That previously recurrent tumors were larger and demonstrated a more extensive subclinical extension compared with primary tumors emphasizes the importance of initial tumor eradication with margin control.

Basal Cell Carcinoma Treated With Mohs Surgery in Australia. II. Outcome at 5-Year Follow-up

Leibovitch I, Huilgol SC, Selva D, et al (Univ of Adelaide, Australia; Wakefield Clinic, Adelaide, Australia; Skin and Cancer Found Australia, Sydney)
J Am Acad Dermatol 53:452-457, 2005   16–28

Background.—Long-term follow-up is essential to evaluate the role of Mohs micrographic surgery (MMS) in the treatment for cutaneous basal cell carcinoma (BCC).

Objective.—Our purpose was to report the 5-year follow-up outcome of patients treated with MMS for BCC.

Method.—This prospective, multicenter case series included all patients in Australia treated with MMS for BCC, who were monitored by the Skin and Cancer Foundation between 1993 and 2002. Parameters recorded were patient demographics, duration of tumor, site, preoperative tumor size, recurrences before MMS, histologic classification of malignancy, postoperative defect size, and 5-year recurrence after MMS.

Results.—Three thousand three hundred seventy (3370) patients (1594 female and 1776 male patients) completed a 5-year follow-up period. Fifty-six percent of the tumors were primary and 44% were previously recurrent. Most of them (98.4%) were located on the head and neck, and the most common histologic subtypes were nodulocystic (29.3%) and infiltrating (28.3%). Recurrence at 5 years was diagnosed in 1.4% of primary and in 4% of recurrent tumors. Previous tumor recurrence ($P < .001$), longer tumor duration before MMS ($P = .015$), infiltrating histology ($P = .13$), and more levels for tumor ($P < .001$) were the main predictors for tumor recurrence after MMS.

Limitation.—Data were missing for some outcome measures.

Conclusion.—The low 5-year recurrence rate of BCC with MMS emphasizes the importance of margin-controlled excision.

▶ This large and well-documented series (Abstracts 16–27 and 16–28) included many patients with primary and recurrent BCCs—many in anatomically critical areas. Many of the patients presented with clinically challenging tumors. The success of MMS for both primary and recurrent tumors is again demonstrated and parallels the results seen in similar studies that have long been considered the benchmarks of documenting the successful track record of the Mohs technique.[1,2]

J. Cook, MD

References

1. Rowe DE, Carroll RJ, Day CL Jr: Long-term recurrence rates in previously untreated (primary) basal cell carcinoma: Implications for patient followup. *J Dermatol Surg Oncol* 15:315-328, 1989.
2. Rowe DE, Carroll RJ, Day CL Jr: Mohs surgery is the treatment of choice for recurrent (previously treated) basal cell carcinoma. *J Dermatol Surg Oncol* 15:424-431, 1989.

Cutaneous Squamous Cell Carcinomas Treated With Mohs Micrographic Surgery in Australia. I. Experience Over 10 Years

Leibovitch I, Huilgol SC, Selva D, et al (Univ of Adelaide, Australia; Wakefield Clinic, Adelaide, Australia; Skin and Cancer Found Australia, Sydney)
J Am Acad Dermatol 53:253-260, 2005　　　　　　　　16–29

Background.—Only a few reports have been published on the long-term outcome of surgical excision of cutaneous squamous cell carcinoma (SCC).

Objective.—Our purpose was to report the clinical findings and 5-year recurrence rate of all patients with cutaneous SCC treated with Mohs micrographic surgery (MMS) in Australia between 1993 and 2002.

Method.—This prospective, multicenter case series included all patients with SCC who were monitored by the Skin and Cancer Foundation. The main outcome measures were patient demographics, reason for referral, duration of tumor, site, preoperative tumor size, postoperative defect size, recurrences before MMS, histological subtypes, and 5-year recurrence after MMS.

Results.—The case series comprised 1263 patients (25.7% female and 74.3% male; $P < .0001$) with a mean age of 66 ± 13 years. In 61.1% of cases the lesion was a primary tumor, and in 38.9% it was a recurrent tumor. Most of the tumors (96.5%) were on the head and neck area. Recurrent tumors were larger than primary tumors ($P < .0001$), had a larger postexcision defect ($P < .0001$), required more levels of excision ($P < .0001$), and had more cases of subclinical extension ($P = .002$). Recurrence after MMS was diagnosed in 15 of the 381 patients (3.9%) who completed the 5-year follow-up after MMS. The recurrence rate was 2.6% in patients with primary SCC and 5.9% in patients with previously recurrent SCC ($P < .001$).

Conclusion.—This large prospective series of SCC managed by MMS is characterized by a high percentage of high-risk tumors. The low 5-year recurrence rate with MMS emphasizes the importance of margin-controlled excision.

Cutaneous Squamous Cell Carcinoma Treated With Mohs Micrographic Surgery in Australia. II. Perineural Invasion

Leibovitch I, Huilgol SC, Selva D, et al (Univ of Adelaide, Australia; Wakefield Clinic, Adelaide, Australia; Skin and Cancer Found Australia, Sydney)
J Am Acad Dermatol 53:261-266, 2005   16–30

Background.—Perineural invasion (PNI) is an important histologic factor that plays a significant role in cutaneous tumors' aggressiveness.

Objectives.—We sought to evaluate the incidence, features, and outcomes of cutaneous squamous cell carcinoma with PNI in patients treated with Mohs micrographic surgery (MMS).

Method.—This prospective, multicenter, case series included all patients in Australia treated with MMS for squamous cell carcinoma with PNI who were monitored by the Skin and Cancer Foundation Australia between 1993 and 2002. The parameters recorded were patient demographics, duration of tumor, site, preoperative tumor size, recurrence before MMS, histologic subtypes, postoperative defect size, and recurrence at 5 years after MMS.

Results.—Seventy patients were given a diagnosis of PNI. PNI was more common in men (77.1%) and in previously recurrent tumors ($P = .04$). The moderately and poorly differentiated histologic subtypes were more likely to be associated with PNI ($P < .0001$). Tumor sizes before excision, postoperative defect sizes, subclinical extension, and mean number of MMS levels were significantly larger in cases with PNI compared with cases without PNI ($P < .0001$, $P < .0001$, $P = .002$, and $P < .0001$, respectively). Most patients with PNI (52.9%) were treated with adjunctive radiotherapy. In all, 25 patients completed a 5-year follow-up post-MMS, and two of them (8.0%) were given a diagnosis of recurrence.

Conclusion.—Although PNI is an uncommon feature of cutaneous squamous cell carcinoma, when present, it is associated with larger, more aggressive tumors, and the risk of recurrence is higher. This emphasizes the importance of tumor excision with margin control and long-term patient monitoring.

▶ These 2 articles (Abstracts 16–29 and 16–30) again demonstrate the success of MMS in the treatment of cutaneous SCC. The biological aggressiveness of SCC may increase significantly with failed initial or subsequent treatments. Recurrent SCC and perineural SCC may prove to be clinically aggressive neoplasms with a significant incidence of tumor dissemination and its attendant morbidity or mortality. This underscores the importance of successful initial treatment of cutaneous SCC. This article echoes the findings of previously published studies that demonstrate the success of the Mohs technique.

J. Cook, MD

Curettage Prior to Mohs' Micrographic Surgery for Previously Biopsied Nonmelanoma Skin Cancers: What Are We Curetting? Retrospective, Prospective, and Comparative Study

Jih MH, Friedman PM, Goldberg LH, et al (DermSurgery Associates, Houston)
Dermatol Surg 31:10-15, 2005   16–31

Background.—Curettage prior to excision and Mohs' micrographic surgery for nonmelanoma skin cancer is performed based on the assumption that the curette will remove softer, more friable tumor-infiltrated dermis and leave structurally intact normal skin. This assumption, however, has not been objectively examined in the dermatologic surgery literature.

Objective.—We performed a study to examine the ability of curettage to selectively remove and delineate nonmelanoma skin cancer prior to Mohs' micrographic surgery.

Methods.—The study included 150 previously biopsied basal cell and squamous cell carcinomas less than 1.5 cm in size. We conducted (1) a retrospective study of 50 tumors curetted prior to Mohs' surgery by a surgeon who routinely curettes preoperatively; (2) a prospective study in which a surgeon who routinely does not curette preoperatively curetted 50 tumors prior to Mohs' surgery; and (3) a comparative historical group of 50 noncuretted tumors treated with Mohs' surgery by the latter surgeon. All curetted tissue was evaluated histologically.

Results.—Only 50% of the curetted tissue demonstrated the presence of tumor in the curettings, but in 76% of these, the curette left residual tumor at the surgical margins. Of the other 50% in which the curette removed only non-cancer-containing skin, 34% had tumor present at the surgical margin. Overall, the curette removed tumor, leaving no residual tumor at the surgical margins in only 12% of lesions. Comparison with historical noncuretted tumors operated on by the same surgeon showed that curettage did not affect the mean number of stages or the proportion of tumors requiring more than one stage for histologic clearance.

Conclusion.—Although curettage may be helpful in debulking friable skin prior to Mohs' micrographic surgery, it does not reliably delineate the extent of a tumor.

► There are 2 groups of Mohs surgeons—those who curette and those who do not. I changed and joined the latter group several years ago. I now do not curette before the initiation of Mohs surgery, and I agree with the findings presented by these authors. In my opinion, curettage may unnecessarily enlarge the size of the defect, particularly in significantly sun-damaged skin.

J. Cook, MD

What Is the Microscopic Tumor Extent Beyond Clinically Delineated Gross Tumor Boundary in Nonmelanoma Skin Cancers?

Choo R, Woo T, Assaad D, et al (Univ of Toronto; Mayo Clinic, Rochester, Minn)
Int J Radiat Oncol Biol Phys 62:1096-1099, 2005   16–32

Purpose.—To quantify the microscopic tumor extension beyond clinically delineated gross tumor boundary in nonmelanoma skin cancers.

Methods and Materials.—A prospective, single arm, study. Preoperatively, a radiation oncologist outlined the boundary of a gross lesion, and drew 5-mm incremental marks in four directions from the delineated border. Under local anesthesia, the lesion was excised, and resection margins were assessed microscopically by frozen section. Once resection margins were clear, the microscopic tumor extent was calculated using the presurgical incremental markings as references. A potential relationship between the distance of microscopic tumor extension and other variables was analyzed.

Results.—A total of 71 lesions in 64 consecutive patients, selected for surgical excision with frozen-section-assisted assessment of resection margins, were accrued. The distance of microscopic tumor extension beyond a gross lesion varied from 1 mm to 15 mm, with a mean of 5.2 mm (Table 2). A margin of 10 mm was required to provide a 95% chance of obtaining clear resection margins. The microscopic tumor extent was positively correlated with the size of gross lesion, but not with other variables.

Conclusions.—The distance of microscopic tumor extension beyond a gross nonmelanoma skin cancer was variable, with a mean of 5.2 mm. Such

TABLE 2.—Maximal Microscopic Tumor Extent Beyond Gross Tumor

	Sclerosing BCC (n = 38)	Other Type BCC (n = 19)	SCC (n = 14)
Mean (mm)	5.0	5.3	5.7
Mean for entire cohort (n = 71): 5.2 mm			
Range			
1 mm	2 (5.2%)	0 (0%)	0 (0%)
2-3 mm	10 (26.3%)	7 (36.8%)	3 (21.4%)
4-5 mm	14 (36.8%)	5 (26.3%)	3 (21.4%)
6-7 mm	6 (15.8%)	4 (21.1%)	5 (35.7%)
8-9 mm	5 (13.2%)	0 (0%)	2 (14.3%)
≥10 mm	1 (2.6%)	3 (15.8%)	1 (7.1%)
Size of gross tumor (≤2 cm vs. >2 cm)			
≤2 cm	3.8 mm	4.2 mm	4.3 mm
>2 cm	6.1 mm	7.1 mm	6.3 mm
Primary vs. recurrent			
Primary	5.1 mm	4.5 mm	4.9 mm
Recurrent	4.8 mm	6.6 mm	6.6 mm
Number of surgical attempts required to obtain clear margins			
1 attempt	3.4 mm	3.5 mm	4.6 mm
≥2 attempts	5.5 mm	5.7 mm	6.9 mm

Abbreviations: BCC = basal cell carcinoma; SCC = squamous cell carcinoma.
(Reprinted from Choo R, Woo T, Assaad D, et al: What is the microscopic tumor extent beyond clinically delineated gross tumor boundary in nonmelanoma skin cancers? *Int J Radiat Oncol Biol Phys* 62:1096-1099, 2005. Copyright 2005, with permission from Elsevier Science.)

information is critical for the proper radiation planning of skin cancer therapy.

▶ In order to cure skin cancer with radiation therapy, one must know how much of a margin of clinically normal surrounding skin to include in the radiation field. This study attempts to answer this question through the use of routine surgical excision with frozen section control. Margins of 2 to 3 mm were used for the initial excision of the lesions. Many of the lesions studied would have been considered high-risk lesions based on their size, histology, recurrence, and nature. Of these lesions, 70.4% required at least one reexcision to obtain clear margins. The mean subclinical extension was 5.2 mm, with a range of 1 to 15 mm. The only variable correlating with the degree of subclinical spread was a size greater than 2 cm. It was determined that a margin of 10 mm would have been necessary to obtain clear margins in 95% of cases. No similar assessment of deep margins was carried out. This study provides useful information not only for the radiation oncologist, but it also demonstrates the variable subclinical spread of high-risk nonmelanoma skin cancers. Thus, to enhance tissue conservation, it suggests that Mohs surgery would be preferable to arbitrary resection of these lesions with a 1-cm margin. From the standpoint of cure, studies need to be done comparing Mohs micrographic surgery to routine surgical removal with frozen section control, although historically Mohs surgery has yielded superior results.

P. G. Lang, Jr, MD

Peritumoral Fibrosis in Basal Cell and Squamous Cell Carcinoma Mimicking Perineural Invasion: Potential Pitfall in Mohs Micrographic Surgery
Hassanein AM, Proper SA, Depcik-Smith ND, et al (Univ of Florida, Gainesville; Ctr for Dermatology and Skin Surgery, Tampa, Fla)
Dermatol Surg 31:1101-1106, 2005   16–33

Background.—Perineural invasion (PI) in cutaneous basal cell carcinoma (BCC) and squamous cell carcinoma (SCC) is linked to an aggressive course. We describe a histologic mimic for PI that we termed *peritumoral fibrosis* (PF).

Objective.—To describe the morphologic changes associated with PF and to determine the incidence of PF and PI in Mohs frozen sections of BCC and SCC.

Material and Methods.—All cases of BCC and SCC that were treated by Mohs micrographic surgery (MMS) at the Skin and Cancer Center, University of Florida College of Medicine, Gainesville, Florida, and the Center for Dermatology and Skin Surgery, Tampa, Florida, during the period from January 1, 2003, to August 1, 2004, were reviewed for the presence of PI and PF. The latter was defined as the presence of concentric layers of fibrous tissue that either surround and/or were surrounded by tumor formations mimicking perineural or intraneural invasion. Seven hundred six cases of BCC and 264 cases of SCC were surveyed. Eleven cases (10 BCC and 1 SCC) with equivocal areas were destained, and immunohistochemical staining with S-100 protein was performed, proving actual PI in all of these cases. Available original hematoxylin-eosin biopsy slides were correlated with the MMS frozen sections.

Results.—PF was noticed in 4.5% of SCCs and 5.8% of BCCs. The incidence of unequivocal PI was noted to be 2.6% in SCC and 2.1% in BCC.

Conclusion.—We describe a specific pattern of fibrosis noted in BCC and SCC that we called PF. It shows concentric layers of fibrous tissue surrounding and/or surrounded by tumor formations and resembles carcinomatous perineural and/or intraneural invasion. Moreover, PF was found to be a sensitive marker for PI. Mohs micrographic surgeons should be aware of this phenomenon to avoid triggering unnecessary steps in managing these cases, such as irradiation.

▶ Perineural tumors can be quite difficult to trace out and at times may require the use of immunostains or permanent sections. In this report, the authors discuss 3 histologic entities that can mimic perineural involvement and with which Mohs surgeons should be familiar: (1) PF, (2) re-excision PI, and (3) epithelial sheath neuroma. The emphasis of the article is on PF. Unfortunately, the photomicrographs do not illustrate very well the authors' contention that PF can mimic PI.

P. G. Lang, Jr, MD

High Recurrence Rates of Squamous Cell Carcinoma After Mohs' Surgery in Patients With Chronic Lymphocytic Leukemia

Mehrany K, Weenig RH, Pittelkow MR, et al (Mayo Clinic, Rochester, Minn)
Dermatol Surg 31:38-42, 2005   16–34

Background.—Cutaneous cancers exhibit a much higher incidence in patients with chronic lymphocytic leukemia than in nonleukemic patients. Squamous and basal cell carcinomas also exhibit greater subclinical tumor extension in patients with chronic lymphocytic leukemia.

Objective.—The purpose of this study was to estimate and compare the recurrence rates of squamous cell carcinoma after Mohs' surgery in patients with chronic lymphocytic leukemia compared with those in controls and to evaluate differences among squamous cell carcinoma size and histologic grade.

Methods.—We retrospectively assessed the clinical histories, postoperative notes, and surgical photographs of patients with chronic lymphocytic leukemia and controls matched (2:1) for age, sex, and surgical year. Both patients and controls underwent Mohs' surgery for squamous cell carcinoma of the head and neck at the Mayo Clinic between March 1988 and April 1999.

Results.—Twenty-eight patients who underwent Mohs' surgery for 57 squamous cell carcinomas had 7 recurrences. The cumulative incidence of recurrence on a per-tumor basis was 4.3% at 1 year, 14.8% at 3 years, and

19.0% at 5 years. Squamous cell carcinoma was seven times more likely to recur in patients with chronic lymphocytic leukemia than in controls ($p = .003$). The distribution of tumor histologic grade was not significantly different between patients and controls ($p = .39$). Maximum preoperative tumor diameters were clinically similar between patients and controls (median 15 mm vs 14 mm; $p = .04$).

Conclusion.—The recurrence rates of squamous cell carcinoma were significantly higher in patients with chronic lymphocytic leukemia. Squamous cell carcinomas in patients with chronic lymphocytic leukemia did not exhibit a significant difference in histologic grade or clinical difference in preoperative tumor size. Close surveillance for squamous cell carcinoma recurrence is warranted in patients with chronic lymphocytic leukemia.

▶ SCCs tend to be significantly more biologically aggressive in patients with chronic lymphocytic leukemia. The treating physician must take this into account when considering the various treatment options.

J. Cook, MD

Interstitial Brachytherapy of Periorificial Skin Carcinomas of the Face: A Retrospective Study of 97 Cases

Rio E, Bardet E, Ferron C, et al (CRLCC-Nantes-Atlantique, Saint Herblain, France; CHU Hôtel Dieu, Saint Herblain, France)
Int J Radiat Oncol Biol Phys 63:753-757, 2005   16–35

Purpose.—To analyze outcomes after interstitial brachytherapy of facial periorificial skin carcinomas.

Patients and Methods.—We performed a retrospective analysis of 97 skin carcinomas (88 basal cell carcinomas, 9 squamous cell carcinomas) of the nose, periorbital areas, and ears from 40 previously untreated patients (Group 1) and 57 patients who had undergone surgery (Group 2). The average dose was 55 Gy (range, 50–65 Gy) in Group 1 and 52 Gy (range, 50–60 Gy) in Group 2 (mean implantation times: 79 and 74 hours, respectively). We calculated survival rates and assessed functional and cosmetic results *de visu*.

Results.—Median age was 71 years (range, 17–97 years). There were 29 T1, 8 T2, 1 T3, and 2 Tx tumors in Group 1. Tumors were <2 cm in Group 2 (Table 1). Local control was 92.5% in Group 1 and 88% in Group 2 (median follow-up, 55 months; range, 6–132 months). Five-year disease-free survival was better in Group 1 (91%; range, 75–97) than in Group 2 (80%; range, 62–90; $p = 0.23$). Of the 34 patients whose results were reassessed, 8 presented with pruritus or epiphora; 1 Group 2 patient had an impaired eyelid aperture. Cosmetic results were better in Group 1 than in Group 2 with, respectively, 72% (8/11) vs. 52% (12/23) good results and 28 (3/11) vs. 43% (10/23) fair results.

Conclusions.—Brachytherapy provided a high level of local control and good cosmetic results for facial periorificial skin carcinomas that pose prob-

TABLE 1.—Patient and Tumor Characteristics

	First-Line Brachytherapy (Group 1; n = 40)	Brachytherapy After Surgery (Group 2; n = 57)
Site		
Nose	25 (62.5)	32 (56)
Tip	10	18
Lateral side	8	10
Bridge	5	3
Nostril	2	1
Periorbital zone	13 (32.5)	17 (30)
Inner canthus	10	10
Lower lid	3	7
Pinna	2 (5)	8 (14)
Concha	1	4
Tragus	1	1
Retroauricular groove	0	3
Histology		
Basal cell carcinoma	35	53
Sclerodermiform subtype	7	8
Squamous cell carcinoma	5	4
Stage*		All 57 <2 cm
T1N0	29 (72.5)	in diameter
T2N0	8 (20)	
T3N0	1 (2.5)	
TxN0	2 (5)	

Numbers in brackets are percentages.
*According to TNM classification.
(Reprinted from Rio E, Bardet E, Ferron C, et al: Interstitial brachytherapy of periorificial skin carcinomas of the face: A retrospective study of 97 cases. *Int J Radiat Oncol Biol Phys* 63:653-757, 2005. Copyright 2005, with permission from Elsevier Science.)

lems of surgical reconstruction. Results were better for untreated tumors than for incompletely excised tumors or tumors recurring after surgery.

▶ Radiation therapy is a reasonable choice for treating basal carcinoma and squamous cell carcinoma in patients who are elderly, patients who are poor surgical candidates, or those who do not wish to undergo the complex or extensive reconstructive surgery that is often necessary in patients with periorificial tumors. When patients are referred for radiation therapy, they usually undergo external radiation, often with electron beams. However, another form of radiation therapy is the use of implants, in this case ^{192}Ir wires. This form of radiation treatment is known as interstitial brachytherapy. In this study, interstitial brachytherapy provided a local control rate of 92.5% for small periorificial basal and squamous cell carcinomas and a control rate of 88% for incompletely excised or recurrent tumors. There was no correlation between control rate and the histology of the tumor. Although the authors are somewhat vague about the long-term cosmetic and functional outcome of treatment, it appears that overall the results were quite acceptable. However, telangiectasia was common and several patients with periocular tumors developed functional impairments.

P. G. Lang, Jr, MD

Radiation Therapy for Bowen's Disease of the Skin

VanderSpek LAL, Pond GR, Wells W, et al (Univ of Toronto)
Int J Radiat Oncol Biol Phys 63:505-510, 2005   16–36

Purpose.—To assess the clinical outcome in the radiation therapy (RT) of squamous carcinoma in situ of the skin (Bowen's disease). We focused on the local control rate and the toxicity according to the biologically effective dose (BED).

Methods and Materials.—A retrospective review was performed on 44 patients with Bowen's disease treated at Princess Margaret Hospital from April 1985 to November 2000. RT was the primary treatment for 32 patients, whereas 12 received RT for residual disease after local ablative therapy. Lesions were located as follows: scalp, 9 patients (20%); face, 12 (27%); trunk, 6 (14%), extremity, 12 (27%), perianal, 3 (7%), and penis, 2 (5%). Orthovoltage X-rays were used in the majority (39 of 44, 89%). There was no standard fractionation regimen: some physicians prescribed high doses, as for invasive skin cancer, whereas others prescribed lower doses because of the noninvasive nature of the disease, a sensitive anatomic location (e.g., extremity), or large treatment area. Because of the variations in fractionation regimens, BED was used as a common metric for biologic effect in the comparison of different regimens and analyzed for correlation with recurrence and toxicity. Local control was defined as the lack of persistent or recurrent disease at the treated site for the follow-up period. Grade 4 toxicity was defined as necrosis (cartilage/bone damage) and/or ulceration for a duration of >3 months.

Results.—The mean patient age was 67.7 years, and the male/female ratio was 29:15. The median pretreatment lesion size was 2.65 cm^2 (range, 0.07-34.56 cm^2). Complete remission was achieved in 42 patients, with follow-up unavailable for the remaining 2 patients. Subsequently, 3 patients experienced recurrences at 0.2, 1.1, and 1-1.5 years after complete remission. One recurrence was Bowen's disease (local); the others were squamous cell carcinoma (one local, one marginal). Four patients experienced a new squamous lesion at a distant cutaneous site. As of last follow-up, 32 patients (73%) were known to be alive. Median follow-up was 2.6 years (range, 0-11.8 years). All but 3 patients were disease-free at last follow-up, 1 of whom died with distant, but not local disease. The 5-year overall survival rate was 68%. Biologically effective dose was not associated with recurrence. The crude local control rate was 93%. There was a trend toward higher radiation doses for smaller pretreatment tumor and field sizes. The BED did not correlate with Grade 4 toxicity; however, the three cases of Grade 4 toxicity occurred in patients treated with hypofractionated regimens (dose per fraction >4 Gy) for extremity lesions.

Conclusions.—Radiation therapy is an effective treatment option for Bowen's disease of the skin. Local recurrences seem to be equally low in patients treated with high- and low-dose regimens. Avoiding hypofractionated

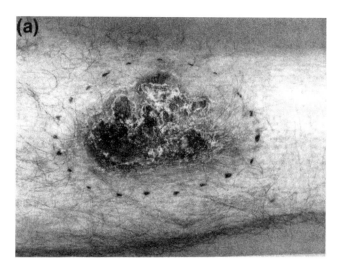

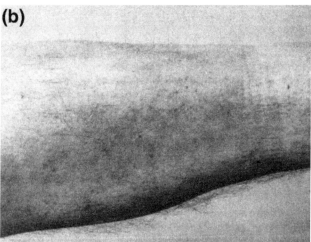

FIGURE 1.—(a) A 66-year-old man with Bowen's disease of the leg, 4 cm × 6 cm, located over the tibia, before radiotherapy. (b) Complete remission of the lesion after treatment with 25 Gy in 10 fractions (125-kV beam; source–skin distance, 50 cm; half-value layer, 3.5 mm Al). Mild pigmentation and telangiectasia were seen 3 years after treatment. (Reprinted from VanderSpek LAL, Pond GR, Wells W, et al: Radiation therapy for Bowen's disease of the skin. *Int J Radiat Oncol Biol Phys* 63:505-510, 2005. Copyright 2005, with permission from Elsevier Science.)

regimens (dose per fraction >4 Gy) in extremity locations might reduce the risk of Grade 4 toxicity (Fig 1).

▶ Unquestionably, the treatment of choice for Bowen's disease is excision. For large lesions, lesions in cosmetically sensitive or anatomically difficult areas, or lesions in patients who are not surgical candidates, a nonsurgical approach may be considered. Although RT is an option, application of imiquimod may be much cheaper and more convenient.[1] Obviously, the comparative therapeutic efficacy of these 2 modalities is unknown.

B. H. Thiers, MD

Reference

1. Mackenzie-Wood A, Kossard S, de Launey J, et al: Imiquimod 5% cream in the treatment of Bowen's disease. *J Am Acad Dermatol* 44:462-470, 2001.

Topical 5-Fluorouracil in the Management of Extensive Anal Bowen's Disease: A Preferred Approach
Graham BD, Jetmore AB, Foote JE, et al (Shawnee Mission Med Ctr, Kan; North Kansas City Hosp, Mo; Mid Missouri Dermatology, Columbia, Mo)
Dis Colon Rectum 48:444-450, 2005 16–37

Purpose.—An alternative approach to anal Bowen's disease was investigated. The use of topical 5 percent 5-fluorouracil for large lesions and surgical excision of small lesions were evaluated.

Methods.—A prospective study was undertaken for anal Bowen's disease in 11 patients over a six-year period. Before therapy all patients underwent anal mapping biopsy and colonoscopy. For one-half circumferential disease or greater, patients underwent topical 5 percent 5-fluorouacil therapy for 16 weeks. For smaller involvement, wide surgical excision was performed. All patients underwent anal mapping biopsy one year after completion of therapy.

Results.—Of 11 patients, 8 (5 male) received 16 weeks of topical 5 percent 5-fluorouacil therapy. Three patients (3 female) underwent surgical excision for localized disease. All but one patient, who was HIV positive, were free of Bowen's disease one year after completion of therapy. One patient underwent total excision of a residual microinvasive squamous carcinoma after circumferential Bowen's disease had resolved. One patient received eight additional weeks of topical 5-fluorouacil therapy for incomplete resolution. All patients were followed yearly, with a mean follow-up of 39 months and a range of 12 to 74 months. There have been no recurrences. There were no long-term side effects or morbidity from topical 5-fluorouacil or local excision. All colonoscopies were normal.

Conclusion.—Topical 5 percent 5-fluorouacil therapy is a safe and effective method to treat anal Bowen's disease. Wide local excision is appropriate for smaller, isolated areas of disease. Anal Bowen's disease was not associated with colonic or other neoplasms.

▶ This report documents the efficacy of topical 5% 5-fluorouracil in the treatment of extensive anal Bowen's disease. Unfortunately, the cohort studied was relatively small, and other possible treatment approaches (eg, topical imiquimod, photodynamic therapy, etc) were not included. Nevertheless, topical

5% 5-fluorouracil may be a viable alternative to surgery for patients with large lesions.

B. H. Thiers, MD

Identification of Muir–Torre Syndrome Among Patients With Sebaceous Tumors and Keratoacanthomas: Role of Clinical Features, Microsatellite Instability, and Immunohistochemistry

Ponti G, Losi L, Di Gregorio C, et al (Univ of Modena and Reggio Emilia, Italy; Carpi Gen Hosp, Modena, Italy; Catholic Univ, Rome)

Cancer 103:1018-1025, 2005   16–38

Background.—The Muir–Torre syndrome (MTS) is an autosomal-dominant genodermatosis characterized by the presence of sebaceous gland tumors, with or without keratoacanthomas, associated with visceral malignancies. A subset of patients with MTS is considered a variant of the hereditary nonpolyposis colorectal carcinoma, which is caused by mutations in mismatch-repair genes. The objective of the current study was to evaluate whether a combined clinical, immunohistochemical, and biomolecular approach could be useful for the identification of Muir–Torre syndrome among patients with a diagnosis of sebaceous tumors and keratoacanthomas.

Methods.—The authors collected sebaceous skin lesions and keratoacanthomas recorded in the files of the Pathology Department of the University of Modena during the period 1986-2000. Through interviews and examination of clinical charts, family trees were drawn for 120 patients who were affected by these skin lesions.

Results.—Seven patients also were affected by gastrointestinal tumors, thus meeting the clinical criteria for the diagnosis of MTS. In the MTS families, a wide phenotypic variability was evident, both in the spectrum of visceral tumors and in the type of skin lesions. Microsatellite instability was found in five MTS patients: These patients showed concordance with immunohistochemical analysis; moreover, a constitutional mutation in the *MSH2* gene was found in 1 patient. Lack of expression of *MSH2/MSH6* or *MLH1* proteins was evident in the skin lesions and in the associated internal malignancies of 3 patients and 2 patients with MTS, respectively.

Conclusions.—The clinical, biomolecular, and immunohistochemical characterization of sebaceous skin lesions and keratoacanthomas may be used as screening for the identification of families at risk of MTS, a disease that is difficult to recognize and diagnose.

▶ Because sebaceous tumors are rare in the general population, their diagnosis warrants a search for an underlying internal malignancy. Ponti et al present biomolecular and immunohistochemical data to aid in the identification of families with suspected MTS. These patients should undergo regular clinical and endoscopic evaluations to allow for the early diagnosis of any associated internal malignancies.

B. H. Thiers, MD

Proliferating Pilar Tumors: A Clinicopathologic Study of 76 Cases With a Proposal for Definition of Benign and Malignant Variants
Ye J, Nappi O, Swanson PE, et al (Dahl-Chase Pathology Associates, Bangor, Me; Cardarelli Hosp, Naples, Italy; Univ of Washington, Seattle; et al)
Am J Clin Pathol 122:566-574, 2004   16–39

Introduction.—We studied proliferating pilar tumors (PPTs) to establish histologic criteria that could predict behavior. We reviewed all cases in our consultation files (1989-2000) and evaluated 76 cases with meaningful follow-up information. Histologic examination involved attention to tumor silhouette, degree of nuclear atypia, mitotic activity, necrosis, and perineurial or angiolymphatic invasion. Tumors were stratified as follows: group 1 PPTs, circumscribed silhouettes with "pushing" margins, modest nuclear atypia, and an absence of pathologic mitoses, necrosis, and invasion of nerves or vessels; group 2 PPTs, similar to group 1 but manifested irregular, locally invasive silhouettes with involvement of the deep dermis and subcutis; group 3, invasive growth patterns, marked nuclear atypia, pathologic mitotic forms, and geographic necrosis, with or without involvement of nerves or vascular structures. Recurrence occurred in none of 48 group 1 PPTs; 3 (15%) of 20 group 2 PPTs had local regrowth; 4 (50%) of 8 of group 3 PPTs recurred and/or metastasized to regional lymph nodes. The differences between groups 1 and 3 and between 2 and 3 were statistically significant (P = .0002, P <.05, respectively). It seems justifiable to regard group 1 PPTs as benign, group 2 as having potential for locally aggressive growth, and group 3 also as having metastatic potential. The latter 2 categories might be equated with low and high grades of malignancy among PPTs of the skin.

▶ What is the malignant potential of a PPT? PPT, atypical fibroxanthoma, and dermatofibrosarcoma protuberans, among others, are cutaneous neoplasms that usually behave in a biologically benign way but in some instances have been documented to metastasize. However, criteria for determining which lesions are more likely to metastasize have not been developed.

This study shows that there may be histologic criteria to determine which PPTs have the potential for metastasis and thus warrant more aggressive therapy. In this study, invasive growth patterns, marked nuclear atypia, pathologic mitotic forms, and geographic necrosis were features that signaled the potential for metastasis.

J. C. Maize, MD

Role of Multiple Scouting Biopsies Before Mohs Micrographic Surgery for Extramammary Paget's Disease

Appert DL, Otley CC, Phillips PK, et al (Mayo Clinic, Rochester, Minn)
Dermatol Surg 31:1417-1422, 2005

16–40

Background.—Extramammary Paget's disease (EMPD) frequently extends subclinically, resulting in high recurrence rates after surgical excision. Mohs micrographic surgery (MMS) improves cure rates but may require time-consuming reexcision of subclinical extension. A mechanism to estimate the location and extent of subclinical extension would be helpful.

Objective.—To describe and evaluate a technique for multiple scouting biopsies before MMS for EMPD.

Method.—A retrospective review of patients at Mayo Clinic who had multiple scouting biopsies before MMS for EMPD without dermal invasion.

Technique.—The clinical extent of EMPD is identified. The scouting biopsy sites are determined and documented with photographs. The scouting biopsy specimens are sent for permanent sections. The results of the scouting biopsies help guide the extent of the initial Mohs layer. The tumor is cleared with MMS. An additional 1 mm peripheral margin of tissue is usually submitted for permanent sections.

Results.—Multiple scouting biopsies were done in five patients. Four of the five patients had at least one true-positive result. At least one true-negative result was obtained in all five patients. Two patients had at least one false-negative result.

Conclusion.—Multiple scouting biopsies before MMS for EMPD without dermal invasion can be a beneficial adjuvant technique.

▶ Even Mohs surgery struggles in the successful extirpation and long-term cure of patients with EMPD. For Mohs surgery to be successful in the resection of any neoplasm, the tumor must be clearly visible and spread in a contiguous fashion. The debate continues about the contiguous spread of this neoplasm. Nevertheless, scouting biopsies obtained before the initiation of surgical efforts may assist the physician in counseling the patient about surgical and nonsurgical treatment alternatives as well as in recruiting the support of other colleagues in urology, gynecology, and so forth. Nonsurgical treatment alternatives for EMPD (eg, topical 5-fluorouracil or imiquimod) may limit the extent of the required surgical intervention.

J. Cook, MD

Management of Superficial Leiomyosarcoma: A Retrospective Study of 10 Cases

Tsutsumida A, Yoshida T, Yamamoto Y, et al (Hokkaido Univ, Sapporo, Japan)
Plast Reconstr Surg 116:8-12, 2005   16–41

Background.—Superficial leiomyosarcoma is a rare soft-tissue tumor. Management of this tumor, including pathological evaluations and therapies, is not clearly defined in the existing literature.

Methods.—Ten patients with superficial leiomyosarcoma treated in our institutes were recalled and scheduled for examination. Assessments were carried out according to clinical characteristics, therapies used, histological grade (based on the grading system of the Fédération Nationale des Centres de Lutte Contre Le Cancer), tumor-node-metastasis stage (using the American Joint Committee on Cancer staging system), recurrences rates, state of metastases, and the current condition of each patient.

Results.—No local recurrences or distant metastases were seen in eight patients with low-grade and early-stage disease, whereas two patients with high-grade and advanced-stage disease had recurrence and one of these two patients died of the disease.

Conclusions.—This study indicates that evaluations using the Fédération Nationale des Centres de Lutte Contre Le Cancer grading system and the American Joint Committee on Cancer tumor staging system were useful. The authors advocate that surgical treatment of low-grade cutaneous leiomyosarcoma by complete excision with a narrow margin is adequate. For low-grade and early-state subcutaneous or soft-tissue leiomyosarcoma, wide excision with a minimum 2-cm lateral margin and one-tissue barrier deep margin is recommended. Management of high-grade leiomyosarcomas is still difficult; adequate wide excision may be the only option.

▶ The title of this article is somewhat misleading in that a superficial leiomyosarcoma usually refers to a lesion arising in the dermis that has an excellent prognosis, in contrast to a subcutaneous leiomyosarcoma that arises in the subcutaneous tissue and is associated with a higher incidence of metastasis. This group of patients was fairly heterogeneous, but all appeared to have deeply invasive tumors. Based on the American Joint Committee on Cancer staging system for soft tissue sarcomas, none of the 8 patients with stage IA disease experienced a recurrence, whereas the 2 patients with stage III disease experienced a recurrence or developed distant metastases. Thus, the authors found staging or grading these tumors was quite helpful from a prognostic standpoint; unfortunately, other than routine surgical excision, they had nothing to offer high-risk patients since radiation therapy and chemotherapy are of questionable benefit. They recommend at least 2-cm excision margins. Although Mohs surgery has been reported to be effective for the superficial variant of leiomyosarcoma, it remains to be determined whether it is more efficacious for stage III disease than is traditional surgical excision.

P. G. Lang, Jr, MD

Sirolimus for Kaposi's Sarcoma in Renal-Transplant Recipients

Stallone G, Schena A, Infante B, et al (Univ of Bari, Italy; Univ of Foggia, Italy)
N Engl J Med 352:1317-1323, 2005   16–42

Background.—Recipients of organ transplants are susceptible to Kaposi's sarcoma as a result of treatment with immunosuppressive drugs. Sirolimus (rapamycin), an immunosuppressive drug, may also have antitumor effects.

Methods.—We stopped cyclosporine therapy in 15 kidney-transplant recipients who had biopsy-proven Kaposi's sarcoma and began sirolimus therapy. All patients underwent an excisional biopsy of the lesion and one biopsy of normal skin at the time of diagnosis. A second biopsy was performed at the site of a previous Kaposi's sarcoma lesion six months after sirolimus therapy was begun. We examined biopsy specimens for vascular endothelial growth factor (VEGF), Flk-1/KDR protein, and phosphorylated Akt and p70S6 kinase, two enzymes in the signaling pathway targeted by sirolimus.

Results.—Three months after sirolimus therapy was begun, all cutaneous Kaposi's sarcoma lesions had disappeared in all patients. Remission was confirmed histologically in all patients six months after sirolimus therapy was begun. There were no acute episodes of rejection or changes in kidney-graft function. Levels of Flk-1/KDR and phosphorylated Akt and p70S6 kinase were increased in Kaposi's sarcoma cells. The expression of VEGF was increased in Kaposi's sarcoma cells and even more so in normal skin cells around the Kaposi's sarcoma lesions.

Conclusions.—Sirolimus inhibits the progression of dermal Kaposi's sarcoma in kidney-transplant recipients while providing effective immunosuppression.

▶ The antiangiogenic effects of sirolimus (rapamycin) were described in an article[1] reviewed in the 2003 YEAR BOOK OF DERMATOLOGY AND DERMATOLOGIC SURGERY. The dual role of the drug as an antirejection agent and as an inhibitor of the progression of Kaposi's sarcoma in kidney transplant recipients suggests its possible use in other situations in which transplant patients are at high risk of a tumor recurrence or primary cancer. As stated differently by Dantal and Soulillou[2] in an accompanying editorial, the results raise "the possibility that equilibrium between efficient immunosuppression and control over the development of cancer may be attainable."

B. H. Thiers, MD

References

1. Guba M, Von Breitenbuch P, Steinbauer M, et al: Rapamycin inhibits primary and metastatic tumor growth by antiangiogenesis: Involvement of vascular endothelial growth factor. *Nat Med* 8:128-135, 2002.
2. Dantal J, Soulillou J-P: Immunosuppressive drugs and the risk of cancer after organ transplantation (editorial). *N Engl J Med* 352:1371-1373, 2005.

Skin Metastases From Unknown Origin: Role of Immunohistochemistry in the Evaluation of Cutaneous Metastases of Carcinoma of Unknown Origin

Azoulay S, Adem C, Pelletier FLE; et al (Groupe Hospitalier Pitié Salpêtrère, Paris)

J Cutan Pathol 32:561-566, 2005   16–43

Introduction.—Determining the primary origin of skin metastases might be a challenging issue for pathologists, especially when there is no primary history or when this history is unavailable. The poor specificity of morphological appreciation is challenging, emphasizing the need for ancillary studies. We have retrieved 44 cases of skin metastases from our pathology files. Paraffin blocks were collected and homemade tissue arrays were made. We have tried to assess the primary origin based on morphological data alone, and then using 13 antibodies (cytokeratins (CK) 5/6, 7, 19, 20, thyroid transcription factor-1, carcinoembryonic antigen, PS100, tumor-associated glycoprotein 72, BerEP4, estrogen receptor (ER), progesterone receptor (PR), CD10, and E-cadherin). Most metastases in our series were from breast (13) and colorectal cancers (six) as they are the main clinical activity in our hospital. Only 44% of cases were correctly assessed based on the sole morphology, emphasizing the need for ancillary studies. CK 20, ER, and PR were the most helpful markers to determine the primary origin of skin metastases by highlighting colorectal origin and mammary origin, respectively. By far, clinical information and morphological evaluation are more reliable than the use of ancillary techniques, which have to be used in the absence of the former one and the poor differentiation of the latter ones.

▶ Carcinomas metastatic to the skin may sometimes demonstrate organizational and cytologic features that are typical of the primary neoplasm, such as mucin-containing goblet cells in metastatic colon carcinoma or differentiation of ducts in breast carcinoma. However, when the metastasis is undifferentiated it is often a challenge to determine the site of the primary carcinoma. These authors investigated the value of a panel of immunohistochemical studies in an attempt to pinpoint the site of origin of carcinomas metastatic to the skin. The majority of the metastases were from colon carcinoma or breast carcinoma, as would be expected, since these are the most common primary carcinomas. CK 20 was highly specific for colorectal metastasis, although its sensitivity was not high (60%). CK 20 may also label metastatic neuroendocrine tumors, but the neuroendocrine cells typically show a perinuclear dot rather than diffuse staining of the cytoplasm as in colorectal carcinoma. The authors also found that ER and PR staining were strongly specific for breast carcinoma. Sensitivities were 50% for ER and 42% for PR. Surprisingly the authors did not test for Her-2 as a marker for breast cancer. Her-2–positive breast carcinomas typically lack staining for ER and PR. The other 10 antibodies out of the 13 antibodies in the panel used by the authors were either not sensitive or not specific or not found helpful in determining the site of origin of undifferentiated metastatic carcinoma to the skin. Therefore, in the evaluation of undifferentiated metastatic carcinoma to the skin, a select antibody panel that includes CK 20, ER, and PR may prove helpful in determining the site of origin of the primary tumor. The authors also emphasize the importance of clinical information, particularly the patient's history with regard to known cancer. In my own experience as a dermatopathologist, it is surprising how frequently important information that is known to the attending physician is not included on the pathology request form.

J. C. Maize, MD

17 Nevi and Melanoma

Melanocytic Nevi of the Breast: A Histologic Case-Control Study
Rongioletti F, Urso C, Batolo D, et al (Univ of Genoa, Italy; SM Annunziata Hosp, Florence, Italy; Univ of Messina, Italy; et al)
J Cutan Pathol 31:137-140, 2004   17–1

Background.—Melanocytic nevi in the genital, acral, and flexural sites often display clinical and histologic features that may simulate melanoma. We verified whether this is the case also for nevi of the breast.

Methods.—Eleven dermatopathologists, from nine Italian Institutions, collected the specimens of melanocytic lesions from the breast and other body sites, excluding the acral, genital, and flexural areas, as controls. Cases and controls were matched for sex and age. All nevi were observed 'blindly' and simultaneously by all participants. For each lesion, 10 histological parameters were analyzed: asymmetry, absence of lateral demarcation of melanocytes, lentiginous proliferation, nested and dyshesive pattern, intraepidermal melanocytes above the basal layer, involvement of the hair follicle, absence of maturation of dermal melanocytes, melanocytic atypia, fibroplasia of the papillary dermis, and lymphocytic dermal infiltrate. Each parameter was scored 2 when present and 1 when absent or not valuable. A total score was calculated for each lesion. Results were statistically analyzed by the chi-square test and the Mann-Whitney U-test.

Results.—One hundred and one nevi came from the breast area and 97 from elsewhere. Breast nevi exhibited significantly more atypical features than nevi from other sites. In particular, breast nevi with intraepidermal melanocytes, melanocytic atypia, and dermal fibroplasia were significantly more numerous. We did not find any sexual difference.

Conclusions.—To avoid undue concerns, dermatopathologists should be aware that melanocytic nevi of the breast may show a high degree of atypical features.

▶ Previous studies have documented that melanocytic nevi on certain anatomical sites may show features that make them difficult to distinguish from melanoma. Acral nevi and nevi of the genitalia, especially the vulva, are perhaps the best characterized in this regard. Other studies have shown that nevi from flexural sites—including the axilla, inguinal creases, umbilicus, pubis, scrotum, and perianal areas—may show features similar to those of nevi on the genitalia.

Rongioletti et al add nevi of the breasts to the growing list of "special sites." Some pathologists would also add the scalp and ears to that list. So, where may ordinary nevi be found? Skin of the face, neck, torso other than the breasts, and the extremities other than acral areas seem to be body sites where no special anatomical influences exist. However, the trunk is the most common site for "dysplastic" (Clark) nevi, and the face and lower extremities are the most common sites for Spitz nevi. One might conclude, with some support from the literature, that every body site is a special site!

J. C. Maize, MD

Melanocytic Nevi in Very Young Children: The Role of Phenotype, Sun Exposure, and Sun Protection
Whiteman DC, Brown RM, Purdie DM, et al (Queensland Inst of Med Research, Brisbane, Australia)
J Am Acad Dermatol 52:40-47, 2005   17–2

Background.—Melanocytic nevi are strongly associated with cutaneous melanoma, yet little is known about factors influencing nevus development in the first years of life.

Objective.—We sought to identify phenotypic and environmental factors associated with nevus counts in very young children.

Methods.—In a cluster prevalence survey, full body nevus counts and phenotypic assessments were conducted on 193 children aged 1 to 3 years. Information on each child's sun exposure and sun protection practices was obtained through parental questionnaire.

Results.—High total nevus counts were associated with heavy facial freckling, time spent outdoors on weekends in summer, and Caucasian ethnicity. Low nevus counts were associated with dark skin color, ability to tan, and frequent application of sunscreen. Frequent wearing of hats was specifically associated with low nevus counts on the face, but not at other sites.

Conclusions.—Nevi are common at a very young age among children in Queensland, Australia, and are associated with sun exposure and freckling. Diligent sun protection practices appear to reduce nevus burden, even after accounting for the effects of phenotype and sun exposure factors. Primary prevention strategies aimed at reducing sun exposure in very early life may be effective in reducing nevus prevalence and melanoma risk.

Site-Specific Protective Effect of Broad-Spectrum Sunscreen on Nevus Development Among White Schoolchildren in a Randomized Trial

Lee TK, Rivers JK, Gallagher RP, et al (Univ of British Columbia, Vancouver, Canada; Simon Fraser Univ, Burnaby, Canada)
J Am Acad Dermatol 52:786-792, 2005   17–3

Background.—Melanocytic nevus density is a strong risk factor for cutaneous malignant melanoma. Reducing the number of nevi in children may reduce the risk of their developing melanoma as adults.

Objective.—We sought to assess the effect of sunscreen use on nevus development by anatomic sites and by nevi of different sizes for white schoolchildren in a randomized trial.

Methods.—We compared the new nevus count between the sunscreen intervention group (n = 145) and the control group (n = 164) by anatomic site.

Results.—Children randomized to the sunscreen group had significantly fewer new nevi on the trunk than children in the control group. The differences were more pronounced among the freckled children than children with no freckles.

Limitations.—Potential limitations to this study include relatively small numbers of enrolled children, and a follow-up period of only 3 years.

Conclusion.—Sunscreen use attenuated new nevus development on intermittently sun-exposed body sites for white schoolchildren, particularly among the freckled children.

▶ Studies such as these (Abstracts 17–2 and 17–3) continue to document that sun protection, including sunscreen use, decreases the number of melanocytic nevi in fair skinned children who freckle. Because a decreased number of nevi may be associated with a decreased incidence of melanoma, sun protection should continue to be encouraged in young children, particularly in those who freckle.

S. Raimer, MD

Variability in Nomenclature Used for Nevi With Architectural Disorder and Cytologic Atypia (Microscopically Dysplastic Nevi) by Dermatologists and Dermatopathologists

Shapiro M, Chren M-M, Levy RM, et al (Univ of Pennsylvania, Philadelphia; Univ of California at San Francisco; Harvard Med School, Boston)
J Cutan Pathol 31:523-530, 2004   17–4

Background.—Although a nevus with the microscopic features of a "dysplastic nevus" is commonly seen, the nomenclature used to describe such a lesion has been thought to be inconsistent. A 1992 National Institutes of Health (NIH) Consensus Conference sought to unify nomenclature and suggested that the term "nevus with architectural disorder" be used along with a comment on melanocytic atypia.

Methods.—We performed a cross-sectional mail survey to determine preferred terminology as well as the level of adherence to the NIH-recommended nomenclature. All 856 active members of the American Society of Dermatopathology (ASDP) and 1100 (13.0%) of the 8471 active members of the American Academy of Dermatology (AAD) were surveyed.

Results.—Five hundred and thirty-three ASDP members and 483 AAD members who fulfilled eligibility criteria completed the questionnaire. The term "dysplastic nevus" was favored by the largest number of responders (favored by 39.1% of ASDP members and 62.3% of AAD members), while the 1992 NIH Consensus Conference-recommended terminology was the second most popular term (25.3% of ASDP and 15.1% of AAD members). Dermatopathologists (OR = 1.9, p = 0.0001) and those who had dual training in dermatology and dermatopathology (OR = 1.6, p = 0.02 for ASDP members; OR = 2.3, p = 0.02 for AAD members) were more likely to adhere to the 1992 NIH Consensus Conference nomenclature.

Conclusions.—Despite attempts to unify nomenclature for microscopically dysplastic nevi through the NIH Consensus Conference, wide variation in terminology persists.

▶ An NIH Consensus Development Conference on early melanoma was convened in 1992. The NIH Consensus Development Panel made recommendations for the nomenclature to be used for describing so-called dysplastic nevi histopathologically. The panel recommended use of the term "nevus with architectural disorder and cytologic atypia." Shapiro et al surveyed members of the American Society of Dermatopathology to assess the terminology used in their practices for the diagnosis of such nevi. The survey had an unusually high rate of responders, which is indicative of the turmoil that still surrounds the nosology as well as the terminology for the nevi originally described in the B-K kindred with familial melanomas. Despite the fact that all parameters indicate that the NIH Development Conference on early melanoma was one of the most successful consensus conferences ever given at the NIH, there is no consensus among practitioners of dermatopathology with regard to the terminology that is used for diagnosing so-called dysplastic nevi.

Dermatologists do not have difficulty reaching consensus on how to name other diseases. Therefore, the lack of consensus on terminology for so-called dysplastic nevi revolves more around concepts of disease than of terminology. Because of the continued confusion as to what to call these lesions, there is still no consensus on how to manage them. Some dermatologists still feel compelled to re-excise any "dysplastic nevi" that extend to the biopsy specimen margin. Others believe them to be just a variant of normal and do not pursue reexcision unless the clinical appearance of the lesion is of great concern. In the current medicolegal environment, it is unlikely that the advocates of the term of "dysplastic nevus" would be willing to abandon that nomenclature because of the belief that it provides them with some protection in the event of a bad outcome. Thus, dermatologists who practice must continue to rely on their expertise in clinicopathologic correlation to determine the best treatment for each individual patient.

J. C. Maize, MD

Use of Bayes Rule and MIB-1 Proliferation Index to Discriminate Spitz Nevus From Malignant Melanoma

Vollmer RT (Duke Univ, Durham, NC)
Am J Clin Pathol 122:499-505, 2004

17–5

Introduction.—Differentiating Spitz nevus from malignant melanoma is difficult and controversial. Despite helpful lists of differential diagnostic features, uncertainty about the diagnosis often provokes some to stain the tumor for MIB-1 antibody to Ki-67 and measure the proliferation index (PI) of the tumor. Of the many reports about MIB-1 PI in Spitz nevi and melanoma, none have consolidated the information to provide guidelines for the predictive probability that a lesion is a Spitz nevus, given that the MIB-1 PI falls into a certain interval. The present study used previously published data and exponential and gamma probability density functions to model statistical distributions of PI, respectively, in Spitz nevi and melanomas and Bayes rule to estimate the predictive probability that a lesion is a Spitz nevus, given an observed PI. Results indicate that PIs more than 10% favor a melanoma diagnosis and PIs less than 2%, Spitz nevus. PI values between 2% and 10% yield various predictive values for Spitz nevus, depending on the a priori probability that the lesion is a Spitz nevus. The algorithm tabulates guidelines for the predictive probabilities of Spitz nevus given an observed PI.

The Spectrum of Spitz Nevi: A Clinicopathologic Study of 83 Cases

Ferrara G, Argenziano G, Soyer HP, et al (Gaetano Rummo Gen Hosp, Benevento, Italy; Second Univ of Naples, Italy; Univ of Tor Vergata, Rome; et al)
Arch Dermatol 141:1381-1387, 2005

17–6

Objective.—To achieve a clinicopathologic classification of Spitz nevi by comparing their clinical, dermoscopic, and histopathologic features.

Design.—Eighty-three cases were independently reviewed by 3 histopathologists and preliminarily classified into classic or desmoplastic Spitz nevus (CDSN, n = 11), pigmented Spitz nevus (PSN, n = 14), Reed nevus (RN, n = 16), or atypical Spitz nevus (ASN, n = 14); the remaining 28 cases were then placed into an intermediate category (pigmented Spitz-Reed nevus, PSRN) because a unanimous diagnosis of either PSN or RN was not reached.

Setting.—University dermatology and pathology departments and general hospital pathology departments.

Patients.—A sample of subjects with excised melanocytic lesions.

Main Outcome Measure.—Frequency of dermoscopic patterns within the different histopathologic subtypes of Spitz nevi.

Results.—Overlapping clinical, dermoscopic, and histopathologic findings were observed among PSN, RN, and PSRN, thereby justifying their inclusion into the single PSRN diagnostic category. Asymmetry was the most frequent indicator of histopathologic ASN (79%; n = 11); in only 4 cases did dermoscopic asymmetry show no histopathologic counterpart, and in those cases the discrepancy was probably the result of an artifact of the gross sampling technique carried out with no attention to the dermoscopic features.

Conclusions.—Among Spitz nevi, histopathologic distinction between PSN and RN is difficult, not reproducible, and may be clinically useless. A simple clinicopathologic classification of these neoplasms might therefore be structured as CDSN, PSRN, and ASN. Asymmetry should be assessed using both dermoscopic and histopathologic analysis, and reliability in histopathologic diagnosis may be enhanced by the simultaneous evaluation of the corresponding dermoscopic images.

▶ Dermatologists and dermatopathologists have relied on microscopic morphologic criteria to distinguish Spitz nevi from melanoma. Since the introduction of diagnostic immunocytochemistry there has been an ongoing effort to find immunohistochemical features that would help differentiate the 2 conditions. MIB-1 is a formalin stable epitope of Ki-67. There have been a number of studies in the literature that indicate that melanomas show a statistically significantly higher percentage of cells that label for Ki-67 than do the cells of a benign melanocytic nevus. Studies that have specifically focused on Spitz nevus have also shown that Spitz nevi usually show a significantly lower labeling index for Ki-67. The issue at hand is how one integrates this information into the diagnostic criteria for distinguishing between Spitz nevi and malignant melanoma.

Bayes theorem is the fundamental mathematical law that determines what degree of confidence we may have in various possible conclusions based on the body of evidence available. It helps us update or revise beliefs in light of new evidence. The report by Vollmer (Abstract 17–5) shows how to integrate the data obtained from the Ki-67 labeling index into the diagnostic algorithm for distinguishing Spitz nevus from malignant melanoma. In those cases of classic Spitz nevi that show all the classic criteria, the Ki-67 labeling index is not needed. However, in the borderline cases it may be a useful adjunct to differential diagnosis. Comparative genomic hybridization enables determination of the molecular footprint that characterizes Spitz nevus; however, it is not readily available. Until the newer molecular techniques become more prevalent, any additional diagnostic study, including data from Ki-67 immunostaining, is welcome by dermatologists and pathologists to allow more accurate differentiation of difficult melanocytic lesions. This article gives practical advice on how to utilize that information.

J. C. Maize, MD

Large or Multiple Congenital Melanocytic Nevi: Occurrence of Cutaneous Melanoma in 1008 Persons
Bett BJ (Nevus Network, West Salem, Ohio)
J Am Acad Dermatol 52:793-797, 2005   17–7

Background.—There is a dearth of information regarding the occurrence of cutaneous melanoma in a large cohort of persons with large congenital melanocytic nevi (LCMN) or multiple congenital melanocytic nevi (MCMN).

Objective.—The purpose of this article is to report our experience with 1008 persons having LCMN and MCMN.

Methods.—Information was evaluated that was obtained from a database of persons with LCMN or MCMN voluntarily submitted by the affected persons to a nevus support group, the Nevus Network.

Results.—Of those with garment LCMN, 2.9% developed cutaneous melanoma associated with 0.8% deaths. Of those with LCMN on the head or extremity, 0.3% developed cutaneous melanoma associated with no deaths to date. Of the small number with MCMN without a giant nevus, 6.7% developed cutaneous melanoma.

Limitations.—Attending physician confirmation of submitted information was unavailable.

Conclusions.—LCMN and MCMN were associated with a low occurrence of cutaneous melanoma in our group.

▶ It is fairly well accepted that the risk of melanomas developing in small or medium-sized congenital nevi is not sufficient to justify their prophylactic removal. At the same time, it is believed that LCMN should be removed because of a significant risk of the development of melanoma; however, the magnitude of this risk has varied from study to study. Bett derived data from the Nevus Network support group. In patients with "garment-type" CMN, 2.9% developed a melanoma. In one third of those patients, the melanomas developed before the age of 1.5 years. Except for 1 patient, it was believed that an attempt at prophylactic removal of the lesion (a procedure that can be technically difficult or take several years to accomplish) would not have affected the risk of melanoma. Patients with MCMN and patients with LCMN of the head and extremities had only a 0.3% incidence of melanoma. As noted by previous investigators, melanomas may arise deep within the nevus and, thus, superficial removal of CMN does not prevent the development of melanoma. Finally, in 1 patient, melanoma developed in a satellite lesion, which is an occurrence that has not been reported previously.

P. G. Lang, Jr, MD

Sun Exposure and Mortality From Melanoma
Berwick M, Armstrong BK, Ben-Porat L, et al (Univ of New Mexico, Albuquerque; Univ of Sydney, Australia; Mem Sloan-Kettering Cancer Ctr, New York; et al)
J Natl Cancer Inst 97:195-199, 2005   17–8

Background.—Melanoma incidence and survival are positively associated, both geographically and temporally. Solar elastosis, a histologic indicator of cutaneous sun damage, has also been positively associated with melanoma survival. Although these observations raise the possibility that sun exposure increases melanoma survival, they could be explained by an association between incidence and early detection of melanoma. We therefore evaluated the association between measures of skin screening and death from cutaneous melanoma.

Methods.—Case subjects (n = 528) from a population-based study of cutaneous melanoma were followed for an average of more than 5 years. Data, including measures of intermittent sun exposure, perceived awareness of the skin, skin self-screening, and physician screening, were collected during in-person interviews and review of histopathology and histologic parameters (i.e., solar elastosis, Breslow thickness, and mitoses) for all of the lesions. Competing risk models were used to compute risk of death (hazard ratios [HRs], with 95% confidence intervals [CIs]) from melanoma. All statistical tests were two-sided.

Results.—Sunburn, high intermittent sun exposure, skin awareness histories, and solar elastosis were statistically significantly inversely associated with death from melanoma. Melanoma thickness, mitoses, ulceration, and anatomic location on the head and neck were statistically significantly positively associated with melanoma death. In a multivariable competing risk analysis, skin awareness (with versus without, HR = 0.5, 95% CI = 0.3 to 0.9, P = .022) and solar elastosis (present versus absent, HR = 0.4, 95% CI = 0.2 to 0.8, P = .009) were strongly and independently associated with melanoma death after adjusting for Breslow thickness, mitotic index, and head and neck location, which were also independently associated with death.

Conclusions.—Sun exposure is associated with increased survival from melanoma.

▶ This study of 528 melanoma patients over 5 years found that increased sun exposure correlated with increased survival. This appears to be totally counterintuitive as studies have consistently found sun exposure to be a major risk factor for development of this tumor. The authors suggest that sunlight-induced vitamin D, which can help regulate cell growth and accelerate apoptosis, may be a factor. They also hypothesize that solar elastosis may provide a physical barrier to help prevent tumor cells from spreading into the lymphatics and beyond.

B. H. Thiers, MD

Association of UV Index, Latitude, and Melanoma Incidence in Nonwhite Populations—US Surveillance, Epidemiology, and End Results (SEER) Program, 1992 to 2001
Eide MJ, Weinstock MA (Brown Univ, Providence, RI)
Arch Dermatol 141:477-481, 2005   17–9

Objective.—To estimate the association between UV index, latitude, and melanoma incidence in different racial and ethnic populations in a high-quality national data set.

Design.—Descriptive study.

Setting.—Eleven US cancer registries that constitute the Surveillance, Epidemiology, and End Results Program (SEER-11).

Patients.—Patients with malignant melanoma of the skin reported between 1992 and 2001.

Main Outcome Measures.—Pearson correlation coefficients and regression coefficients were used to estimate the relationship of age-adjusted melanoma incidence rates (2000 US standard population) with the UV index or latitude within racial and ethnic groups.

Results.—A higher mean UV index was significantly associated with an increase in melanoma incidence only in non-Hispanic whites ($r = 0.85$, $P = .001$), although a nonsignificant association was noted in Native Americans ($r = 0.42$, $P = .20$). Negative, but not significant, correlations with incidence were observed in blacks ($r = -0.53$, $P = .10$), Hispanics ($r = -0.43$, $P = .19$), and Asians ($r = -0.28$, $P = .41$). Latitude also had a significant correlation with incidence only in non-Hispanic whites ($r = -0.85$, $P = .001$). A substantial portion of the variance in registry incidence in non-Hispanic whites could be explained by the UV index ($R^2 = 0.71$, $P = .001$).

Conclusions.—Melanoma incidence is associated with increased UV index and lower latitude only in non-Hispanic whites. No evidence to support the association of UV exposure and melanoma incidence in black or Hispanic populations was found.

▶ A disproportionate number of melanomas in dark-skinned individuals occur on acral areas, which often receive minimal sun exposure. Thus, it would appear somewhat puzzling that some prior studies have suggested a correlation between sun exposure and the development of melanoma in nonwhite individuals. This did not appear to be the case in this report from the SEER program. Eide and Weinstock found no correlation between the UV index or latitude and the development of melanoma in nonwhites. However, these 2 variables did correlate with the development of melanoma in whites.

P. G. Lang, Jr, MD

Public Awareness About Risk Factors Could Pose Problems for Case-Control Studies: The Example of Sunbed Use and Cutaneous Melanoma
de Vries E, Boniol M, Severi G, et al (Erasmus MC, Rotterdam, The Netherlands; INSERM U 590, Lyon, France; Internatl Agency for Research on Cancer, Lyon, France; et al)
Eur J Cancer 41:2150-2154, 2005   17–10

Background.—Case-control studies are especially helpful to investigate relatively rare disorders, require a shorter time and smaller samples than cohort studies, and cost less to perform. They have the drawback of possible bias, including recall bias and bias with respect to who chooses or refuses to participate. When the general public has received a fair amount of general information about potential or established risk factors for a disease, bias can be particularly prevalent. A case-control study was undertaken to assess the link between sunbed exposure and melanoma risk in Europe.

Methods.—Data came from 597 patients with melanoma (cases) and 622 controls aged 18 to 50 years from Sweden, The Netherlands, the United Kingdom, Belgium, and France. Cases were recruited through hospitals or population-based cancer registries. Controls came from population registries, general practitioner patient lists, door-to-door searches, or newspaper advertisements. Cases and controls were interviewed about their sunbathing habits and use of sunbeds. Skin type, eye and hair color, and presence of freckles were noted. Nevus counts were obtained for both arms of each subject. Confounding variables included skin type, exposure to natural sunlight, and protective measures taken before diagnosis.

Results.—The prevalence of sunbed use varied widely in both cases and controls, with considerable but nonsignificant differences in the odds ratio (OR) of each country. Among controls, France had a low sunbed use of 19%, and Sweden had the highest at 86%. In Sweden, The Netherlands, and England, the incidence of melanoma is high, so extensive health campaigns about skin cancers have been produced. As a result, the normal population's knowledge about melanoma risk factors was also most likely high. Sun exposure and melanoma risk were negatively related. The adjusted OR for ever and never sunbathing and melanoma was 0.87, which differs from published data. The reported relationships between skin phototype and interviewer-determined hair color were confirmed. The adjusted OR for skin type I versus skin type IV was 2.6 and that for red or blond versus brown or black hair was 2.0. Sunbathing's apparent protective effect with respect to melanoma was attributed to underreporting of sunbathing by cases. People with melanoma had more nevi on both arms than controls. Among controls, sun exposure before 15 years of age and nevus count for episodes of sunburn during childhood were positively associated. Reported sunbathing in adults with melanoma was inversely but not significantly related to nevus count. When reported sunbathing took place during the warmest hours of the day, the negative association with nevus count was stronger. Cases had a stronger negative link in this parameter than controls. However, increased sun exposure can make nevi resolve faster in adults, so those with higher sun exposure could have lower nevus counts. Despite information provided on sun exposure and melanoma, more than half of the patients with melanoma in The Netherlands did not believe that their melanoma was related to sun exposure, so they may have underestimated true exposure. If this held for the other countries, both sun exposure and sunbed use were likely underreported.

Conclusions.—Both cases and controls underreported sun exposure, but the cases showed more serious underreporting. Sunbed use cannot be ruled out as a risk factor for melanoma or as a protective factor because of the potential biases in recruitment and recall in this study.

A Multicentre Epidemiological Study on Sunbed Use and Cutaneous Melanoma in Europe

Bataille V, Boniol M, De Vries E, et al (Wolfson Inst of Preventive Medicine, London; INSERM U 590, Lyon, France; Erasmus Univ Med Ctr, Rotterdam, The Netherlands; et al)
Eur J Cancer 41:2141-2149, 2005   17–11

Introduction.—A large European case–control study investigated the association between sunbed use and cutaneous melanoma in an adult population aged between 18 and 49 years. Between 1999 and 2001 sun and sunbed exposure was recorded in 597 newly diagnosed melanoma cases and 622 controls in Belgium, France, The Netherlands, Sweden and the UK. Fifty three percent of cases and 57% of controls ever used sunbeds. The overall adjusted odds ratio (OR) associated with ever sunbed use was 0.90 (95% CI: 0.71-1.14). There was a South-to-North gradient with high prevalence of sunbed exposure in Northern Europe and lower prevalence in the South (prevalence of use in France 20%, OR: 1.19 (0.68-2.07) compared to Sweden, prevalence 83%, relative risk 0.62 (0.26-1.46)). Dose and lag-time between first exposure to sunbeds and time of study were not associated with melanoma risk, neither were sunbathing and sunburns (adjusted OR for mean number of weeks spent in sunny climates >14 years: 1.12 (0.88-1.43); adjusted OR for any sunburn >14 years: 1.16 (0.9-1.45)). Host factors such as numbers of naevi and skin type were the strongest risk indicators for melanoma. Public health campaigns have improved knowledge regarding risk of UV-radiation for skin cancers and this may have led to recall and selection biases in both cases and controls in this study. Sunbed exposure has become increasingly prevalent over the last 20 years, especially in Northern Europe but the full impact of this exposure on skin cancers may not become apparent for many years.

▶ Sunbed use has increased dramatically over the years, and, as noted by the authors, its full impact on cutaneous health may not yet be appreciated. Although the authors were unable to document an association between sunbed use and melanomas, the latency period before tumor development is unknown. With the increased prevalence of sunbed use and the availability of more potent devices, exposed patients will need careful monitoring on a regular basis.

B. H. Thiers, MD

Cutaneous Melanoma in Postmenopausal Women After Nonmelanoma Skin Carcinoma: The Women's Health Initiative Observational Study

Rosenberg CA, Khandekar J, Greenland P, et al (Evanston Northwestern Healthcare, Ill; Northwestern Univ, Chicago; Fred Hutchinson Cancer Research Ctr, Seattle)
Cancer 106:654-663, 2006   17–12

Background.—An elevated risk for cutaneous melanoma has been reported in individuals with nonmelanoma skin carcinoma (NMSC), but to the authors' knowledge, this association has not been prospectively studied in a large, multigeographic population of postmenopausal women.

Methods.—The association between NMSC and the incidence of cutaneous melanoma was assessed in the Women's Health Initiative Observational Study involving 67,030 non-Hispanic white postmenopausal women ages 50-79 years and who were free of prior other cancers at baseline. Cancer history, demographics, and previous and current risk exposures were determined by questionnaires at baseline and follow-up. Participants' reports of incident cutaneous melanoma collected annually were confirmed by physician review of medical records. Cox proportional hazards analyses were used to assess the relation of prior NMSC with incident cutaneous melanoma.

Results.—In age-adjusted analysis, women with a history of NMSC but no other malignancy (n = 5552) were found to be 2.41 times more likely to develop cutaneous melanoma over a mean 6.5 years compared with women who had no history of NMSC (95% confidence interval [95% CI], 1.82-3.20). In a multivariate analysis, women with a history of NMSC and no other cancer history at baseline were 1.70 times more likely to develop cutaneous melanoma compared with women without NMSC (95% CI, 1.18-2.44).

Conclusion.—The results of the current study provide evidence and further define the magnitude of increased risk for cutaneous melanoma in postmenopausal non-Hispanic white women with a history of NMSC.

▶ In older white postmenopausal women, a history of NMSC appears to be an independent risk factor for melanoma, regardless of sun exposure. These patients are especially good candidates for regular skin examinations.

B. H. Thiers, MD

Malignant Melanoma in Pregnancy: A Population-Based Evaluation

O'Meara AT, Cress R, Xing G, et al (Univ of California, Sacramento; Public Health Inst, Sacramento, Calif; Health Information Solutions, Rocklin, Calif)
Cancer 103:1217-1226, 2005   17–13

Background.—For many years, there has been controversy in the medical community regarding the correlation of female hormonal factors with the outcome of women with malignant melanoma. There have been multiple reports that women with high hormone states, such as pregnancy, had thicker tumors and/or a worse prognosis compared with a group of control women.

Methods.—The authors used a database that contained maternal and neonatal discharge records from the entire state of California from 1991 to 1999 and linked those records to the California Cancer Registry, which maintains legally mandated records of all cancers reported in California during the same time period. Four hundred twelve women with malignant melanoma diagnosed during or within 1 year after pregnancy were identified (145 antepartum, 4 at delivery, and 263 postpartum) and were compared with a group of age-matched, nonpregnant women with melanoma (controls). The database captured only pregnancies at ≥ 20 weeks of gestation.

Results.—When comparing women who had pregnancy-associated melanoma with the control group, the authors found no difference in the distribution of disease stage (82.0% of pregnant and postpartum women had localized melanoma vs. 81.9% of control women) or the tumor thickness (mean: 0.77 mm for pregnant women, 0.90 mm for postpartum women, and 0.81 mm for the control group). In a multiple regression model that controlled for age, race, stage, and tumor thickness, pregnancy had no impact on survival in women with melanoma. Lymph node assessment and positivity of lymph nodes also were equivalent between the two groups. Maternal and neonatal outcomes did not differ between pregnant women with melanoma and control women who were pregnant and had no history of malignancy. Small numbers of women with advanced melanoma and the inability to capture melanoma that occurred in pregnancies that were lost or were terminated prior to 20 weeks limited the conclusions primarily to women with localized melanoma.

Conclusions.—In this large, population-based study of pregnant women in California from 1991 to 1999 with malignant melanoma, there were no data found to support a more advanced stage, thicker tumors, increased metastases to lymph nodes, or a worsened survival. The outcome for women with localized melanoma associated with pregnancy was excellent. Maternal and neonatal outcomes also were equivalent to those of pregnant women without melanoma.

▶ Some prior data have indicated that pregnancy may have an adverse effect on melanoma outcome. However, this study, along with other recent studies, suggests that this is not the case. Unlike some previous series, the pregnant women reported here did not have thicker lesions. There also did not appear to be an increased incidence of melanoma in this population. Neither the disease nor its appropriate treatment appeared to adversely affect the pregnancy or the fetus.

P. G. Lang, Jr, MD

Malignant Melanoma in Childhood and Adolescence: Report of 13 Cases

Jafarian F, Powell J, Kokta V, et al (Univ of Montreal)
J Am Acad Dermatol 53:816-822, 2005   17–14

Introduction.—We reviewed all cases of malignant melanoma in children younger than 17 years of age who were evaluated at Sainte Justine Hospital, a tertiary care pediatric center, between 1980 and 2002. The medical records and histologic features of all cases were reviewed. Thirteen cases were identified, 4 boys and 9 girls. Fifty-three percent of patients were prepubescent. None of the patients had a predisposing condition (eg, giant congenital nevi, dysplastic nevus syndrome, or xeroderma pigmentosum). One patient had had chemoradiotherapy previously for an undifferentiated pleuropulmonary malignant tumor (blastoma) and another patient had Down syndrome. The most frequent reason for initial consultation was a recent increase in size of the lesion. Three patients had pyogenic granuloma–like lesions. Eighty-five percent of the observed melanomas were nodular in type. Tumor thickness ranged from 0 to 6 mm with a median and mean thickness of 2.8 and 3.2 mm, respectively. The overall 5-year survival rate was 58.8%. Lack of awareness and delay in diagnosis may lead to a higher incidence of thick and intermediate melanoma in children. Because it appears that the majority of melanomas in childhood and adolescence occur de novo, clinicians should consider this condition in the differential diagnosis of any suspect lesion in children and adolescents even without an identified predisposing factor.

▶ Even though melanoma is uncommon in childhood and adolescence, the tumor appears to be as aggressive in this age group as it is in adults. In this series of 13 cases, the tumors were relatively thick at diagnosis, likely because malignancy was not suspected in these young patients. Excision of any clinically suspicious lesion, even in children, is recommended to preclude delay in diagnosis and treatment.

S. Raimer, MD

Increased Incidence of Melanoma in Renal Transplantation Recipients

Hollenbeak CS, Todd MM, Billingsley EM, et al (Penn State College of Medicine, Hershey, Pa; Skin Cancer Ctr of Northern Virginia, Sterling; Lehigh Valley Hosp, Allentown, Pa)
Cancer 104:1962-1967, 2005   17–15

Background.—It is well established that the incidence of nonmelanoma skin carcinoma is increased in renal transplantation recipients. However, existing studies are not in agreement over whether patients who undergo transplantation have an increased risk of melanoma. The objective of this study was to estimate the risk of melanoma among immunosuppressed renal transplantation recipients and to determine whether that risk is associated with patient and transplantation characteristics.

Methods.—The authors studied 89,786 patients who underwent renal transplantation between 1988 and 1998 using the United States Renal Data System. Age standardized (to the United States 2000 population) incidence rates for melanoma were computed as diagnoses per 100,000 population and were compared with rates from the Surveillance, Epidemiology, and End Results (SEER) data. Incidence rates also were stratified to examine differences by age and gender.

Results.—Of the 89,786 patients who underwent transplantation, 246 patients developed melanoma. The age-adjusted incidence rate of melanoma among renal transplantation recipients was 55.9 diagnoses per 100,000 population. This represented an increase in age-adjusted, standardized risk that was 3.6 times greater than the SEER population. Stratified analysis suggested that the risk of melanoma accelerated in male transplantation recipients as age increased, but the risk leveled off with age among female transplantation recipients. Finally, there was a trend for patients who experienced at least 1 acute rejection episode to develop melanoma (odds ratio = 1.34; $P = 0.059$).

Conclusions.—Renal transplantation recipients were nearly 3.6 times more likely to develop melanoma than the general population. Physicians who care for renal transplantation recipients should be vigilant in screening for melanoma.

▶ The incidence of melanoma appears to be especially high in immunosuppressed renal transplant recipients. These patients should not only undergo regular examination by a dermatologist but should also be instructed on routine self-examination of their skin.

B. H. Thiers, MD

Clinicopathological Features of and Risk Factors for Multiple Primary Melanomas

Ferrone CR, Porat LB, Panageas KS, et al (Mem Sloan-Kettering Cancer Ctr, New York)
JAMA 294:1647-1654, 2005   17–16

Context.—The incidence of multiple primary melanomas ranges from 1.3% to 8.0% in large retrospective reviews; however, the impact of certain risk factors is not understood.

Objectives.—To determine the incidence of multiple primary melanomas (MPM) from a prospective, single-institution, multidisciplinary database, and to describe the clinical and pathological characteristics and risk factors specific to these patients.

Design and Setting.—Review of a prospectively maintained database at Memorial Sloan-Kettering Cancer Center in New York, NY.

Patients.—A total of 4484 patients diagnosed with a first primary melanoma between January 1, 1996, and December 31, 2002.

Main Outcome Measures.—Incidence of and risk factors for MPM.

Results.—Three hundred eighty-five patients (8.6%) had 2 or more primary melanomas, with an average of 2.3 melanomas per MPM patient. Seventy-eight percent had 2 primary melanomas. For 74% of patients, the initial melanoma was the thickest tumor. Fifty-nine percent presented with their second primary tumor within 1 year. Twenty-one percent of MPM patients had a positive family history of melanoma compared with only 12% of patients with a single primary melanoma (SPM) (*P*<.001). Thirty-eight percent of MPM patients had dysplastic nevi compared with 18% of SPM patients (*P*<.001). The estimated cumulative 5-year risk of a second primary tumor for the entire cohort was 11.4%, with almost half of that risk occurring within the first year. For patients with a positive family history or dysplastic nevi, the estimated 5-year risk of MPM was significantly higher at 19.1% and 23.7%, respectively. The most striking increase in incidence for the MPM population was seen for development of a third primary melanoma from the time of second primary melanoma, which was 15.6% at 1 year and 30.9% at 5 years.

Conclusions.—The incidence of MPM is increased in patients with a positive family history and/or dysplastic nevi. These patients should undergo intensive dermatologic screening and should consider genetic testing.

▶ This article is a good review of the risk factors associated with MPM. The overall incidence of MPM was 8.6%, and the 5-year cumulative risk for a patient developing a second melanoma was 11.4%. Both the presence of dysplastic nevi and a family history of melanoma increased the likelihood of a patient developing additional melanomas. As previously reported, subsequent melanomas tended to be thinner. Whether this is caused by increased surveillance or the tendency to develop less-aggressive tumors is unclear since the thickness of the initial melanoma in patients with MPM was thinner than in those with a single melanoma. Similar speculations could also be addressed in patients with dysplastic nevi, who tended to have thinner lesions. It had always been this reviewer's understanding that patients with MPM often developed their initial melanoma at a younger age, but in this study, except for patients with dysplastic nevi, patients with MPM tended to be older.

P. G. Lang, Jr, MD

High Constant Incidence Rates of Second Cutaneous Melanomas
Levi F, Randimbison L, Te V-C, et al (Institut Universitaire de Médecine Sociale et Préventive, Lausanne, Switzerland)
Int J Cancer 117:877-879, 2005   17–17

Introduction.—The incidence of most epithelial cancers rises with a power of age. However, second breast cancers have a high constant incidence independent of age. The skin is one of the few other sites allowing examination of age incidence curves of second neoplasms of the same organ. We considered the risk of second primary cutaneous malignant melanoma (CMM) in a population-based series of 3,439 first CMM registered and followed-up between 1974 and 2003 in the Swiss Cantons of Vaud and Neuchâtel (about 786,000 inhabitants). A total of 43 cases of second CMM were observed vs. 9.3 expected, corresponding to a standardized incidence ratio (SIR) of 4.6. The SIR was 8.5 under age 50, 5.7 at age 50-59 and 3.5 at age 60 or over. At 20 years, the cumulative risk of second CMM was 5%. Age-specific incidence rates of second primary CMM did not vary across age groups 30-39 through 80+, ranging between 1 and 2.5 per 1,000 person-years. Thus, the risk of CMM is substantially increased in subjects diagnosed with a CMM, and the relative risk is greater at younger age and declines with advancing age. The high constant incidence curve of second CMM is compatible with the occurrence of a single mutational event in a population of susceptible individuals.

▶ This article emphasizes the need for careful monitoring of patients with a previously diagnosed melanoma. The relative risk of a second melanoma appears to be greater at a younger age and declines with time.

B. H. Thiers, MD

Incidence of Noncutaneous Melanomas in the U.S.

McLaughlin CC, Wu X-C, Jemal A, et al (New York State Dept of Health, Albany; Louisiana State Univ, New Orleans; American Cancer Society, Atlanta, Ga; et al)
Cancer 103:1000-1007, 2005   17–18

Background.—Description of the epidemiology of noncutaneous melanoma has been hampered by its rarity. The current report was the largest in-depth descriptive analysis of incidence of noncutaneous melanoma in the United States, using data from the North American Association of Central Cancer Registries.

Methods.—Pooled data from 27 states and one metropolitan area were used to examine the incidence of noncutaneous melanoma by anatomic subsite, gender, age, race, and geography (northern/southern and coastal/noncoastal) for cases diagnosed between 1996 and 2000. Percent distribution by stage of disease at diagnosis and histology were also examined.

Results.—Between 1996 and 2000, 6691 cases of noncutaneous melanoma (4885 ocular and 1806 mucosal) were diagnosed among 851 million person-years at risk. Ocular melanoma was more common among men compared with women (6.8 cases per million men compared with 5.3 cases per million women, age-adjusted to the 2000 U.S. population standard), whereas mucosal melanoma was more common among women (2.8 cases per million women compared with 1.5 cases per million men). Rates of ocular melanoma among whites were greater than eight times higher than among blacks. Rates of mucosal melanoma were approximately two times higher among whites compared with blacks.

Conclusions.—In contrast to cutaneous melanoma, there was no apparent pattern of increased noncutaneous melanoma among residents of southern or coastal states, with the exception of melanoma of the ciliary body and iris. Despite their shared cellular origins, both ocular and mucosal melanomas differ from cutaneous melanoma in terms of incidence by gender, race, and geographic area.

▶ This large population-based study gives a good perspective on the epidemiology and incidence of noncutaneous melanoma in the United States. Like cutaneous melanoma, ocular and mucosal melanomas are more common in whites than in blacks, but the difference for mucosal melanomas is much less. Ocular melanoma may have more in common with cutaneous melanoma than mucosal lesions in that it may be sun related and influenced by genetic factors as well as the presence of numerous nevi. Mucosal melanomas are often advanced at the time of diagnosis and thus are associated with a poor prognosis.

P. G. Lang, Jr, MD

Development of Prognostic Factors and Survival in Cutaneous Melanoma Over 25 Years: An Analysis of the Central Malignant Melanoma Registry of the German Dermatological Society

Buettner PG, Leiter U, Eigentler TK, et al (James Cook Univ, Townsville, Australia; Eberhard-Karls-Univ of Tuebingen, Germany)
Cancer 103:616-624, 2005   17–19

Background.—Recent studies revealed that incidence rates of cutaneous melanoma (CM) were leveling off predominantly among younger people and patterns suggested birth-cohort effects. The current study analyzed the development of prognostic factors and survival in incident CM over 25 years.

Methods.—All 45,483 patients with incident CM diagnosed between 1976 and 2000 recorded by the German Central Malignant Melanoma Registry were considered. Linear and logistic regression analyses were used to judge time trends. Trends of survival rates were tested with the multivariate Cox model.

Results.—Median tumor thickness decreased from 1.81 mm in 1976 to 0.53 mm in 2000 ($P < 0.0001$). The percentages of in situ and level II CM increased, respectively ($P < 0.0001$). The percentage of ulcerated CM decreased ($P < 0.0001$). The percentage of superficial spreading melanoma increased, whereas the percentage of nodular melanoma decreased ($P < 0.0001$). These time trends were all significant in the strata of gender, however, male patients presented in general with more advanced disease. Between 1976 and 2000, the average patient got older ($P < 0.0001$). The percentage of patients diagnosed with the primary tumor alone increased ($P < 0.0001$). Across the 25 years of observation, adjusted survival rates did not increase for females ($P = 0.1561$) but they increased for males ($P < 0.0001$).

Conclusions.—The data demonstrated a strong trend towards prognostically more favorable CM most likely due to earlier diagnosis. Men and older people should be the focus of health promotion activities as they presented with more advanced disease.

▶ This study from Germany is consistent with observations worldwide. Because of public education and increased public awareness, melanomas are being diagnosed at an earlier stage. Consequently, overall survival is improving, especially in women. However, men, especially those older than 55 years, continue to present with thick lesions and more advanced disease, which negatively affects survival.

P. G. Lang, Jr, MD

Estimates of Stage-Specific Survival Are Altered by Changes in the 2002 American Joint Committee on Cancer Staging System for Melanoma
Ben-Porat L, Panageas KS, Hanlon C, et al (Mem Sloan-Kettering Cancer Ctr, New York)
Cancer 106:163-171, 2006   17–20

Background.—The objectives of the current study were to examine how the estimated stage-specific survival is altered in the 2002 American Joint Committee on Cancer (AJCC) melanoma staging system compared with the 1997 AJCC staging system and to contrast the predictive accuracy of the 2 staging systems.

Methods.—There were 5847 consecutive melanoma patients who presented to Memorial Sloan-Kettering Cancer Center from 1996 to 2004 and who were entered prospectively into a data base. These patients were staged according to both the 1997 and 2002 AJCC staging criteria. Overall survival estimates were determined using the Kaplan-Meier method. The overall predictive accuracy of the two staging systems was compared using concordance estimation.

Results.—In total, 1035 patients were shifted to a lower stage in the 2002 staging system, whereas only 15 patients were upstaged. The number of patients with Stage I melanoma increased by 697 under the 2002 system ($n = 2166$ patients) compared with the 1997 system ($n = 1463$ patients). Because of the changes in 2002, the estimated 5-year overall survival for patients with Stage II melanoma decreased considerably, from 79% (1997) to 64% (2002). With the initiation of subgroups in 2002, it became apparent that patients with Stage III melanoma were very heterogeneous in terms of their survival probabilities (5-yr overall survival ranged from 70% in patients with Stage IIIA disease to 24% in patients with Stage IIIC disease). Furthermore, in the 2002 system, there was substantial prognostic overlap between Stage II and Stage III. Despite the increased complexity of the 2002 system, the 2 staging systems had similar concordance estimates: 58% for the 1997 staging system compared with 58% (ignoring the subgroups) and 59% (with subgroups) for the 2002 system.

Conclusions.—Estimates of stage-specific survival were altered substantially by the changes made in the 2002 AJCC staging system for melanoma, particularly for Stage II. Stage subgroups that were added in the 2002 system resulted in a large diversity of risk within Stage III. This must be taken into account to stratify patients properly for clinical trials. The increased complexity of the 2002 system did not improve its predictive ability over the simpler 1997 system, highlighting the importance of developing individualized risk-prediction models.

▶ The revision of a staging system should hopefully help better predict survival in patients with a malignancy. This was the AJCC's goal when it developed a new staging system for melanoma in 2002. However, as this study demonstrates, the goal remains elusive. Despite its increased complexity, the 2002 staging system is no better than the simpler 1997 staging system in predicting disease outcome. Because of the shortcomings of an overall staging system, the authors suggest that a prognostic algorithm, which incorporates many variables, is more suitable for predicting disease outcome in any given individual.

P. G. Lang, Jr, MD

Limitations of Dermoscopy in the Recognition of Melanoma

Skvara H, Teban L, Fiebiger M, et al (Univ of Vienna; Emco Privatklinik, Bad Dürrnberg, Salzburg, Austria)
Arch Dermatol 141:155-160, 2005   17–21

Objective.—To compare dermoscopic features of melanocytic nevi with those of early melanomas that were not excised initially because of their uncharacteristic clinical and dermoscopic appearance.

Design.—Retrospective study of the baseline images of 325 melanocytic skin lesions that were observed by digital dermoscopy and finally excised because of changes over time.

Setting.—A dermatologic clinic and a dermatologic department at a university hospital.

Main Outcome Measures.—Comparison of baseline images of melanomas and melanocytic nevi by pattern analysis, the ABCD rule of dermoscopy, and the 7-point checklist.

Results.—Baseline dermoscopic images of 262 melanocytic nevi and 63 melanomas from 315 patients were included in the analysis. The patterns of dermoscopic features observed in the baseline images of melanocytic lesions finally diagnosed as melanomas during follow-up did not differ substantially from the patterns observed in the baseline images of melanocytic nevi. Pattern analysis, the ABCD rule of dermoscopy, and the 7-point checklist failed to achieve adequate diagnostic accuracy for melanoma. In retrospect, no dermoscopic feature or pattern of features could be identified that reliably differentiated between melanomas and melanocytic nevi at the time of the first presentation.

Conclusion.—Dermoscopy depends on the appearance of classic dermoscopic features and is therefore limited in the diagnosis of very early and mainly featureless melanomas.

▶ Prior studies have suggested that dermoscopy, when utilized by clinicians experienced in the use of this diagnostic aid, can significantly increase the ability to diagnose early melanoma. In contrast, this study suggests that there is a significant subset of in situ and invasive melanomas that early on do not meet the dermoscopic criteria for the diagnosis of melanoma, but which can be subsequently diagnosed through the use of stored serial digital dermoscopic images. Total body photography has proved to be quite useful in following patients who are at significant risk for the development of melanoma. This study suggests that the use of stored digital dermoscopic images in patients with selected suspicious pigmented lesions might be another useful aid to diagnose melanoma in its early stage.

P. G. Lang, Jr, MD

Skin Biopsy Rates and Incidence of Melanoma: Population Based Ecological Study
Welch HG, Woloshin S, Schwartz LM (Dept of Veterans Affairs Med Ctr, White River Junction, Vt)
BMJ 331:481, 2005   17–22

Objectives.—To describe changes in skin biopsy rates and to determine their relation with changes in the incidence of melanoma.
Design.—Population based ecological study.
Setting.—Nine geographical areas of the United States.
Participants.—Participants of the Surveillance Epidemiology and End Results (SEER) programme aged 65 and older.
Main Outcome Measures.—For the period 1986 to 2001, annual skin biopsy rates for each surveillance area from Medicare claims and incidence rates for melanoma for the same population.
Results.—Between 1986 and 2001 the average biopsy rate across the nine participating areas increased 2.5-fold among people aged 65 and older (2847 to 7222 per 100,000 population). Over the same period the average incidence of melanoma increased 2.4-fold (45 to 108 per 100,000 population). Assuming that the occurrence of true disease was constant, the extra number of melanoma cases that were diagnosed after carrying out 1000 additional biopsies was 12.6 (95% confidence interval 11.2 to 14.0). After controlling for a potential increase in the true occurrence of disease, 1000 additional biopsies were still associated with 6.9 (3.1 to 10.8) extra melanoma cases diagnosed. Stage specific analyses suggested that 1000 biopsies were associated with 4.4 (2.1 to 6.8) extra cases of in situ melanoma diagnosed and 2.3 (0.0 to 4.6) extra cases of local melanoma, but not with the incidence of advanced melanoma. Mortality from melanoma changed little during the period.

Conclusion.—The incidence of melanoma is associated with biopsy rates. That the extra cases diagnosed were confined to early stage cancer while mortality remained stable suggests overdiagnosis—the increased incidence being largely the result of increased diagnostic scrutiny and not an increase in the incidence of disease.

▶ There has been much debate about whether there has been a true increase in the incidence of melanoma. These authors used Medicare data to propose that more melanomas are being diagnosed because more biopsies are being performed. There is no question that physicians nowadays are more likely to biopsy suspicious pigmented lesions, and this likely contributes at least partially to the "increased" incidence of melanoma. Increased public education and awareness also certainly contribute to this increase. Nonetheless, there is little doubt in this reviewer's mind, based on years of observation, that there has been a true increase in the incidence of melanoma. Finally, this reviewer would take issue with the assertion that because the mortality rate has not increased, these early lesions are biologically benign. Although the risk of early lesions causing death is small, there is no question that with the passage of time they can evolve into life-threatening malignancies. Early detection is therefore of paramount importance.

P. G. Lang, Jr, MD

Subepidermal Cleft Formation as a Diagnostic Marker for Cutaneous Malignant Melanoma
Braun-Falco M, Friedrichson E, Ring J (Technische Universität München, Germany)
Hum Pathol 36:412-415, 2005   17–23

Introduction.—Cleft formation has been postulated as a clue to the histopathological diagnosis of malignant melanoma (MM). The frequency and reliability of clefts as a diagnostic criterion remain to be determined. We reviewed 503 cases of histologically proven MM searching for clefting between the epidermal layer and underlying MM. Cleft was defined as a separation of at least 0.3 mm in length. Conspicuous cleft formation was present in 120 (24%) of 503 MMs. The presence of clefts was not associated with age or sex of the patients, but showed a slight predilection for the back, a slightly higher prevalence in superficial spreading type of MM and for tumors with a Breslow thickness between 1 and 2 mm. Morphologically, clefts could be separated in 3 different types: linear (37.5%), single-nest (10.9%), and multi-nest (51.6%) (Fig 2; see color plate XIII). In comparison, among 939 benign melanocytic lesions including 100 Spitz or Reed nevi, only 9 exhibited clefts longer than 0.3 mm (<1%). One was an atypical compound nevus; all others were Spitz nevi, with the majority exhibiting an arched morphology above 1 or 2 large round nests. The relative frequency of cleft formation allowed a highly significant differentiation between MM and benign

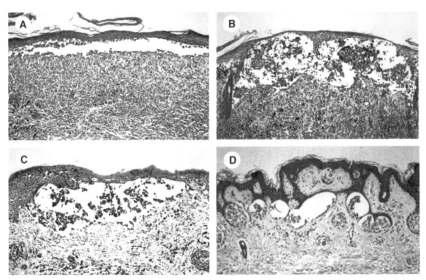

FIGURE 2.—Morphologic variants of cleft formation among malignant melanoma and benign melanocytic lesions. (A) Linear cleft (1.5 mm) in SSM (tumor thickness 0.8 mm, Clark level III). (B) Multi-nest cleft (0.5 mm) in NM (tumor thickness 1.1 mm, Clark level III). (C) Single-nest cleft (1.1 mm) in NM (tumor thickness 1.4 mm, Clark level IV). (D) A 0.35-mm-long cleft within an atypical compound nevus (all hematoxylin and eosin, original magnification ×100). (Courtesy of Braun-Falco M, Friedrichson E, Ring J: Subepidermal Cleft Formation as a Diagnostic Marker for Cutaneous Malignant Melanoma. *Hum Pathol* 36:412-415, 2005.)

melanocytic lesions. Clefts are a reliable diagnostic criterion in favor of MM.

▶ Dermatologists are very familiar with the cleft that occurs between the epidermis and dermis in lichen planus. The cleft results from destruction of the basal zone of the epidermis by the T-cell–mediated immune response in the papillary dermis and at the dermal-epidermal junction. These so-called Max Josef clefts have diagnostic significance. In MM, proliferation of melanocytes as nests and as solitary units along the dermal-epidermal junction when confluent causes dysadhesion between the epidermis and dermis and results in cleft formation when the tissue specimen is processed. Although this microscopic finding was described by Ackerman et al,[1] its significance as a clue to the diagnosis of melanoma has not achieved wide recognition.

Braun-Falco et al tested the hypothesis that cleft formation at the dermal-epidermal junction in melanocytic lesions is a marker for melanoma but not for benign melanocytic proliferations. They found that the sign has a very high degree of significance ($P < 10^{-4}$). Spitz nevi often present the greatest challenge in the differential diagnosis from malignant melanoma. It is common in Spitz nevi to find cleft formation between the epidermis and the nests of large Spitz nevus cells at the dermal-epidermal junction. In this situation, the length of the cleft is critical. Clefts of at least 0.3 mm proved to be the most discriminatory, occurring in melanoma but not in benign melanocytic lesions.

J. C. Maize, MD

Reference

1. Ackerman AB, Jacobson M, Vitale P: Clue 34. In Ackerman AB, Jacobson M, Vitale P (eds): *Clues to diagnosis in dermatopathology,* Chicago, 1991, ASCP Press, p 133-136.

Increasing Incidence of Lentigo Maligna Melanoma Subtypes: Northern California and National Trends 1990–2000

Swetter SM, Boldrick JC, Jung SY, et al (Veterans Affairs Palo Alto Health Care System, Calif; Stanford Univ, Calif)
J Invest Dermatol 125:685-691, 2005   17–24

Introduction.—Worldwide, lentigo maligna melanoma (LMM) comprises 4%-15% of cutaneous melanoma and occurs less commonly than superficial spreading or nodular subtypes. We assessed the incidence of melanoma subtypes in regional and national Surveillance, Epidemiology, and End Results (SEER) cancer registry data from 1990 to 2000. Because 30%-50% of SEER data were not classified by histogenetic type, we compared the observed SEER trends with an age-matched population of 1024 cases from Stanford University Medical Center (SUMC) (1995-2000). SEER data revealed lentigo maligna (LM) as the most prevalent in situ subtype (79%-83%), and that LMM has been increasing at a higher rate compared with other subtypes and to all invasive melanoma combined for patients aged 45-64 and ≥65 y. The SUMC data demonstrated LM and LMM as the only subtypes increasing in incidence over the study period. In both groups, LM comprised ≥75% of *in situ* melanoma and LMM ≥27% of invasive melanoma in men 65 y and older. Regional and national SEER data suggest an increasing incidence of LM and LMM, particularly in men ≥age 65. An increased incidence of LM subtypes should direct melanoma screening to heavily sun-exposed sites, where these subtypes predominate.

▶ One wonders whether the findings reflect the increased longevity and the increased leisure time available in our society. LM and LMM typically occur on chronically sun-exposed areas and are likely linked to cumulative sun exposure. This contrasts to superficial spreading melanoma and nodular melanoma, which more typically occur on the trunk and extremities, and reflect intermittent intense rather than chronic cumulative exposure to UV light. The findings reported by Swetter et al are unlikely to be limited to northern California, and suggest that we all should be more attuned to the presence of atypical pigmented lesions in chronically sun-exposed areas.

B. H. Thiers, MD

Variation in the Diagnosis, Treatment, and Management of Melanoma In Situ: A Survey of US Dermatologists

Charles CA, Yee VSK, Dusza SW, et al (Mem Sloan-Kettering Cancer Ctr, New York; New York Univ School of Medicine)
Arch Dermatol 141:723-729, 2005   17–25

Objective.—To assess current practices of US dermatologists regarding the diagnosis, treatment, and management of melanoma in situ (MIS).

Design.—Survey.

Participants.—A total of 1200 dermatologists randomly selected from the American Board of Medical Specialists Directory of Board Certified Medical Specialists.

Main Outcome Measures.—Results based on 597 questionnaires returned.

Results.—The overall response rate was 63% (597 of 945 eligible participants). To aid in clinical assessment, respondents reported using a magnifying lens (57.4%) and dermoscopy (17.4%). Most dermatologists preferred excisional and saucerization biopsies as the method of choice for sampling. A large percentage of physicians (78.9%) preferentially used dermatopathologists for the evaluation of the majority of pigmented lesions. Although most respondents would not unquestioningly accept a benign pathology diagnosis when there was a clinical suspicion of MIS, 16.1% would accept a pathologist's diagnosis without further action. There was no consensus on the appropriate surgical margins or depth of excision for MIS. Of the respondents who characterized MIS as premalignant and malignant, 63.2% and 46.4%, respectively, did not know what percentage of MISs would progress to metastatic disease if left untreated.

Conclusions.—Considerable variability exists in the clinical concept and management of MIS. Dermoscopy is underutilized. The true nature of the evolution of MIS is unknown. Surgical margins and depth of excision need to be standardized to help dermatologists manage disease. Further research in the specific area of MIS is warranted to develop clear guidelines in the management and prevention of further disease.

▶ Although the authors commented on the relative underutilization of dermoscopy, it could also be argued that any atypical-appearing lesion deserves an excisional biopsy, no matter what its dermatoscopic appearance.

B. H. Thiers, MD

Treatment of Lentigo Maligna (Melanoma In Situ) With the Immune Response Modifier Imiquimod

Wolf IH, Cerroni L, Kodama K, et al (Med Univ of Graz, Austria; Hokkaido Univ, Sapporo, Japan)
Arch Dermatol 141:510-514, 2005   17–26

Background.—Surgical excision is the treatment of choice for lentigo maligna (LM), or melanoma in situ. Topical application of imiquimod, a local immune response modifier, is a novel therapeutic approach that leads to LM tumor clearance. This pilot, open-label, nonrandomized study evaluates the efficacy of imiquimod in patients with LM and other systemic problems that make them poor surgical risks.

Observations.—Six biopsy-proven cases of LM from 5 patients (age range, 67-80 years) in whom standard surgical therapy was contraindicated were enrolled in the study. Five tumors were located on the face and 1 on the right shoulder. Imiquimod was used as a 5% cream once a day for a maximum of 13 weeks. Immediate clinical responses and follow-up, as well as histopathologic changes and immunohistologic parameters (in 2 patients), were analyzed. The complete response rate for all LM cases was 100%. Time to complete clearing varied from 5 to 13 weeks based on both clinical and histopathologic findings. The inflammatory infiltrate following imiquimod treatment consisted of T-helper lymphocytes mixed with a significant number of cytotoxic cells and monocytes or macrophages. These results indicate that imiquimod induces a cytotoxic T-cell-mediated immune response. In all patients, erythema and erosions occurred at the treated area 2 to 4 weeks after initiation of imiquimod therapy. The patients have been followed up for 3 to 18 months without evidence of recurrences.

Conclusions.—Topical imiquimod appears to be an excellent therapeutic option for LM. Close evaluation of patients, including posttherapy histopathologic investigation, is essential. Imiquimod can be added to the list of therapeutic approaches for carefully selected patients with LM.

► Topical imiquimod appears to be evolving as a treatment alternative for LM. As is the case with basal cell carcinoma, the reported results are not on a par with those of surgical intervention, which will remain the treatment of choice. Nevertheless, there may be patients in whom a surgical approach is not practical, and such individuals may be good candidates for topical treatment. In addition, future studies may be done to assess the role of topical imiquimod in preventing recurrence of previously excised LM.

B. H. Thiers, MD

Follicular Malignant Melanoma: A Variant of Melanoma to Be Distinguished From Lentigo Maligna Melanoma

Hantschke M, Mentzel T, Kutzner H (Dermatopathologische Gemeinschaftpraxis, Friedrichshafen, Germany)
Am J Dermatopathol 26:359-363, 2004   17–27

Introduction.—Follicular malignant melanoma can be regarded as a rare and unique presentation of melanoma. It is characterized by a deep-seated follicular structure in which atypical melanocytes extend downward along the follicular epithelium and permeate parts of the follicle as well as the adjacent dermis. The clinical diagnosis of follicular malignant melanoma may be difficult because the tumor mostly resembles a comedo or a pigmented cyst. We studied five cases of follicular malignant melanoma in which the patients were between 61 and 82 years old. Three lesions were localized on the nose, one on the cheek, and one on the back of the neck. Clinically, all five cases measured distinctly less than 0.5 cm in size. While lentigo maligna is traditionally known as a pigmented macule in actinically damaged skin that gradually evolves in a slow process before invasive growth, three follicular malignant melanomas had developed in relatively short timeframes of 9 months to 1½ years. In all five cases the inconspicuous clinical appearance did not herald a malignant melanoma with invasive growth. Follicular malignant melanoma underlines the importance of a correct excision technique with subsequent histologic workup and diagnosis. Superficial shave excision or even laser treatment in these specific cases may lead to a fatal prognosis for the patient.

▶ The authors call attention to an unusual growth pattern of melanoma in which there is colonization of only a small area of the epidermis, but there is extensive involvement of follicular epithelium. The importance of this variant is the fact that invasion may occur from a site deep in the hair follicle and that the appropriate measurement is not from the surface in a vertical dimension but from the follicle in a radial dimension. From a clinician's viewpoint, it is essential to know that this phenomenon exists because these small lesions might be easily confused with blue nevi, which are relatively common on the head and neck area of middle-aged and elderly adults.

J. C. Maize, MD

Microstaging Accuracy After Subtotal Incisional Biopsy of Cutaneous Melanoma

Karimipour DJ, Schwartz JL, Wang TS, et al (Univ of Michigan, Ann Arbor; Univ of Alabama at Birmingham)
J Am Acad Dermatol 52:798-802, 2005   17–28

Background.—A significant portion of cutaneous melanoma may remain after subtotal incisional biopsy. The accuracy of microstaging and impact on clinical practice in this scenario are unknown.

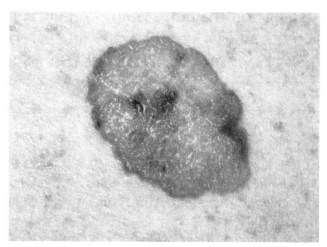

FIGURE 1.—Initial small punch biopsy specimen of 2.5- × 3-cm back lesion was interpreted as severely atypical melanocytic proliferation, consistent with melanoma in situ. Complete excision revealed melanoma, Breslow depth of 1.4 mm. Of interest, a 6-mm punch biopsy specimen from central black component during complete excision revealed melanoma, 0.5 mm thick. (Reprinted by permission of the publisher from Karimipour DJ, Schwartz JL, Wang TS, et al: Microstaging accuracy after subtotal incisional biopsy of cutaneous melanoma. *J Am Acad Dermatol* 52:798-802, 2005. Copyright 2005 by Elsevier.)

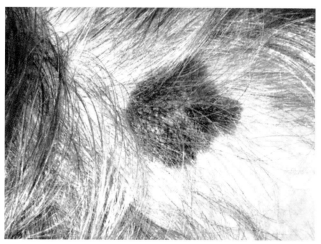

FIGURE 2.—Initial small punch biopsy specimen of 2.6- × 2.5-cm scalp lesion was interpreted as melanoma in situ. Complete excision revealed melanoma, Breslow depth 0.98 mm (adnexal extension to 1.90 mm, Clark level V) with regression. Of interest, a 6-mm punch biopsy specimen from the blackest and most elevated component during complete excision revealed melanoma in situ. (Reprinted by permission of the publisher from Karimipour DJ, Schwartz JL, Wang TS, et al: Microstaging accuracy after subtotal incisional biopsy of cutaneous melanoma. *J Am Acad Dermatol* 52:798-802, 2005. Copyright 2005 by Elsevier.)

Objective.—Our purpose was to examine microstaging accuracy of an initial incisional biopsy with a significant portion of the clinical lesion remaining ($\geq 50\%$).

Methods.—Patients with cutaneous melanoma, diagnosed by incisional biopsy with $\geq 50\%$ of the lesion remaining, were prospectively evaluated for microstaging accuracy, comparing initial Breslow depth (BD1) to final depth (BD2) after excision of the residual lesion. Impact on prognosis and treatment was also evaluated.

Results.—Two hundred fifty of 1783 patients (14%) presented with $\geq 50\%$ residual clinical lesion after incisional biopsy. The mean BD1 was 0.66 mm; the mean BD2, 1.07 mm ($P = .001$). After complete excision of the residual lesion, upstaging occurred in 21% and 10% became candidates for sentinel node biopsy.

Conclusion.—An incisional biopsy with $\geq 50\%$ clinical lesion remaining afterward may be inadequate for accurate microstaging of melanoma. This scenario is relatively uncommon but clinically significant (Figs 1 and 2; see color plate XIV).

▶ The authors found that the vast majority of suspected melanomas were biopsied either by punch or shave technique. For both dermatologists and nondermatologists, fewer than 10% of biopsy specimens were elliptical incisions or excisions. The risk with the punch technique is that the thickest portion of the lesion is not sampled, and the risk with a shave is that the invasive component of the lesion is transected. Therefore, both techniques may underestimate the thickness of a lesion. In this study, 14% of patients had more than 50% of the residual lesion remaining after incisional biopsy. The mean Breslow thickness was 0.66 mm in the original biopsy specimen versus 1.07 mm in the definitive excisional specimen. This difference is highly statistically significant. After complete excision, 21% of the patients with more than 50% of the lesion remaining after the original biopsy were upstaged, and 10% became candidates for sentinel node biopsy. The authors conclude that excision of the entire lesion should be performed whenever possible to obtain the most accurate microstaging information. They also point out that wide local excision based on inadequate microstaging might affect patient care by interfering with the patient's eligibility for sentinel lymph node biopsy. This study reminds us of the importance of selecting the correct biopsy technique to acquire the information that is necessary for the management of the patient's disease, whether it be a cutaneous neoplasm or an inflammatory dermatosis.

J. C. Maize, MD

Histopathologic Excision Margin Affects Local Recurrence Rate: Analysis of 2681 Patients With Melanomas ≤2 mm Thick

McKinnon JG, Starrit EC, Scolyer RA, et al (Univ of Calgary, Alberta, Canada; Univ of Sydney, New South Wales, Australia; Royal Prince Alfred Hosp, Camperdown, New South Wales, Australia)
Ann Surg 241:326-333, 2005   17–29

Objective.—Prospective trials have shown that 1-cm and 2-cm margins are safe for melanomas <1 mm thick and ≥1 mm thick, respectively. It is unknown whether narrower margins increase the risk of LR or mortality.

Summary Background Data.—To determine the relationship between histopathologic excision margin, local recurrence (LR) and survival for patients with melanomas ≤2 mm thick.

Methods.—Data were extracted from the Sydney Melanoma Unit database for all patients with cutaneous melanoma ≤2 mm thick, diagnosed up to 1996. Patients with positive excision margins or follow-up <12 months were excluded, leaving 2681 for analysis. Outcome measures were LR (recurrence <5 cm from the excision scar), in-transit recurrence, and disease-specific survival. Factors predicting LR and overall survival were tested with Cox proportional hazards analysis.

Results.—Median follow-up was 83.8 months. LR was identified in 55 patients (median time to recurrence, 37 months). At 120 months, the actuarial LR rate was 2.9%. Five-year survival after LR was 52.8%. In multivariate analysis, only margin of excision and tumor thickness were predictive of LR (both $P = 0.003$). When all patients with a margin <0.8 cm in fixed tissue (corresponding to a margin of <1 cm in vivo) were excluded from analysis, margin was no longer significant in predicting LR. Thickness, ulceration, and site were predictive of survival, but margin was not ($P = 0.49$).

Conclusions.—Histopathologic margin affects the risk of LR. However, if the in vivo margin is ≤1 cm, it no longer predicts risk of LR. Patient survival is not affected by margin.

▶ The authors demonstrate that for patients with melanomas 2 mm thick or less, the risk of LR is small and inversely related to the margin of excision. However, if an in vivo margin of at least 1 cm (corresponding to a histopathologic margin of 0.8 cm) is achieved, this relationship is lost. Moreover, there was no identifiable relationship between margin width and survival. The data suggest that once a certain excision margin is achieved (in this case, 1 cm), further excision of normal tissue has no effect on the rate of LR. The findings support the safety of a 1-cm margin for melanomas that are 1- to 2-mm thick.

B. H. Thiers, MD

Cutaneous Head and Neck Melanoma Treated With Mohs Micrographic Surgery

Bricca GM, Brodland DG, Ren D, et al (Skin Cancer Surgery Ctr, Sacramento, Calif; Univ of Pittsburgh, Pa; Pittsburgh, Pa)
J Am Acad Dermatol 52:92-100, 2005   17–30

Background.—Previous studies show that Mohs micrographic surgery is a viable treatment option for cutaneous melanoma. The head and neck region represents an anatomic location of historically high recurrence/metastasis rates and poor survival rates.

Objective.—Our purpose was to determine the safety and efficacy of Mohs micrographic surgery for the treatment of primary cutaneous melanoma of the head and neck.

Methods.—A consecutive sample of 625 patients referred for treatment of primary cutaneous melanoma of the head and neck comprised the study group. Mean follow-up for the group was 58.0 months. All melanomas were excised using Mohs micrographic surgery and surgical margin examination was performed using frozen section tissue in all cases. After stratification using updated American Joint Commission for Cancer (AJCC) Breslow thickness criteria, the Kaplan-Meier method was used to calculate 5-year local recurrence rates, metastasis rates, and disease specific survival rates. Tumors were then re-stratified by earlier Breslow thickness criteria for comparison to historical controls for local recurrence rates, metastasis rates, and disease-specific survival rates. Recommendations for predetermined excision margins were proposed and were based on the surgical margin widths that achieved complete melanoma removal in 97% of the cases in this study.

Results.—Mohs micrographic surgery for the treatment of head and neck melanoma achieved five-year local recurrence rates, metastasis rates, and disease specific survival rates comparable to or better than historical controls after Breslow thickness stratification. The size of the surgical margin required for complete excision was significantly related to tumor thickness but not tumor size or specific location.

Conclusion.—Mohs micrographic surgery is an effective treatment modality for primary cutaneous melanoma, and may contribute to favorable outcomes especially on the head and neck where extensive sub-clinical spread is relatively common.

▶ This large study documents the success of Mohs micrographic surgery for the resection of malignant melanoma of the head and neck. The authors here used exclusively frozen section analysis. It should be noted that there is some controversy about whether frozen sections are accurate for the histopathologic interpretation of melanoma resection margins.

The data presented here certainly support the use of frozen sections during Mohs surgery for melanoma. Nevertheless, one should understand that the use of frozen sections during Mohs surgery for melanoma requires a very skilled Mohs surgeon and a technically proficient Mohs laboratory (frozen sections for melanoma are typically cut 2-4 μm thick).

J. Cook, MD

Follow-up in Patients With Localised Primary Cutaneous Melanoma

Francken AB, Bastiaannet E, Hoekstra HJ (Univ of Groningen, The Netherlands)

Lancet 6:608-621, 2005   17–31

Introduction.—Follow-up services for patients with localised cutaneous melanoma are widely discussed but there is no international consensus. Our aim was to discuss frequency and duration of follow-up, type of health professional involved, optimum intensity of routine investigation, and patients' satisfaction with follow-up. Searches of the published work were directed at publications between January, 1985, and February, 2004 on recurrences, subsequent primary melanoma, routine tests, and patients' satisfaction. In a selection of 72 articles, 2142 (6.6%) recurrences were reported, 62% of which were detected by the patients themselves. 2.6% of patients developed a subsequent primary melanoma. Most investigators do not support high-intensity routine follow-up investigations. Of the various follow-up investigations requested by physicians, only medical history and physical examination seem to be cost effective. Lymph-node sonography seems to be a promising method for detection, although survival benefit remains to be proven. Patients were found to be anxious about follow-up visits, although other research showed that provision of information to patients was much appreciated. Published work on the follow-up of patients with cutaneous melanoma has mainly been retrospective and descriptive. Recommendations can be given with only a low grade of evidence. For meaningful guidelines to be developed, prospective, high-quality methodological research is needed.

▶ Many aspects of melanoma management are controversial, including recommended surveillance of patients with American Joint Committee on Cancer stage I and II disease. It has been shown that patients are as likely to detect recurrent disease as their physicians are, and except for one study that showed that physicians are more likely to detect asymptomatic recurrent disease there has been no demonstrated survival advantage based on who detects the recurrence. However, it has been shown that physicians are more likely to detect a second primary lesion that is usually thin and thus should have a good prognosis. The reported risk of developing a second primary melanoma has ranged from 2% to 7%. Most studies have recommended that the history and physical exam are the most important investigations to perform at follow-up with respect to detecting recurrent disease, and that the routine ordering of laboratory tests, including chest radiographs, is not cost effective and does not correlate with improved survival, as there is no effective treatment for disseminated disease. In some studies, lymph node sonography has been shown to be worthwhile for detecting regional recurrences, but again it remains to be determined whether this investigation is cost effective or improves survival. Unfortunately, most of the data on follow-up recommendations are based on retrospective analyses, and there is a need for well-designed and controlled prospective studies that address this issue. Until these are performed, there will continue to be a great deal of variability in how frequently and by what means clinicians monitor their stage I and II melanoma patients. Not usually considered is patient expectations, that is, how would they feel if their physicians did not ask them to return for routine follow-up visits or saw them infrequently and never ordered any laboratory tests? What are the medicolegal ramifications? Finally, there are patients with limited metastatic disease who experience significant survival after resection of a single metastatic focus or after biochemotherapy.

P. G. Lang, Jr, MD

Detection of Lymphatic Invasion in Primary Melanoma With Monoclonal Antibody D2-40: A New Selective Immunohistochemical Marker of Lymphatic Endothelium

Niakosari F, Kahn HJ, Marks A, et al (Univ of Toronto)
Arch Dermatol 141:440-444, 2005   17–32

Objectives.—To identify the presence of lymphatic invasion in primary cutaneous melanoma using monoclonal antibody D2-40, a marker of lymphatic endothelium, and to correlate the presence of lymphatic invasion with other clinicopathologic characteristics of the tumors.

Design.—Retrospective melanoma case series study comparing conventional hematoxylin-eosin staining with D2-40 immunostaining for detection of lymphatic invasion.

Setting.—Departments of Pathology and Dermatology, Sunnybrook and Women's College Health Sciences Center, University of Toronto, Toronto, Ontario. Patients Forty-four consecutive cases of primary cutaneous melanoma with a tumor thickness greater than 0.75 mm were examined for presence of lymphatic invasion.

Results.—Seven (16%) of 44 melanomas showed the presence of lymphatic invasion under immunostaining with D2-40. In 2 cases, subepidermal lymphatic involvement was present; in 5 cases lymphatic invasion was noted within the tumor, including 1 case of additional lymphatic invasion at the invasive edge of the tumor. Lymphatic invasion was not detected on routine hematoxylin-eosin staining. We observed a trend in the association between lymphatic invasion and 2 markers of tumor aggressiveness, namely, a deeper Clark level and increased frequency of ulceration, which suggests that lymphatic invasion detected with D2-40 may indicate a poor prognosis.

Conclusions.—Immunostaining with D2-40 increases the frequency of detection of lymphatic invasion relative to conventional hematoxylin-eosin staining in primary melanoma. Future outcome data will determine the prognostic significance of lymphatic invasion detected by D2-40 immuno-staining.

▶ The addition of this immunostain allowed detection of occult lymphatic invasion by melanoma that was not seen with conventional staining. It will be interesting to determine whether lymphatic invasion detected by D2-40 immunostaining affects long-term prognosis.

J. Cook, MD

Is Ultrasound Lymph Node Examination Superior to Clinical Examination in Melanoma Follow-up? A Monocentre Cohort Study of 373 Patients
Machet L, Nemeth-Normand F, Giraudea B, et al (Centre Hospitalier Universitaire, Tours Cedex, France)
Br J Dermatol 152:66-70, 2005   17–33

Background.—There is still lack of consensus regarding the most effective follow-up for stage I and II melanoma patients although some consensus conferences have provided guidelines stating that clinical examination should be the standard.

Objectives.—Our aim was to study the value of adding ultrasound lymph node examination (7.5 MHz) to the routine clinical examination recommended by French guidelines in melanoma follow-up.

Methods.—A cohort of melanoma patients was enrolled between 1 July 1995 and 1 July 2000 in a follow-up protocol including clinical examination performed four times a year for thick melanomas (Breslow index ≥ 1.5 mm) and twice a year for thin melanomas (Breslow index < 1.5 mm) according to French guidelines, and ultrasound lymph node examination performed every 6 months for thick melanomas and every year for thin melanomas. Follow-up was continued up to 1 July 2003. When clinical or ultrasound examination indicated signs of node recurrence, surgical biopsy of the involved node was performed. When ultrasound examination was only suspicious, another ultrasound examination was performed within the following 3 months. The results of both clinical and ultrasound examinations were compared with histopathology examination when node biopsy was performed.

Results.—Ultrasound follow-up was performed for 373 patients (213 females and 160 males). Mean age at diagnosis of melanoma was 59 years (range 14-90, SD 15). In total, 1909 ultrasound examinations combined with clinical examination were analysed. Node biopsy was performed in 65 patients and demonstrated melanoma metastases in 54. Sensitivity of clinical examination and ultrasound examination was 71.4%[95% confidence interval (CI) 55.4-84.3] and 92.9 (95% CI 80.5-98.5), respectively, $P = 0.02$. Specificity of clinical examination and ultrasound examination was 99.6% (95% CI 99.2-99.8) and 97.8% (95% CI 97.0-98.4), respectively. Despite this apparent superiority of ultrasound examination over palpation, only 7.2% of the patients really benefited from ultrasound examination (earlier lymph node metastasis detection or avoidance of unnecessary surgery), while 5.9% had some deleterious effect from ultrasound examination (unnecessary stress caused by repetition of ultrasound examination for benign lymph nodes, useless removal of benign lymph node).

Conclusions.—This study confirms the greater sensitivity of ultrasound examination to clinical examination in the diagnosis of node metastases from cutaneous melanoma. However, the place of ultrasound in routine follow-up is at least questionable as only a very small proportion of patients (1.3%) really benefited from adding ultrasound examination to clinical examination.

▶ In the United States, US is not commonly used to assess regional nodes in patients with cutaneous melanoma. However, some studies from Europe have suggested that US is an excellent method to monitor melanoma patients and to detect early lymph node involvement. In this study from France, the authors assessed the value of US for patients with cutaneous melanoma. US was more sensitive but less specific than palpation for detecting lymph node enlargement. Moreover, only 1.3% of patients truly benefited from US when compared to clinical examination.

P. G. Lang, Jr, MD

Mitotic Rate as a Predictor of Sentinel Lymph Node Positivity in Patients With Thin Melanomas

Kesmodel SB, Karakousis GC, Botbyl JD, et al (Univ of Pennsylvania, Philadelphia)
Ann Surg Oncol 12:449-458, 2005   17–34

Background.—Lymphatic mapping and sentinel lymphadenectomy (LM/SL) provide important prognostic information for patients with early-stage melanoma. Although the use of this technique in patients with thin melanomas (≤1.00 mm) is not routine, risk factors that may predict sentinel lymph node (SLN) positivity in this patient population are under investigation. We sought to determine whether mitotic rate (MR) is associated with SLN positivity in thin-melanoma patients and, therefore, whether it may be used to risk-stratify and select patients for LM/SL.

Methods.—Clinical and histopathologic variables were reviewed for 181 patients with thin melanomas who underwent LM/SL from January 1996 through January 2004. Univariate and multivariate logistic regression analyses were performed to identify factors associated with SLN positivity. Risk groups were defined on the basis of the development of a classification tree.

Results.—The overall SLN positivity rate was 5%. All patients with positive SLNs had an MR of >0. By univariate analysis, MR and thickness were significant predictors of SLN positivity. The association between MR and SLN positivity remained significant controlling for each of the other variables evaluated. On the basis of a classification tree, patients with an MR > 0 and tumor thickness ≥.76 mm were identified as a higher-risk group, with an SLN positivity rate of 12.3%.

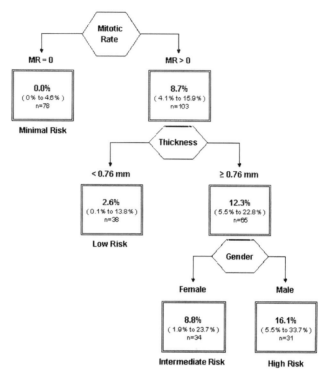

FIGURE 1.—Risk groups defined for sentinel lymph node positivity based on the development of a classification tree. Four risk groups were identified: (1) minimal risk: MR of 0 (SLN positivity rate, .0%); (2) low risk: MR >0, thickness <.76 mm (2.6%); (3) intermediate risk: MR >0, thickness ≥.76 mm, and female sex (8.8%); and (4) high risk: MR >0, thickness ≥.76 mm, and male sex (16.1%). *Abbreviations: SLN,* Sentinel lymph node; *MR,* mitotic rate. (Courtesy of Kesmodel SB, Karakousis GC, Botbyl JD, et al: Mitotic rate as a predictor of sentinel lymph node positivity in patients with thin melanomas. *Ann Surg Oncol* 12(6):449-458, 2005.).

Conclusions.—In patients with thin melanomas, MR > 0 seems to be a significant predictor of SLN positivity that may be used to risk-stratify and select patients for LM/SL. To confirm these results, the predictive value of MR for SLN positivity needs to be validated in other populations of thin-melanoma patients (Fig 1).

▶ In some studies, the MR associated with a melanoma has been found to be an important variable in determining whether a patient is at significant risk of developing recurrent disease. The cutoff point for this MR, however, has varied from study to study. In this study, an MR >0 was associated with SLN positivity, irrespective of other histologic variables, in a group of patients with thin melanomas (≤1.0 mm) demonstrating a vertical growth phase. Moreover, if patients were further stratified based on sex and tumor thickness (≥.76 mm or <.76 mm), 4 groups of patients varying in risk for SLN positivity could be identified, ranging from minimal risk (0% positivity) to high risk (16.1%). If this finding is confirmed by other studies, the MR in combination with other clinical and histologic variables may allow us to better select which patients with thin melanomas should undergo SLN biopsy.

P. G. Lang, Jr, MD

The Importance of Total Number of Sentinel Lymph Nodes in Patients With Stage N0 Cutaneous Melanoma

Stewart LE, Tyler DS, Vollmer RT (Duke Univ, Durham, NC)
Am J Clin Pathol 124:77-82, 2005

17–35

Introduction.—Staging of malignant melanoma now relies routinely on the sentinel node (SN) technique. On average, 2.1 SNs are removed per patient. Nevertheless, despite the success of the SN technique, approximately 10% of patients with negative SNs experience metastatic recurrence. Because a prior theoretical analysis using Poisson and Bayes probability models suggested that limited sampling of SNs could cause false-negative results, we undertook this study to see whether the subset of patients with negative SN and only 1 or 2 nodes examined have a shorter time to recurrence than patients with 3 or more nodes examined and found to be negative. Our study cases comprised 178 melanoma cases with SN biopsy: positive SN, 47; negative SN and fewer than 3 nodes examined, 68; and negative SN and more than 2 nodes examined, 63. Patients with negative SNs and fewer than 3 examined had disease-free survival intermediate between patients with positive SNs and those with negative SNs and more than 2 examined ($P = .013$). These results suggest that among patients with negative SNs, those with fewer than 3 nodes examined have greater risk for recurrence (Table 2).

▶ The false-negative rate for sentinel lymph nodes biopsies (SLNB) is approximately 10%. Although the SLNB technique for melanoma has been fairly well standardized, there is enough variability that the number of SLNs ultimately harvested can vary from patient to patient or surgeon to surgeon. This, in theory, could have an impact on the reliability of the SLNB as a prognostic indicator. In this study it was demonstrated that the harvesting of at least 3 SLNs was associated with an overall lower incidence of recurrence, as well as lower incidence of recurrence in the nodal basin previously sampled, when patients had a negative SLNB. If confirmed, this study would suggest that from a prognostic standpoint not only is it important to have a negative SLNB, it is also important to have sampled at least 3 SLNs.

P. G. Lang, Jr, MD

TABLE 2.—Comparison of Key Variables by SN Category

Variable	SN Negative		SN Positive	P
	>2 Nodes Sampled	<3 Nodes Sampled	Any No. of Nodes Sampled	
No. of patients	63	68	47	—
Mean age (y)	47	46	48	>.8
No. (%) females	34 (54)	26 (38)	13 (28)	>.1
Mean thickness (mm)	1.86	1.82	2.69	>.6
Median Clark level	4	4	4	>.9
No. (%) with ulcerated tumor	14 (22)	12 (18)	13 (28)	>.4
No. (%) with recurrence	2 (3)	10 (15)	16 (34)	
No. (%) with nodal recurrence	1 (50)	4 (40)	4 (25)	—
Mean time to recurrence (mo)	85.6	68.9	47.8	.013

SN, sentinel node.

*Statistical testing was done to compare only the results between the 2 groups with negative SNs. For categorical variables such as female sex, Clark level, and ulceration, the θ^2 test was used; for age and thickness, the Kruskal-Wallis rank test; and for time to recurrence, the log-rank test.

(Courtesy of Stewart LE, Tyler DS, Vollmer RT: The Importance of Total Number of Sentinel Lymph Nodes in Patients With Stage N0 Cutaneous Melanoma. Am J Clin Pathol 124:77-82, 2005. Copyright 2005 by the American Society of Clinical Pathologists. Reprinted with permission.)

Outcome in 846 Cutaneous Melanoma Patients From a Single Center After a Negative Sentinel Node Biopsy

Yee VSK, Thompson JF, McKinnon JG, et al (Royal Prince Alfred Hosp, Camperdown, New South Wales, Australia; Univ of Sydney, New South Wales, Australia)
Ann Surg Oncol 12:429-439, 2005   17–36

Background.—A negative sentinel node biopsy (SNB) implies a good prognosis for melanoma patients. The purpose of this study was to determine the long-term outcome for melanoma patients with a negative SNB.

Methods.—Survival and prognostic factors were analyzed for 836 SNB-negative patients. All patients with a node field recurrence were reviewed, and sentinel node (SN) tissue was reexamined.

Results.—The median tumor thickness was 1.7 mm, and 23.8% were ulcerated. The median follow-up was 42.1 months. Melanoma specific survival at 5 years was 90%, compared with 56% for SN-positive patients ($P < .001$). On multivariate analysis, only thickness and ulceration retained significance for disease-free and disease-specific survival. Five-year survival for patients with nonulcerated lesions was 94% vs. 78% with ulceration. Eighty-three patients (9.9%) had a recurrence. Twenty-seven patients developed recurrence in the regional node field, and in 22 of these, it was the first recurrence site. Six developed local recurrence, 17 an in-transit metastasis, and 58 distant disease. The false-negative rate was 13.2%. SN slides and tissue blocks were further examined in 18 patients with recurrence in the node field, and metastatic disease was found in 3 of them.

Conclusions.—This large, single-center study confirms that patients with a negative SNB have a significantly better prognosis than those with positive SNs. In those with a negative SNB, primary tumor thickness and ulceration are independent predictors of survival. Incorrect pathologic diagnosis contributed to only a minority of the false-negative results in this study.

▶ Since its early description by Morton and colleagues, the sentinel lymph node biopsy (SLNB) technique for melanomas has undergone several modifications. Early on, elective lymph node dissections were done concomitantly to determine whether this procedure was a reliable predictor of regional lymph node involvement. After a sufficient amount of data were generated, it was suggested that the SLNB was a reliable predictor of regional lymph node involvement and that patients with negative SLNB findings did not require a complete node dissection. Since the initial investigations, several studies have re-examined this issue to determine the false-negative rate for SLNB. This article comes from one of the larger melanoma centers in the world. In 836 patients with negative SLNB results, the investigators found that only 2.6% had a recurrence in their previously sampled nodal basin. In several cases, re-examination of the sentinel node revealed tumor tissue that had not been detected by the pathologist. Other possible explanations included a lack of experience of the surgeon and the use of blue dye alone. The sentinel nodes were not re-examined with the use of more advanced molecular techniques.

Although patients with negative SLNB results fared better than those with positive SLNB results, they still were subject to the risk of a tumor recurrence, not only in terms of nodal disease but also in-transit disease and the possibility of a distant recurrence. Thickness and ulceration of the primary lesion were important prognostic variables in determining the risk of recurrence and death in patients with negative SLNB results.

P. G. Lang, Jr, MD

Sentinel Node Biopsy for Early-Stage Melanoma: Accuracy and Morbidity in MSLT-I, an International Multicenter Trial

Morton DL, and the Multicenter Selective Lymphadenectomy Trial Group (John Wayne Cancer Inst, Santa Monica, Calif)
Ann Surg 242:302-313, 2005   17–37

Objective.—The objective of this study was to evaluate, in an international multicenter phase III trial, the accuracy, use, and morbidity of intraoperative lymphatic mapping and sentinel node biopsy (LM/SNB) for staging the regional nodal basin of patients with early-stage melanoma.

Summary Background Data.—Since our introduction of LM/SNB in 1990, this technique has been widely adopted and has become part of the American Joint Committee on Cancer (AJCC) staging system. Eleven years ago, the authors began the international Multicenter Selective Lymphadenectomy Trial (MSLT-I) to compare 2 treatment approaches: wide excision (WE) plus LM/SNB with immediate complete lymphadenectomy (CLND) for sentinel node (SN) metastases, and WE plus postoperative observation with CLND delayed until the subsequent development of clinically evident nodal metastases.

Methods.—After each center achieved 85% accuracy of SN identification during a 30-case learning phase, patients with primary cutaneous melanoma (≥ 1 mm with Clark level $\geq$III, or any thickness with Clark level $\geq$IV) were randomly assigned in a 4:6 ratio to WE plus observation (WEO) with delayed CLND for nodal recurrence, or to WE plus LM/SNB with immediate CLND for SN metastasis. The accuracy of LM/SNB was determined by comparing the rates of SN identification and the incidence of SN metastases in the LM/SNB group versus the subsequent development of nodal metastases in the regional nodal basin of those patients with tumor-negative SNs. Early morbidity of LM/SNB was evaluated by comparing complication rates between the 2 treatment groups. Trial accrual was completed on March 31, 2002, after enrollment of 2001 patients.

Results.—Initial SN identification rate was 95.3% overall: 99.3% for the groin, 95.3% for the axilla, and 84.5% for the neck basins. The rate of false-negative LM/SNB during the trial phase, as measured by nodal recurrence in a tumor-negative dissected SN basin, decreased with increasing case volume at each center: 10.3% for the first 25 cases versus 5.2% after 25 cases. There were no operative mortalities. The low (10.1%) complication rate after LM/

SNB increased to 37.2% with the addition of CLND; CLND also increased the severity of complications.

Conclusions.—LM/SNB is a safe, low-morbidity procedure for staging the regional nodal basin in early melanoma. Even after a 30-case learning phase and 25 additional LM/SNB cases, the accuracy of LM/SNB continues to increase with a center's experience. LM/SNB should become standard care for staging the regional lymph nodes of patients with primary cutaneous melanoma.

▶ This article simply confirms what other studies have shown, that is, SNB requires experience to correctly identify the SN but is a safe procedure with low morbidity rates. In experienced hands, the false-negative rate can be as low as 1.7%. In contrast to other anatomic sites, the head and neck area appears to present more difficulty in identifying the SN. Although this article does not answer whether an SNB, followed by a complete lymph node dissection, conveys any survival advantage, it does demonstrate that when a wait-and-see policy is adopted and the patient subsequently develops clinical nodal involvement, more removed lymph nodes will contain tumor.

P. G. Lang, Jr, MD

Clinical Significance of Occult Metastatic Melanoma in Sentinel Lymph Nodes and Other High-Risk Factors Based on Long-term Follow-up
Leong SPL, Kashani-Sabet M, Desmond RA, et al (Univ of California, San Francisco; Univ of Alabama at Birmingham)
World J Surg 29:683-691, 2005   17–38

Introduction.—Selective sentinel lymphadenectomy (SSL) following preoperative lymphoscintigraphy is the most significant recent advance in the management of patients with primary melanoma. This study evaluates the prognostic value of sentinel lymph node (SLN) status and other risk factors in predicting survival and recurrence in patients with primary cutaneous melanoma. From October 1993 to July 1998 a series of 412 patients with primary invasive melanoma underwent SSL at the UCSF/Mt. Zion Melanoma Center. The outcome of 363 evaluable patients is summarized in this study. The factors related to survival and disease recurrence were analyzed by Cox proportional hazard regression models. The overall incidence of patients with positive SLNs was 18%. Over a median follow-up of 4.8 years, the overall mortality rate in patients with primary cutaneous melanoma was 18.7%, and 74 recurrences occurred (20.4%). Mortality was significantly related to SLN status [HR = 2.06; 95% confidence interval (CI) 1.18, 3.58], angiolymphatic invasion (HR = 2.21; 95% CI 1.08, 4.55), ulceration (HR = 1.79; 95% CI 1.02, 3.15), mitotic index (HR = 1.38; 95% CI 1.01, 1.90), and tumor thickness (HR = 2.20, 95% CI 1.21, 3.99). Factors significantly related to disease-free survival included SLN status (HR = 2.09; 95% CI 1.31, 3.34), tumor thickness (HR = 1.89; 95%. CI 1.20,2.98), and age (HR = 1.26 95% CI 1.08, 1.47). SLN status was the most significant

TABLE 4.—Summary of Outcomes of Melanoma Patients Undergoing Selective SLN Dissection

Study	Year	No.	Median Follow-Up	Outcome	Significant Factors for Survival
Gadd [18]	1999	89 SLN−	23 Months	12% recurrence in SLN-group	None (small numbers)
Gershenwald	1999	85 SLN+; 495 SLN−	40 Months	3-years disease-free survival SLN+ 55.8%; 3-years disease-free survival SLN-88.5%; 3-year ysurvival SLN + 69.9%	Tumor thickness, Clark level > III, ulceration, and SLN status
Essner [17]	1999	42 SLN+	45 Months SLN	3-year survival SLN+ 96.8%; 5-year survival SLN+ 64%	Tumor thickness, Clark level > III, and SLN status
		225 SLN−; 22 ELND+; 235 ELND−	169 Months ELND	5-year survival ELND+ 45%; SLN+ 38% recurrence; ELND+ 57% recurrence; SLN− 11.5% recurrence; ELND − 14.9% recurrence	N/A because matched study for age, site, and tumor thickness not analyzed. The retrospective study was conducted to compare the efficiency of lymphatic mapping/sentinel lymphadenectomy and elective lymph node dissection.
Clary [16]	2000	31 SLN+; 121 SLN−; 44 ELND+; 285 ELND−	26 Months SLN; 79 Months ELND	3-year disease-free survival SLN 80%; 3-year disease-free survial ELND 71%	SLN: tumor thickness and age; ELND: tumor thickness, ulceration, and Clark level
Cherpelis [13]	2000	51 SLN+; 150 SLN− (all > 3.0 mm)	51 Months	3-year disease-free survival SLN+ 37%; 3-year disease-free survival SLN− 73%; 3-year survival SLN+ 70%; 3-year survival SLN− 82%	Ulceration; Age, tumor thickness, Clark level, and ulceration
Status Muller [15]	2001	52 SLN+; 211 SLN−	48 Months	3-year disease-free survival SLN+ 79%; 3-year disease-free survival SLN+ 95%; 5-year survival SLN+ 49%; 5-year survival SLN− 91%	SLN status, tumor thickness, ulceration, lymphatic invasion, and age
Wagner [28]	2003	85 SLN+	31 Months	31-Month disease-free survival SLN + 36.5%; 31-Month disease-free survival SLN, 12.1%	Tumor thickness, ulceration, SLN status, and number of positive lymph nodes
Leong [29]	2004	323 SLN−; 65 SLN+; 297 SLN−	58 Months	5-year disease-free survival SLN+ 38.1%; 5-year disease-free survival SLN−68.6%; 5-year survival SLN+ 59.9%; 5-year survival SLN− 68.6%	SLN status, tumor thickness, age, and gender; SLN status, tumor thickness, ulceration, lymphatic invasion, and mitotic index

ELND: elective lymph node dissection.

(Courtesy of Leong SPL, Kashani-Saber M, Desmond RA, et al: Clinical significance of occult metastatic melanoma in sentinel lymph nodes and other high-risk factors based on long-term follow-up. *World J Surg* 29:683-681, 2005. Copyright Springer-Verlag.)

factor for melanoma recurrence and death. Other important predictors include tumor thickness, ulceration, lymphatic invasion, and mitotic index (Table 4).

▶ Although the status of the SLN is the most important determinant of recurrence and survival in patients with melanoma, this article demonstrates that other variables are also important, including tumor thickness, ulceration, lymphatic invasion, mitotic index, and age.

P. G. Lang, Jr, MD

Predictors of Nonsentinel Lymph Node Positivity in Patients With a Positive Sentinel Node for Melanoma
Sabel MS, Griffith K, Sondak VK, et al (Univ of Michigan, Ann Arbor)
J Am Coll Surg 201:37-47, 2005   17–39

Background.—Patients found to harbor melanoma micrometastases in the sentinel lymph node (SLN) are recommended to proceed to complete lymph node dissection (CLND), although the majority of patients will have no additional disease identified in the nonsentinel lymph nodes (NSLNs). We sought to assess predictive factors associated with finding positive NSLNs, and identify a subset of patients with low likelihood of finding additional disease on CLND.

Study Design.—We queried our prospective melanoma database for patients from January 1996 to August 2003 with a positive SLN. Univariable logistic regression models were fit for multiple factors and a positive NSLN. To derive a probabilistic model for occurrence of one or more positive NSLN(s), a multivariable logistic model was fit using a stepwise variable selection method.

Results.—Of 980 patients who underwent SLN biopsy for cutaneous melanoma, 232 (24%) had a positive SLN; 221 (23%) followed by CLND. Of these patients, 34 (15%) had one or more positive NSLN(s). In multivariable analysis, male gender (odds ratio [OR] 3.6 [95% CI 1.33, 9.71]; p = 0.01), Breslow thickness (OR 4.58 [95% CI 1.28, 16.36]; p = 0.019), extranodal extension (OR 3.2 [95% CI 1.0, 10.5]; p = 0.05), and three or more positive sentinel nodes (OR 65.81 [95% CI 5.2, 825.7]; p = 0.001) were all associated with the likelihood of finding additional positive nodes on CLND. Of 47 patients with minimal tumor burden in the SLN, only 1 (2%) had additional disease in the NSLN.

Conclusions.—These results provide additional data to plan clinical trials to answer the question of who can safely avoid CLND after a positive SLN. Patients with minimal tumor burden in the SLN might be the most likely group, although defining "minimal tumor burden" must be standardized. Serial sectioning and immunohistochemistry on the NSLN in any "low-risk" group must be performed in a clinical trial to confirm that residual disease is unlikely before avoiding CLND can be recommended.

Sentinel Lymph Node Tumor Load: An Independent Predictor of Additional Lymph Node Involvement and Survival in Melanoma

Vuylsteke RJCLM, Borgstein PJ, van Leeuwen PAM, et al (VU Univ, Amsterdam)

Ann Surg Oncol 12:440-448, 2005

17–40

Background.—Even though 60% to 80% of melanoma patients with a positive sentinel lymph node (SLN) have no positive additional lymph nodes (ALNs), all these patients are subjected to an ALN dissection (ALND) with its associated morbidity. The aim of this study was to predict the absence of ALN metastases in patients with a positive SLN by using features of the primary melanoma and SLN tumor load.

Methods.—Of 71 SLN-positive patients, 52 had metastasis limited to the SLN (group 1), and 19 had ≥ 1 positive ALN after ALND (group 2). The tumor load of the SLN was assessed by measuring the total surface area by computerized morphometry. Breslow thickness, ulceration and lymphatic invasion of the primary tumor, and total SLN metastatic area were tested as covariates predicting the absence of positive ALNs.

Results.—The mean SLN metastatic area was 1.18 mm^2 (group 1) and 3.39 mm^2 (group 2) ($P = .003$) and was the only significant and independent factor after multivariate analysis ($P = .02$). None of the patients with both a Breslow thickness <2.5 mm and an SLN metastatic area <.3 mm^2 had a positive ALN.

Conclusions.—SLN metastatic area can be used to predict the absence of positive ALNs in melanoma patients. In this study, patients with a Breslow thickness <2.5 mm and an SLN tumor load <.3 mm^2 seemed to have no positive ALN and had excellent survival. We hypothesize that this subgroup might not benefit from ALND. Prospective larger trials, using this model and randomizing between ALND and no ALND, should confirm this hypothesis.

▶ Most patients who undergo a CLND after having positive findings on an SLN biopsy (SLNB) will not have involvement of NSLNs and, thus, have been subjected to an unnecessary procedure. Therefore, it would be ideal if one could better predict what patients with positive results on SLNB require a CLND. Several studies have found that the amount of tumor in the SLN correlates with NSLN positivity. In these 2 studies (Abstracts 17–39 and 17–40), it was found that a combination of tumor thickness and the amount of tumor in the SLN was a good predictor of NSLN involvement. Hopefully, these studies will serve as a catalyst for controlled studies that address the question of what subset of patients with positive results on an SLNB require a CLND.

P. G. Lang, Jr, MD

One-Stage Versus Two-Stage Lymph Node Dissection After Investigation of Sentinel Lymph Node in Cutaneous Melanoma: A Comparison of Complications, Costs, Hospitalization Times, and Operation Times

von Känel OEC, Haug M, Pierer G (Kantonsspital Basel, Switzerland)
Eur J Plast Surg 27:347-350, 2005   17–41

Background.—Lymph node metastases that are not causing problems clinically can be detected by sentinel lymph node (SLN) removal and investigation. Performing a frozen section analysis in the same procedure as the removal and dissection of the SLN is not yet an accepted practice. Whether doing this would change the duration of hospital stay, cost, time for the operation, and incidence of complications was assessed.

Methods.—Two patient groups underwent SLN removal and investigation. Group 1 (13 patients) had frozen section analysis of the SLN and dissection of the indicated lymph node basin in a 1-step procedure. Group 2 (13 patients) had the dissection performed in a second operation, for a 2-step procedure. The charts of all patients who had metastatic involvement of the SLN were reviewed retrospectively. The 2 groups were compared on the basis of duration of hospital stay, cost, time for the procedure, and development of complications postoperatively. The waiting time for frozen section analysis was not considered in the 2-step procedure.

Results.—Hospitalization lasted a mean of 14.2 days for patients in group 1 and 23.9 days for those in group 2. Group 2 patients had more complications than group 1 (5 vs 2), but the difference was not significant. No significant difference in operation duration was noted for the 2 groups. The cost per patient was significantly lower for patients in group 1 compared with group 2. The added frozen section analysis and longer period of hospitalization were the principal cost factors that contributed to the difference. The frozen section analysis identified metastatic involvement of the SLN in 13 patients who had dissection of the lymph node basin during the same procedure. In 9 patients, metastases were not detected on frozen section but found after immunohistochemical analysis. Thus, frozen section analysis had a sensitivity of 59%, a specificity of 99%, a positive predictive value of 92.8%, and a negative predictive value of 93.1%.

Conclusions.—Performing frozen section analysis of the SLN and dissection of the lymph node basin in the same procedure produced a shorter hospital stay, lower cost, and a lower rate of complications than performing these in a 2-step approach. The operation time did not differ significantly between the 2 approaches. Frozen section investigation had a sensitivity of 59% in this analysis.

▶ In general, frozen section analysis of SLNs from patients with cutaneous melanoma has not been advocated because of (1) a lack of sensitivity, and (2) the risk of eliminating a microscopic focus of tumor that would have otherwise been detected with permanent sectioning. In this small series of patients, the authors found that the use of frozen sections in conjunction with an immediate node dissection was more cost-effective and decreased the number of days of hospitalization. Although quite specific for the diagnosis of melanoma, the sensitivity of frozen sections was only 59%. While many SLNs judged negative by frozen section technique subsequently will be shown to be positive by permanent sectioning, the concern still remains that frozen sectioning may remove a small focus of melanoma. Unfortunately, we have no data to determine how often this might occur.

P. G. Lang, Jr, MD

Survival in Sentinel Lymph Node–Positive Pediatric Melanoma

Roaten JB, Partrick DA, Bensard D, et al (Univ of Colorado, Denver; Children's Hosp of Denver)
J Pediatr Surg 40:988-992, 2005   17–42

Background.—Sentinel lymph node (SLN) status is the strongest predictor of survival in adult melanoma. However, the prognostic value of SLN status in children and adolescents with melanoma is unknown.

Methods.—Records of 327 patients aged 12 to 86 years undergoing SLN biopsy for melanoma or other melanocytic lesions were reviewed (Table 1). A literature search identified additional patients younger than 21 years undergoing SLN biopsy for the same indications and these patients were combined with our series for meta-analysis (Table 3).

Results.—Sentinel lymph node metastases were found in 8 (40%) of 20 patients aged 12 to 20 years compared with 55 (18%) of 307 adults ($P < .05$). Median follow-up was 35 and 17 months for the groups, respectively. Sentinel lymph node-positive pediatric patients did not recur, whereas 14 (25%) adults recurred within this period. Of the 55 adults, 5 (9.1%) have died of disease. Of the combined SLN-positive children and adolescents from the literature (total n = 25), only a single (4%) child recurred at 6 months. The difference in survival for adult and pediatric patients was significant.

TABLE 1.—Characteristics of Children and Adolescents
Undergoing SLNBX at the University of Colorado

Age (y)	17 ± 3
Male	35 (7)
Preoperative histology	
Melanoma	75 (15/20)
Atypical nevi	25 (5/20)
Beslow depth (mm)	3.2 ± 1.0
Positive sentinel nodes	
Total	40 (8/20)
Melanoma	33 (5/15)
Atypical nevi	60 (3/5)
CLND	35 (7/8)

Data are presented as mean ± SEM or as percentage (n).
(Courtesy of Roaten JB, Partrick DA, Bensard D, et al: Survival in sentinel lymph node–positive pediatric melanoma. *J Pediatr Surg* 40:988-992, 2005.)

TABLE 3.—Comparison of Patients, Tumor Characteristics, and Regional Nodal Status of Adults With Positive SLNBX and Pooled Children and Adolescents With Positive SLNBX

	Ages 12-20 (n = 25)	Age >20 (n = 55)	P
Age (y)	12 ± 1.0	46 ± 1.9	.0001
Male sex	52 (13)	64 (35)	.32
Breslow depth (mm)	4.9 ± 0.9	2.7 ± 0.24	.001
Tumor depth (mm)			
T1 (<1.00)	0 (0)	7 (4)	.17
T2 (1-2)	16 (4)	42 (23)	.002
T3 (2.01-4)	52 (13)	31 (17)	.07
T4 (>4.01)	32 (8)	20 (11)	.2
Nodal stage			
N1 (1 node)	68 (17)	80 (44)	.24
N2 (2-3 nodes)	16 (4)	13 (7)	.69
N3 (≥4 nodes)	16 (4)	7 (4)	.23
Any recurrence	4 (1)	25 (14)	.02
Died of disease	4 (1)	9 (5)	.42
Median follow-up (mo)	24	17	NA

Data are presented as mean ± SEM as percentage (n) or otherwise indicated.
(Courtesy of Roaten JB, Partrick DA, Bensard D, et al: Survival in sentinel lymph node–positive pediatric melanoma. *J Pediatr Surg* 40:988-992, 2005.)

Conclusion.—Pediatric patients have a higher incidence of SLN metastases than adults yet have a lower incidence of recurrence. Sentinel lymph node status does not predict early recurrence in pediatric patients with melanoma or atypical Spitz nevi.

▶ Because the incidence of melanoma in the pediatric population is low, it has not been possible to carry out large, well-controlled studies on the management of melanoma in this age group. Thus, the same guidelines used to manage melanoma in adults are usually used to treat melanoma in pediatric patients. Moreover, a number of children subjected to SLN biopsy do not have histologically confirmed melanomas but instead have atypical Spitz nevi that cannot be distinguished from spitzoid melanoma. When compared with adults, the authors found that pediatric patients had a higher incidence of positive SLN biopsy results (40% vs 18%). However, on average, they also had thicker lesions. Although the number of lesions was small, those with atypical melanocytic lesions had the highest incidence of SLN biopsy positivity (60%). Interestingly, despite the high incidence of SLN biopsy positivity, pediatric patients were less apt to develop recurrences or die from their disease.

P. G. Lang, Jr, MD

Predictors and Natural History of In-Transit Melanoma After Sentinel Lymphadenectomy

Pawlik TM, Ross MI, Johnson MM, et al (Univ of Texas, Houston)
Ann Surg Oncol 12:587-596, 2005   17–43

Background.—In-transit recurrence is a unique and uncommon pattern of treatment failure in patients with melanoma. Little information exists concerning the incidence, predictors, and natural history of in-transit disease since the introduction of sentinel lymph node biopsy (SLNB).

Methods.—Between 1991 and 2001, 1395 patients with primary melanoma underwent SLNB. Univariate and multivariate logistic regression analyses were performed to examine the association among known clinicopathologic factors, in-transit recurrence, and distant metastatic failure after the development of in-transit disease.

Results.—With a median follow-up of 3.9 years, 241 patients (17.3%) experienced disease recurrence, including 91 (6.6%) who developed in-transit recurrence. Independent predictors of in-transit recurrence included age >50 years, a lower extremity location of the primary tumor, Breslow depth, ulceration, and sentinel lymph node (SLN) status. Of the 69 patients who presented with in-transit disease as the sole site of first recurrence, 39 developed distant disease. By univariate analysis, predictors of distant failure among patients with in-transit disease included SLN status, largest metastatic focus in the SLN >2.5 mm^2, subcutaneous location of in-transit disease, in-transit tumor size ≥2 cm, and a disease-free interval before in-transit recurrence of <12 months. In-transit tumor size remained a significant predictor of distant metastasis by multivariate analysis (odds ratio, 9.69).

Conclusions.—The overall incidence of in-transit metastases in patients undergoing SLNB is low and does not seem to have increased since the introduction of the SLNB technique. In-transit recurrence, as well as subsequent distant metastatic failure, can be predicted on the basis of adverse tumor factors and SLN status.

A Sentinel Node Biopsy Does Not Increase the Incidence of In-Transit Metastasis in Patients With Primary Cutaneous Melanoma

van Poll D, Thompson JF, Colman MH, et al (Royal Prince Albert Hosp, Camperdown, New South Wales, Australia; Univ of Sydney, New South Wales, Australia)
Ann Surg Oncol 12:597-608, 2005   17–44

Background.—It has been suggested that performing a sentinel node biopsy (SNB) in patients with cutaneous melanoma increases the incidence of in-transit metastasis (ITM).

Methods.—ITM rates for 2018 patients with primary melanomas ≥1.0 mm thick treated at a single institution between 1991 and 2000 according to 3 protocols were compared: wide local excision (WLE) only (n = 1035),

WLE plus SNB (n = 754), and WLE plus elective lymph node dissection (n = 229).

Results.—The incidence of ITM for the three protocols was 4.9%, 3.6%, and 5 7%, respectively (not significant), and as a first site of recurrent disease the incidence was 2.5%, 2.4%, and 4.4%, respectively (not significant). The subset of patients who were node positive after SNB and after elective lymph node dissection also had similar ITM rates (10.8% and 7.1%, respectively; $P = .11$). On multivariate analysis, primary tumor thickness and patient age predicted ITM as a first recurrence, but type of treatment did not. Patients who underwent WLE only and who had a subsequent therapeutic lymph node dissection (n = 149) had an ITM rate of 24.2%, compared with 10.8% in patients with a tumor-positive sentinel node treated with immediate dissection (n = 102; $P = .03$).

Conclusions.—Performing an SNB in patients with melanoma treated by WLE does not increase the incidence of ITM.

Sentinel Lymphonodectomy Does Not Increase the Risk of Loco-regional Cutaneous Metastases of Malignant Melanomas
Kretschmer L, Beckmann I, Thoms KM, et al (Georg August Univ of Göttingen, Germany)
Eur J Cancer 41:531-538, 2005   17–45

Introduction.—With regard to malignant melanoma, the impact of lymph node surgery on the development of loco-regional cutaneous metastases (LCM) has not yet been adequately addressed. However, this aspect is of interest, since sentinel lymphonodectomy (SLNE) has been suspected of causing LCM by inducing entrapment of melanoma cells. We analysed 244 patients with SLNE and compared the data with 199 patients treated with delayed lymph node dissection (DLND) for clinically palpable metastases. Analysis of both groups commenced at the time of excision of the primary tumour, using the Kaplan-Meier method. LCM that appeared as a first recurrence, as well as the overall probability of developing LCM, were recorded. For sentinel-negative patients with a primary melanoma >1 mm thick, the 5-year probability of developing LCM as a first recurrence was 6.9 ± 0.02% (±standard error of the mean (SEM)). The probability was 17.6 ± 0.03% in the DLND group. Comparing the two node-positive subgroups, the probability of developing LCM as a first recurrence was significantly higher in patients with positive SLNE (27.3 ± 0.05%, $P = 0.03$). However, the 5-year overall probability of developing LCM did not differ significantly in the node-positive groups (33.3% in the DLND group vs. 33.7% in patients with positive sentinel lymph nodes (SLNs)). Since early excision of lymphatic metastases by SLNE avoids nodal recurrences, thereby prolonging the recurrence-free interval, the chance of LCM to manifest as a first recurrence should inevitably increase. However, the overall in-transit probability is not increased after SLNE.

▶ It has previously been suggested that SLNB might result in the entrapment of melanoma cells in afferent lymphatics, thereby increasing the incidence of ITM. Although approaching this hypothesis in slightly different ways, the investigators from each of these studies (Abstracts 17–43 to 17–45) reached the same conclusion: neither the SLNB nor the subsequent complete node dissection that was done in patients with positive findings on SLNB resulted in an increased incidence of ITM. Predictors of ITM included Breslow thickness, lesion ulceration, positive SLNB results, and the location of the lesion on the lower extremity. Of note is that patients who underwent a complete lymph node dissection after positive findings on SLNB had a longer disease-free interval than did patients undergoing a delayed therapeutic lymph node dissection.

P. G. Lang, Jr, MD

The Role of Microsatellites as a Prognostic Factor in Primary Malignant Melanoma

Shaikh L, Sagebiel RW, Ferreira CMM, et al (Univ of California, San Francisco)
Arch Dermatol 141:739-742, 2005   17–46

Objective.—To determine the impact of microsatellites as a prognostic factor in primary cutaneous melanoma.

Design.—Retrospective cohort study.

Setting.—Tertiary referral center.

Patients.—A total of 504 patients with a history of primary melanoma observed for 2 years or having experienced a first relapse.

Main Outcome Measures.—Overall survival (OS) and relapse-free survival (RFS).

Results.—Forty-five patients had evidence of microsatellites in their primary melanoma. Presence of microsatellites significantly correlated with the presence of several other histologic high-risk factors such as tumor thickness, ulceration, Clark level, vascular factors, and mitotic rate. Univariate analysis demonstrated decreased RFS and OS in patients with microsatellites. Presence of microsatellites was associated with increased locoregional metastasis but not distant metastasis. In multivariate analysis, with the inclusion of 6 other clinical and histologic factors, presence of microsatellites was a significant predictor of RFS but not OS. Patients with clinical macrosatellites had a trend toward worsening OS compared with those with microsatellites.

Conclusions.—The presence of microsatellites is intimately tied to other markers of melanoma aggressiveness. Microsatellites appear to predict locoregional relapse and RFS but neither distant metastasis nor OS. These results may have implications for patient care as well as the inclusion of microsatellites in stage III of the current classification.

▶ Microscopic satellites are felt to represent local metastatic spread of tumor. Thus, it is not surprising that these authors found that the presence of microsatellites was associated with regional relapse, that is, macroscopic satellites and nodal metastases. It was a little surprising that the presence of microscopic satellites was not associated with distant metastases; however, this may relate to the fact that patients with only intravascular tumor deposits were not included in the analysis. It was also notable that, in contrast to macroscopic satellites, when other risk factors (tumor thickness, ulceration, mitotic rate, tumor vascularity, the presence of intravascular tumor, and Clark level) were controlled for, the presence of microscopic satellites was independently associated with a decrease in RFS but not OS. At first glance, these observations would appear to have significant therapeutic and prognostic implications. However, since the presence of microscopic satellites correlated with the presence of other significant variables, such as tumor thickness, ulceration, Clark level and vascular invasion, this could simply mean that these patients have such a bad starting prognosis that the presence of microscopic satellites adds little to affect these patients' overall survival.

P. G. Lang, Jr, MD

Is Increased Serum S-100 Protein Concentration a Marker of Metastasis in Malignant Melanoma? A Four-Year Experience Report
Governa M, Dorizzi RM, Gatti S, et al (Verona Hosp, Italy)
Eur J Plast Surg 28:17-20, 2005   17–47

Background.—The incidence of malignant melanoma has significantly increased among the white population in recent years. This neoplasm can metastasize anywhere and is generally incurable once it is disseminated. Follow-up after surgery is disappointing, and about 20% of affected patients die because of tumor metastasis. The development of reliable serum markers to improve early diagnosis and allow monitoring of disease progression is a major goal of clinical and laboratory management of these patients. S-100 is an acidic calcium-binding protein with a molecular weight of 21 kd. Until recently, its specific biological function was unknown; however, it has been shown to increase in CSF and serum after different brain injuries, and its measurement has been proposed in brain-damage assessment. An immediate assay of S-100 serum concentration was performed in patients with melanomas so that patients at high risk of a recurrence could be identified and the prognostic value of rising S-100 levels could be assessed.

Methods.—Over 4 years, the S-100 serum protein concentration was measured in 880 samples obtained from 178 consecutive patients with histologically confirmed malignant melanomas. The S-100 concentration was measured with an assay based on 3 monoclonal antibodies against bovine S-100 protein B-subunit, and an automated chemiluminescence analyzer, a method much faster than available technology, was used. S-100 concentrations were determined in less than 1 hour, which is a time that allows the surgeon to utilize data on S-100 levels in determining the course of patient management and follow-up scheduling.

Results.—Local or distant metastasis was present in 17 of 178 patients (9.5%). In 14 of those 17 patients (82.4%), S-100 levels were higher than 250 ng/L (decision level) when disease progression was detected. In addition, follow-up in 5 patients indicated that a renewed rise in S-100 concentration was reflective of a new tumor recurrence.

Conclusions.—Increases in concentration levels of S-100 are associated with disease progression in patients with malignant melanomas, and these increased levels are often the first symptoms of a recurrence. Assay of S-100 protein concentration before clinical evaluation can greatly improve the management of these patients.

▶ Governa et al found serum S-100 protein concentrations to be a reliable marker of metastasis in patients with malignant melanomas. The previously reported observation that S-100 is not found in melanoma cells until they enter the vertical growth phase suggests a possible role for this protein as a biological marker of tumor aggressiveness. As suggested by the authors, for changes in levels of markers to be useful, they must precede rather than follow conventional methods of detecting disease; this, in turn, would allow for earlier initiation of therapy.[1]

B. H. Thiers, MD

Reference

1. Jury CS, McAllister EJ, Mackie RM: Rising levels of serum S-100 protein precede other evidence of disease progression in patients with malignant melanoma. *Br J Dermatol* 143:269, 2000.

High Serum Levels of Matrix Metalloproteinase-9 and Matrix Metalloproteinase-1 Are Associated With Rapid Progression in Patients With Metastatic Melanoma

Nikkola J, Vihinen P, Vuoristo M-S, et al (Turku Univ, Finland)
Clin Cancer Res 11:5158-5166, 2005   17–48

Purpose.—Matrix metalloproteinases (MMP) are proteolytic enzymes that play an important role in various aspects of cancer progression. In the present work, we have studied the prognostic significance of serum levels of gelatinase B (MMP-9), collagenase-1 (MMP-1), and collagenase-3 (MMP-13) in patients with advanced melanoma.

Experimental Design.—Total pretreatment serum levels of MMP-9 in 71 patients and MMP-1 and MMP-13 in 48 patients were determined by an assay system based on ELISA. Total MMP levels were also assessed in eight healthy controls. The active and latent forms of MMPs were defined by using Western blot analysis and gelatin zymography.

Results.—Patients with high serum levels of MMP-9 ($\geq$376.6 ng/mL; $n = 19$) had significantly poorer overall survival (OS) than patients with lower serum MMP-9 levels ($n = 52$; median OS, 29.1 versus 45.2 months; $P = 0.033$). High MMP-9 levels were also associated with visceral or bone metastasis ($P = 0.027$), elevated serum alkaline phosphatase level ($P = 0.0009$), and presence of liver metastases ($P = 0.032$). Serum levels of MMP-1 and MMP-13 did not correlate with OS. MMP-1 and MMP-9 were found mainly in latent forms in serum, whereas the majority of MMP-13 in serum was active (48 kDa) form. MMP-13 was found more often in active form in patients (mean, 99% of the total MMP-13 level) than in controls (mean, 84% of the total MMP-13 level; $P < 0.0001$). After initiating the therapy, patients with elevated levels of MMP-1 (≥ 29.8 ng/mL, $n = 10$) progressed more rapidly than patients with lower levels (median, 1.9 versus 3.5 months; $P – 0.023$). Serum levels of MMP-9 and MMP-13 did not correlate with the time to progression (TTP). In multivariate analysis with age and gender, MMP-9 or MMP-1 turned out to be independent prognostic factors for OS [$P = 0.039$; hazard ratio (HR), 1.8; 95% confidence interval (95% CI), 1.03-3.3] or TTP ($P = 0.023$; HR, 2.7; 95% CI, 1.15-6.4), respectively.

Conclusions.—Our findings provide evidence that MMP-1, MMP-9, and MMP-13 play important roles at different phases of metastatic melanoma spread and that serum MMP-9, in particular, could have clinical value in identifying patients at high risk for melanoma progression.

▶ The human MMP family has 23 members that are divided into 8 structural classes. The MMPs can also be classified on the basis of substrate specificity and primary structure into subgroups, including collagenases, gelatinases, and stromelysins. The collagenases, which include MMP-1, MMP-8 and MMP-13, are the principal extracellular proteinases, capable of degrading native collagens, and, hence, have been implicated in tumor spread. Nikkola et al provide evidence that these MMPs have important roles at different phases of the metastatic process and that measurement of serum MMP-9, especially, could be of clinical value in identifying patients at high risk of tumor progression.

B. H. Thiers, MD

Elevated Neutrophil and Monocyte Counts in Peripheral Blood Are Associated With Poor Survival in Patients With Metastatic Melanoma: A Prognostic Model

Schmidt H, Bastholt L, Geertsen P, et al (Aarhus Univ, Denmark; Odense Univ, Denmark; Univ of Copenhagen)
Br J Cancer 93:273-278, 2005   17–49

Introduction.—We aimed to create a prognostic model in metastatic melanoma based on independent prognostic factors in 321 patients receiving interleukin-2 (IL-2)-based immunotherapy with a median follow-up time for patients currently alive of 52 months (range 15-189 months). The patients were treated as part of several phase II protocols and the majority received treatment with intermediate dose subcutaneous IL-2 and interferon-α. Neutrophil and monocyte counts, lactate dehydrogenase (LDH), number of metastatic sites, location of metastases and performance status were all statistically significant prognostic factors in univariate analyses. Subsequently, a multivariate Cox's regression analysis identified elevated LDH (P<0.001, hazard ratio 2.8), elevated neutrophil counts (P=0.02, hazard ratio 1.4) and a performance status of 2 (P=0.008, hazard ratio 1.6) as independent prognostic factors for poor survival. An elevated monocyte count could replace an elevated neutrophil count. Patients were assigned to one of three risk groups according to the cumulative risk defined as the sum of simplified risk scores of the three independent prognostic factors. Low-, intermediate- and high-risk patients achieved a median survival of 12.6 months (95% confidence interval (CI), 11.4-13.8), 6.0 months (95% CI, 4.8-7.2) and 3.4 months (95% CI, 1.2-5.6), respectively. The low-risk group encompassed the majority of long-term survivors, whereas the patients in the high-risk group with a very poor prognosis should probably not be offered IL-2-based immunotherapy.

▶ Tumor infiltrating inflammatory cells have been shown to play a pivotal role in tumor progression and dissemination in a wide variety of cancers; indeed, baseline elevated neutrophil and monocyte counts in peripheral blood have been proposed as prognostic factors for a shorter survival duration in patients with metastatic renal cell carcinoma undergoing immunotherapy with IL-2 or α-interferon-2b. Schmidt et al report similar data in patients with metastatic melanomas. They propose a prognostic model, including neutrophil counts, LDH, and performance status, that identifies a low-risk group encompassing the majority of long-term survivors and a high-risk group with a very poor prognosis. They suggest that patients in the latter group should not be offered IL-2–based immunotherapy.

B. H. Thiers, MD

Post-surgery Adjuvant Therapy With Intermediate Doses of Interferon Alfa 2b Versus Observation in Patients With Stage IIb/III Melanoma (EORTC 18952): Randomised Controlled Trial
Eggermont AMM, for the EORTC Melanoma Group (Erasmus Univ, Rotterdam, The Netherlands; et al)
Lancet 366:1189-1196, 2005   17–50

Background.—Individuals affected by melanoma with thick primary tumours or regional node involvement have a poor outlook, with only 30–50% alive at 5 years. High-dose and low-dose interferon alfa have been assessed for the treatment of these patients, with the former having considerable toxicity and a consistent effect on disease free survival, but not on overall survival, and the latter no consistent effect on either. Our aim was, therefore, to assess the effect of two regimens of interferon of intermediate dose versus observation alone on distant metastasis-free interval (DMFI) and overall survival in such patients.

Methods.—We did a randomised controlled trial in 1388 patients who had had a thick primary tumour (thickness ≥4 mm) resected (stage IIb) or regional lymph node metastases dissected (stage III) and had been assigned to 13-months (n=553) or 25 months (n=556) of treatment with subcutaneous interferon alfa 2b, or observation (n=279). Treatment comprised 4 weeks of 10 million units (MU) of interferon alfa (5 days per week) followed by either 10 MU three times a week for 1 year or 5 MU three times a week for 2 years, to a total dose of 1760 MU. Our primary endpoint was DMFI. Analyses were by intent to treat.

Findings.—After a median follow-up of 4.65 years, we had recorded 760 distant metastases and 681 deaths. At 4.5 years, the 25-month interferon group showed a 7.2% increase in rate of DMFI (hazard ratio 0.83, 97.5% CI 0.66–1.03) and a 5.4% improvement in overall survival. The 13-month interferon group showed a 3.2% increase in rate of DMFI at 4.5 years (0.93, 0.75–1.16) and no extension of overall survival. Toxicity was acceptable, with 18% (195 of 1076) of patients going off study because of toxicity or as a result of refusal of treatment because of side-effects.

Interpretation.—Interferon alfa as used in the regimens studied does not improve outcome for patients with stage IIb/III melanomas, and cannot be recommended. With respect to efficacy of the drug, duration of treatment seemed more important than dose, and should be assessed in future trials.

▶ Since the initial study that suggested that high-dose interferon alfa 2b given to high-risk melanoma patients improved disease-free survival and overall survival, there have been no studies on high- or low-dose interferon that have confirmed these findings. In this study, the authors assessed the benefits of intermediate doses of interferon in patients with stages IIb and III disease by using both a 13-month and 25-month regimen. Although better tolerated than high-dose interferon, no significant benefit was observed.

P. G. Lang, Jr, MD

Thalidomide Enhances the Anti-Tumor Activity of Standard Chemotherapy in a Human Melanoma Xenotransplantation Model
Heere-Ress E, Boehm J, Thallinger C, et al (Med Univ of Vienna, Austria; Univ of British Columbia, Vancouver, Canada)
J Invest Dermatol 125:201-206, 2005   17–51

Introduction.—It has been demonstrated that thalidomide's anti-angiogenic properties result in clear anti-tumor activity in a number of human malignancies. We studied thalidomide in a human melanoma severe combined immunodeficiency mouse xenotransplantation model. Thalidomide as a single agent showed a significant tumor reduction of 46% compared with the control group. Thalidomide combined with dacarbazine treatment markedly enhanced the anti-tumor effect of chemotherapy and showed a significant tumor reduction relative to the dacarbazine-only group (61%) and even more tumor reduction (74%) compared with the control group. We also measured clearly reduced levels of tumor necrosis factor-α in the thalidomide-treated group. A significantly lower microvessel density was encountered in the thalidomide treatment groups (thalidomide alone or combined with DTIC), underscoring the anti-angiogenic effect of thalidomide as a single agent as well as in combination with chemotherapy in this model. In line with these results, we observed a nearly 3-fold increase of apoptosis for the combination of thalidomide and DTIC compared with the rate of apoptotic cells in DTIC-only-treated melanoma xenotransplants. These data underline the rationale for combining dacarbazine—a cytotoxic agent—and thalidomide—an anti-angiogenic cytostatic agent—as a promising strategy for the treatment of melanoma.

▶ The logic of combining a cytotoxic agent (dacarbazine) with thalidomide (an antiangiogenic agent) is appealing, although the relevance of the mouse model used to human disease remains problematic.

B. H. Thiers, MD

Wide Excision Without Radiation for Desmoplastic Melanoma
Arora A, Lowe L, Su L, et al (Univ of Michigan, Ann Arbor)
Cancer 104:1462-1467, 2005   17–52

Background.—Adjuvant radiation has been proposed for the treatment of patients with desmoplastic melanoma, who reportedly have local recurrence rates as high as 40–60%. The authors investigated local recurrence rates at a tertiary referral center to determine the success of wide excision alone for patients with desmoplastic melanoma.

Methods.—A review of a prospectively maintained melanoma clinical data base identified 65 patients between March 1997 and March 2004 with pure cutaneous desmoplastic melanoma. Complete surgical, histopathologic, and staging information was collected along with data on outcome, including local, regional, and distant recurrence and survival.

Results.—Similar to previous reports, patients with desmoplastic melanoma had a male-to-female ratio of 2 to 1, a mean age of 65.0 years (range, 31–92 yrs), and the majority of their tumors (55%) were located on the head and neck. The mean Breslow depth at diagnosis was 4.21 mm, with 38% of tumors thicker than 4.0 mm. All patients in this series underwent wide excision without radiation therapy. Surgical margins ≤2 cm were obtained for all trunk and extremity lesions and for 63% of head and neck lesions that measured >1 mm in depth (63%). Margins of 1–2 cm were obtained for the remaining patients. Among 49 patients who had a minimum of 2 years of follow-up (mean, 3.7 yrs), the local recurrence rate was 4% (2 of 49 patients) (Table 2). Seventy-eight percent of the patients studied remained alive with no evidence of disease.

Conclusions.—Local recurrence rates in the current series were considerably lower than the historically reported rates. This finding suggests that, for patients with desmoplastic melanoma, wide local excision with careful at-

TABLE 2.—Recurrence Rates After Definitive Management
of Desmoplastic Melanoma in 49 Patients With a Minimum
of 2 Years of Follow-up

Characteristic	No. of Patients (%)
Location	
Head and neck	26 (53)
Trunk	9 (18)
Upper extremity	10 (20)
Lower extremity	4 (8)
Male:female ratio	2.5:1.0
Age in yrs	
Median	64.3
Range	21-92
Local recurrence rate	2 (4)
Distant recurrences	3 (6)
Died without disease	6 (11)
Two-yr disease-free survival (%)	78

(Courtesy of Arora A, Lowe L, Su L, et al: Wide excision without radiation for desmoplastic melanoma. *Cancer* 104:462-467, 2005. Copyright 2005 American Cancer Society. Reprinted by permission of Wiley-Liss, Inc, a subsidiary of John Wiley & Sons, Inc.)

tention to appropriate margins produces excellent local control rates without the need for adjuvant radiation.

▶ Because of a high reported incidence of recurrence after surgical resection, some authors have suggested that patients with desmoplastic melanoma should routinely receive postoperative radiation therapy. In this study from the University of Michigan, the authors report a local recurrence rate of only 4% when margins of 1 to 2 cm are used to treat this unusual variant of melanoma. Thus, they do not recommend the routine use of radiation therapy but instead suggest that it should be reserved for patients with unresectable disease, those with positive margins that are unresectable, and those patients with locally recurrent disease after excision. Another controversial issue in the management of these patients is whether they should be subjected to sentinel lymph node biopsy since the incidence of positivity is low and recurrence often becomes manifest at a distant site. However, the authors agree with this observation, they still advocate sentinel lymph node biopsy for patients with desmoplastic melanoma. In this series, patients with neurotropism were more likely to have a positive biopsy, but this may have been because they had thicker tumors.

P. G. Lang, Jr, MD

5-Aminolaevulinic Acid Photodynamic Therapy in a Transgenic Mouse Model of Skin Melanoma

Córdoba F, Braathen LR, Weissenberger J, et al (Univ of Bern, Switzerland; Kanazawa Univ, Japan; Nagoya Univ, Japan; et al)
Exp Dermatol 14:429-437, 2005   17–53

Introduction.—Photodynamic therapy (PDT) is widely used to treat preneoplastic skin lesions and non-melanoma skin tumours. Studies analyzing the effects of PDT on malignant melanoma have yielded conflicting results. On the one hand, melanoma cell lines in culture as well as cell lines transplanted into experimental animals were sensitive to PDT. On the other hand, spontaneous melanomas of human patients responded poorly to most PDT regimens tested so far. Here, we analyzed effects of 5-aminolaevulinic acid (5-ALA)-based PDT on melanoma cell lines and on experimental melanomas. To mimic the clinical situation as closely as possible, metallothionein-I/ret (MT-ret) mice, a transgenic model of skin melanoma development, were used. Optimal doses of 5-ALA as well as energy doses and power densities were determined in vitro using a cell line (Mel25) established by us from a melanoma of an MT-ret transgenic mouse as well as commercially available human and mouse melanoma cell lines. Treatment with light irradiation alone had no effect. In combination with 5-ALA, however, this illumination readily induced the death of all mouse and human melanoma cell lines examined. Still, 5-ALA PDT caused only minor focal regressive changes including haemorrhages and fibrosis of MT-ret melanomas in vivo and did not significantly delay tumour growth. These results show that, even though MT-ret melanoma cells are vulnerable to 5-ALA PDT in vitro, malignant MT-ret melanomas in vivo are quite resistant to this type of therapy at doses which are highly effective in vitro.

▶ The results provide a cautionary tale against too quickly extrapolating data from in vitro studies to in vivo conditions.

B. H. Thiers, MD

Familial Cancer Associated With a Polymorphism in *ARLTS1*

Calin GA, Trapasso F, Shimizu M, et al (Thomas Jefferson Univ, Philadelphia; Fox Chase Cancer Ctr, Philadelphia; Univ of Ferrara, Italy; et al)
N Engl J Med 352:1667-1676, 2005   17–54

Background.—The finding of hemizygous or homozygous deletions at band 14 on chromosome 13 in a variety of neoplasms suggests the presence of a tumor-suppressor locus telomeric to the *RB1* gene.

Methods.—We studied samples from 216 patients with various types of sporadic tumors or idiopathic pancytopenia, peripheral-blood samples from 109 patients with familial cancer or multiple cancers, and control blood samples from 475 healthy people or patients with diseases other than cancer. We performed functional studies of cell lines lacking *ARLTS1* expression with the use of both the full-length *ARLTS1* gene and a truncated variant.

Results.—We found a gene at 13q14, *ARLTS1*, a member of the ADP-ribosylation factor family, with properties of a tumor-suppressor gene. We analyzed 800 DNA samples from tumors and blood cells from patients with sporadic or familial cancer and controls and found that the frequency of a nonsense polymorphism, G446A (Trp149Stop), was similar in controls and patients with sporadic tumors but was significantly more common among patients with familial cancer than among those in the other two groups (P=0.02; odds ratio, 5.7; 95 percent confidence interval, 1.3 to 24.8). *ARLTS1* was down-regulated by promoter methylation in 25 percent of the primary tumors we analyzed. Transfection of wild-type *ARLTS1* into A549 lung-cancer cells suppressed tumor formation in immunodeficient mice and induced apoptosis, whereas transfection of truncated *ARLTS1* had a limited effect on apoptosis and tumor suppression. Microarray analysis revealed that the wild-type and Trp149Stop-transfected clones had different expression profiles.

Conclusions.—A genetic variant of *ARLTS1* predisposes patients to familial cancer.

▶ Previous studies have strongly suggested the presence of a tumor suppressor gene on human chromosome 13 in a region within the genome (13q14) that is deleted in a number of neoplastic diseases, including chronic lymphocytic leukemia and prostate cancer. These investigators identified a highly conserved candidate gene in this region (*ARLTS1*) that codes for a member of the Ras superfamily. Examination of a large population of cancer patients and control subjects revealed the occurrence of a single base exchange polymorphism within *ARLTS1* that resulted in production of a truncated protein product. This polymorphism was detected in 2.1% of 475 controls, 3.7% of patients with sporadic tumors, and 5.5% of 109 patients with familial tumors, including melanoma. This increase of the variant in those with familial neoplasia was statistically significant (P = .02). Interestingly, in 1 informative family that included 5 members with a variety of malignancies, including chronic lymphocytic leukemia and lung cancer, the variant was found in all 5 affected individuals. Further studies showed that transfection of *ARLTS1* into a tumor cell line deficient in expression of the gene resulted in increased susceptibility of the cells to apoptosis and also significantly reduced their ability to induce tumors in nude mice. These data indicate that *ARLTS1* functions as a human tumor suppressor gene.

G. M. P. Galbraith, MD

Distinct Sets of Genetic Alterations in Melanoma

Curtin JA, Fridlyand J, Kageshita T, et al (Univ of California, San Francisco; Kumamoto Univ, Japan; Mem Sloan-Kettering Cancer Ctr, New York; et al)
N Engl J Med 353:2135-2147, 2005   17–55

Background.—Exposure to ultraviolet light is a major causative factor in melanoma, although the relationship between risk and exposure is complex. We hypothesized that the clinical heterogeneity is explained by genetically distinct types of melanoma with different susceptibility to ultraviolet light.

Methods.—We compared genome-wide alterations in the number of copies of DNA and mutational status of *BRAF* and *N-RAS* in 126 melanomas from four groups in which the degree of exposure to ultraviolet light differs: 30 melanomas from skin with chronic sun-induced damage and 40 melanomas from skin without such damage; 36 melanomas from palms, soles, and subungual (acral) sites; and 20 mucosal melanomas.

Results.—We found significant differences in the frequencies of regional changes in the number of copies of DNA and mutation frequencies in *BRAF* among the four groups of melanomas. Samples could be correctly classified into the four groups with 70 percent accuracy on the basis of the changes in the number of copies of genomic DNA. In two-way comparisons, melanomas arising on skin with signs of chronic sun-induced damage and skin without such signs could be correctly classified with 84 percent accuracy. Acral melanoma could be distinguished from mucosal melanoma with 89 percent accuracy. Eighty-one percent of melanomas on skin without chronic sun-induced damage had mutations in *BRAF* or *N-RAS*; the majority of melanomas in the other groups had mutations in neither gene. Melanomas with wild-type *BRAF* or *N-RAS* frequently had increases in the number of copies of the genes for cyclin-dependent kinase 4 (*CDK4*) and cyclin D1 (*CCND1*), downstream components of the RAS–BRAF pathway.

Conclusions.—The genetic alterations identified in melanomas at different sites and with different levels of sun exposure indicate that there are distinct genetic pathways in the development of melanoma and implicate *CDK4* and *CCND1* as independent oncogenes in melanomas without mutations in *BRAF* or *N-RAS*.

▶ This fascinating study suggests that the role of UV radiation in the development of melanomas may vary depending on one's genetic makeup and location of the tumor. In an accompanying editorial, Meltzer[1] comments on the consequences of these findings. Questions to be considered include (1) how much will we need to individualize cancer therapy and (2) should cancer treatment be tailored according to the specific pattern of mutations in each patient? He concludes that understanding the vulnerabilities revealed by profiling the DNA of a tumor will be critical to the development of more effective cancer therapies.

B. H. Thiers, MD

Reference

1. Meltzer PS: Genetic diversity in melanoma. *N Engl J Med* 353:2104-2107, 2005.

The Gene Expression Signatures of Melanoma Progression
Haqq C, Nosrati M, Sudilovsky D, et al (Univ of California at San Francisco)
Proc Natl Acad Sci U S A 102:6092-6097, 2005   17–56

Introduction.—Because of the paucity of available tissue, little information has previously been available regarding the gene expression profiles of primary melanomas. To understand the molecular basis of melanoma progression, we compared the gene expression profiles of a series of nevi, primary melanomas, and melanoma metastases. We found that metastatic melanomas exhibit two dichotomous patterns of gene expression, which unexpectedly reflect gene expression differences already apparent in comparing laser-capture microdissected radial and vertical phases of a large primary melanoma. Unsupervised hierarchical clustering accurately separated nevi and primary melanomas. Multiclass significance analysis of microarrays comparing normal skin, nevi, primary melanomas, and the two types of metastatic melanoma identified 2,602 transcripts that significantly correlated with sample class. These results suggest that melanoma pathogenesis can be understood as a series of distinct molecular events. The gene expression signatures identified here provide the basis for developing new diagnostics and targeting therapies for patients with malignant melanoma.

▶ The finding of the gene expression signature of some radial growth phase melanomas in metastatic lesions is disconcerting, and it suggests that some radial growth phase lesions do in fact have metastatic potential. Thus, the simple model of tumor progression from radial to vertical growth phase and, ultimately, to metastatic disease may not be totally valid.

B. H. Thiers, MD

▶ This impressive study was designed to examine the expression of 19,740 individual genes in primary melanoma in radial and vertical growth phases, metastatic melanoma, benign nevi, and normal skin. By using cutting-edge molecular biologic techniques, several expression signatures were clearly identified. For example, transition of melanoma to vertical growth was characterized by loss of expression of α2 and laminin γ2. In several adhesion factors such as integrin α2 addition, expression of cadherin-3 and matrix metalloproteinase-10 were markedly higher in the radial growth phase than in the vertical growth phase ($P < .0005$ and .001, respectively). Furthermore, the signatures differed between types I and II metastatic melanoma. Whereas type II expressed melanoma-associated proteins such as Melan-1, type I was characterized by predominant expression of extracellular matrix and cell adhesion molecules. Further investigation revealed that primary melanoma could be distinguished from benign nevus by differences in expression of more than 1000 genes. The data presented in this article represent an invaluable contribution to the elucidation of the genetic basis of melanoma and future clinical applications in terms of diagnosis, prognosis, and novel therapeutic approaches.

G. M. P. Galbraith, MD

Clinicopathologic Significance of Dysadherin Expression in Cutaneous Malignant Melanoma: Immunohistochemical Analysis of 115 Patients

Nishizawa A, Nakanishi Y, Yoshimura K, et al (Natl Cancer Ctr Research Inst, Tokyo; Hirosaki Univ, Japan)

Cancer 103:1693-1700, 2005   17–57

Background.—The E-cadherin–mediated cell adhesion system is frequently inactivated by multiple mechanisms and is involved in tumor progression in many types of cancer. Recently, the authors reported a novel cell membrane glycoprotein, dysadherin, which has an anti–cell-cell adhesion function and down-regulates E-cadherin.

Methods.—Expression of both dysadherin and E-cadherin was investigated immunohistochemically in 115 patients with cutaneous malignant melanoma to determine the correlation between the 2 molecules and their associations with both patient survival and the clinicopathologic features of the tumors.

Results.—Dysadherin and E-cadherin were expressed at the cell membranes of melanoma cells. Fifty-two percent of the tumors showed dysadherin immunopositivity, and 91% of the tumors showed reduced E-cadherin immunopositivity. There was no significant inverse correlation between dysadherin expression and E-cadherin expression. Increased dysadherin expression was significantly correlated with nodular subtype ($P = 0.042$), Clark level ($P < 0.001$), tumor thickness ($P < 0.001$), ulceration ($P = 0.008$), lymph node metastasis ($P < 0.001$), high TNM classification ($P < 0.001$), and poor patient survival ($P < 0.001$). Multivariate analysis of patient survival revealed that increased dysadherin expression was a significant predictor of poor survival ($P < 0.001$).

Conclusions.—Thus, increased expression of dysadherin was a significant indicator of poor prognosis in patients with cutaneous malignant melanoma.

▶ Nishizawa et al document overexpression of dysadherin in cutaneous melanoma, a phenomenon that appears to be a marker of poor prognosis and tumor aggressiveness. Dysadherin is a cancer-associated cell membrane glycoprotein that downregulates the expression and function of E-cadherin, a protein that promotes cell–cell adhesiveness. Inactivation of E-cadherin leads to dysfunction of the cell–cell adhesion system, promotes detachment of tumor cells from the primary lesion, and may play an important roll in tumor progression and metastasis.

B. H. Thiers, MD

Multiple Markers for Melanoma Progression Regulated by DNA Methylation: Insights From Transcriptomic Studies

Gallagher WM, Bergin OE, Rafferty M, et al (Univ College Dublin; Our Lady's Hosp for Sick Children, Dublin; Spanish Natl Cancer Centre (CNIO), Madrid; et al)
Carcinogenesis 26:1856-1867, 2005   17–58

Introduction.—The incidence of melanoma is increasing rapidly, with advanced lesions generally failing to respond to conventional chemotherapy. Here, we utilized DNA microarray-based gene expression profiling techniques to identify molecular determinants of melanoma progression within a unique panel of isogenic human melanoma cell lines. When a poorly tumorigenic cell line, derived from an early melanoma, was compared with two increasingly aggressive derivative cell lines, the expression of 66 genes was significantly changed. A similar pattern of differential gene expression was found with an independently derived metastatic cell line. We further examined these melanoma progression-associated genes via use of a tailored TaqMan Low Density Array (LDA), representing the majority of genes within our cohort of interest. Considerable concordance was seen between the transcriptomic profiles determined by DNA microarray and TaqMan LDA approaches. A range of novel markers were identified that correlated here with melanoma progression. Most notable was *TSPY*, a Y chromosome-specific gene that displayed extensive down-regulation in expression between the parental and derivative cell lines. Examination of a putative CpG island within the *TSPY* gene demonstrated that this region was hypermethylated in the derivative cell lines, as well as metastatic melanomas from male patients. Moreover, treatment of the derivative cell lines with the DNA methyltransferase inhibitor, 2'-deoxy-5-azacytidine (DAC), restored expression of the *TSPY* gene to levels comparable with that found in the parental cells. Additional DNA microarray studies uncovered a subset of 13 genes from the above-mentioned 66 gene cohort that displayed re-activation of expression following DAC treatment, including *TSPY*, *CYBA* and *MT2A*. DAC suppressed tumor cell growth in vitro. Moreover, systemic treatment of mice with DAC attenuated growth of melanoma xenografts, with consequent re-expression of *TSPY* mRNA. Overall, our data support the hypothesis that multiple genes are targeted, either directly or indirectly, by DNA hypermethylation during melanoma progression.

▶ This study addresses the question of why men are more likely than women to develop more aggressive forms of melanoma. Gallagher et al used gene chip technology to study 66 genes that change as the melanoma moves from a nonaggressive to an aggressive state and found that a common feature among a significant percentage of these genes was that they were chemically altered by DNA methylation. Interestingly, one of the genes turned off by this process is located only on the male Y chromosome, which may explain the more aggressive biological behavior of the tumor in men.

B. H. Thiers, MD

Sequential Immune Escape and Shifting of T Cell Responses in a Long-term Survivor of Melanoma

Yamshchikov GV, Mullins DW, Chang C-C, et al (Univ of Virginia, Charlottesville; Roswell Park Cancer Inst, Buffalo, NY)
J Immunol 174:6863-6871, 2005   17–59

Introduction.—Immune-mediated control of tumors may occur, in part, through lysis of malignant cells by CD8[+] T cells that recognize specific Ag-HLA class I complexes. However, tumor cell populations may escape T cell responses by immune editing, by preventing formation of those Ag-HLA complexes. It remains unclear whether the human immune system can respond to immune editing and recognize newly arising escape variants. We report an example of shifting immune responses to escape variants in a patient with sequential metastases of melanoma and long-term survival after surgery alone. Tumor cells in the first metastasis escaped immune recognition via selective loss of an HLA haplotype (HLA-A11, -B44, and -Cw17), but maintained expression of HLA-A2. In the second metastasis, immune escape from an immunodominant MART-1-specific T cell response was mediated by HLA class I down-regulation, resulting in a failure to present this epitope, but persistent presentation of a tyrosinase-derived epitope. Consequent to this modification in tumor Ag presentation, the dominant CTL response shifted principally toward a tyrosinase-targeted response, even though tyrosinase-specific CTL had been undetectable during the initial metastatic event. Thus, in response to immune editing of tumor cells, a patient's spontaneous T cell response adapted, gaining the ability to recognize and to lyse "edited" tumor targets. The observation of both immune editing and immune adaptation in a patient with long-term survival after surgery alone demonstrates an example of immune system reactivity to counteract the escape mechanism(s) developed by tumor cells, which may contribute to the clinical outcome of malignant disease.

▶ This fascinating report describes the clinical course of melanoma in a single patient over the course of many years and the charting of an extraordinary conflict between the evasion tactics of the tumor and the successful adaptation of the patient's immune system. The patient, who initially presented with melanoma in the absence of detectable metastases, was treated with surgery alone. Five years later, and 6 years thereafter, multiple metastatic lymph nodes were surgically removed and the patient remained subsequently disease free. Long-term investigation of the tumor and the patient response showed that the tumor had altered its immunogenic signature each time that metastatic disease occurred, primarily by loss of expression of cell surface HLA molecules, and the patient had adapted the cytotoxic T-lymphocyte response accordingly. The final antitumor T-cell activity was directed against a previously "hidden" peptide. The patient eventually died of unrelated causes but unknowingly provided compelling evidence that the human immune system can successfully combat neoplastic disease.

G. M. P. Galbraith, MD

Tumor Progression Can Occur Despite the Induction of Very High Levels of Self/Tumor Antigen-Specific CD8$^+$ T Cells in Patients With Melanoma

Rosenberg SA, Sherry RM, Morton KE, et al (NIH, Bethesda, Md)
J Immunol 175:6169-6176, 2005   17–60

Introduction.—The identification of many tumor-associated epitopes as nonmutated "self" Ags led to the hypothesis that the induction of large numbers of self/tumor Ag-specific T cells would be prevented because of central and peripheral tolerance. We report in this study on vaccination efforts in 95 HLA-A*0201 patients at high risk for recurrence of malignant melanoma who received prolonged immunization with the "anchor-modified" synthetic peptide, gp100$_{209-217(210M)}$. Vaccination using this altered peptide immunogen was highly effective at inducing large numbers of self/tumor-Ag reactive T cells in virtually every patient tested, with levels as high as 42% of all CD8$^+$ T cells assessed by tetramer analysis. From 1 to 10% of all CD8$^+$ cells were tumor-Ag reactive in 44% of patients and levels >10% were generated in 17% of patients. These studies were substantiated using the ELISPOT assay and a bulk cytokine release assay. Although our data regarding "tumor escape" were inconclusive, some patients had growing tumors that expressed Ag and HLA-A*0201 in the presence of high levels of antitumor T cells. There was no difference in the levels of antitumor Ag-specific T cells in patients who recurred compared with those that remained disease-free. Thus, the mere presence of profoundly expanded numbers of vaccine-induced, self/tumor Ag-specific T cells cannot by themselves be used as a "surrogate marker" for vaccine efficacy. Further, the induction of even high levels of antitumor T cells may be insufficient to alter tumor progression.

▶ This important study casts a clear light on the often frustrating clinical results of therapeutic vaccination in melanoma patients. Studies of melanoma vaccine strategies are published each year. A recurring finding is a less-than-desirable clinical response rate. In this study, the authors performed repetitive vaccination of 95 high-risk but disease-free melanoma patients. The vaccine consisted of a modified synthetic peptide corresponding to the gp100 self/melanoma epitope given in conjunction with incomplete Freund's adjuvant. The efficacy of the vaccine was exemplified by the production of substantial numbers of tumor-reactive CD8$^+$ T lymphocytes in the majority of patients. However, the induction of these cells did not appear to confer significant protection against disease progression. In fact, tumor recurrence was recorded in 45% to 65% of immunized patients at 3 years. Furthermore, there was no difference in tumor-specific cytotoxic T-cell induction between patients with recurrence and those who remained tumor free. The mechanisms underlying this dichotomy between apparent vaccine efficacy and clinical outcomes are unknown.

G. M. P. Galbraith, MD

The TLR7 Agonist Imiquimod Enhances the Anti-Melanoma Effects of a Recombinant *Listeria monocytogenes* Vaccine

Craft N, Bruhn KW, Nguyen BD, et al (Univ of California, Los Angeles)
J Immunol 175:1983-1990, 2005   17–61

Background.—Many cancer immunotherapies are centered on the activation of CD8 CTL that recognizes specific tumor Ags. Therapies for melanoma in both animal and human studies have included the Ags MART-1, gp100, tyrosinase, tyrosinase-related protein (TRP)[4]-1, and TRP-2. Overcoming self-tolerance is vital to the success of this form of immunotherapy because the target Ags represent immunologic self. CTL-mediated immunity can also be induced by using live bacterial vectors to stimulate the immune system and simultaneously deliver Ags.

One therapeutic strategy is to enhance the function of APCs such as dendritic cells by providing them with tumor Ags along with immunostimulatory signals that induce maturation and augment the APC ability to activate T cells. Whether topical imiquimod, a Toll-like receptor 7 (TLR7) agonist, is effective as an adjuvant during immunization with a live recombinant *Listeria monocytogenes* (rLM) vaccine expressing TRP-2 was investigated.

Methods.—rLM was the virulent parental bacterial strain used for all recombinant constructs. Female C57BL/6 mice were inoculated in the tail vein with 0.1 LD_{50} of each rLM strain in 20 μl of PBS. Boosted immunizations were given 2 to 3 weeks later at a dose of 1.0 LD_{50}. Tumor challenge was conducted with the B16 murine melanoma cell line. Imiquimod was applied daily as a 5% cream to shaved skin at the tumor site or to the flank. Control mice were treated with vehicle control.

Infected mice were sacrificed and liver and spleen were homogenized in 1% Triton X-100/PBS. For survival curves, infected mice were monitored daily for signs of systemic illness.

Results.—Tumors were monitored by bioluminescent imaging. A partial response was noted in 2 separate experiments, but the effects were variable and not statistically significant. However, histologic examination of the tumor sites revealed destruction of tumors in mice that received imiquimod compared with animals that did not. A similar response to lung metastatic tumors was also noted in mice challenged with B16 cells IV and treated topically with imiquimod alone.

Conclusion.—Imiquimod treatment alone was shown to induce partial and variable tumor destruction, both locally and via systemic immunomodulation. Topical imiquimod, a synthetic TLR7 agonist, significantly enhanced the protective antitumor effects of a live, recombinant *Listeria* vaccine against murine melanoma. The protective effect was not dependent on direct application to the tumor and was associated with an increase in tumor-associated and splenic-dendritic cells.

The combination of imiquimod treatment with prior vaccination led to the development of localized vitiligo. Additional studies of the exact mechanisms of tumor protection and bacterial susceptibility are warranted to determine the potential of imiquimod for treatment of neoplastic disease.

▶ Previous studies by these investigators revealed that mice immunized with an rLM expressing TRP-2, a melanoma-associated antigen, developed a TRP-2–specific cytotoxic T-lymphocyte response and a degree of protection against tumor growth from transferred B16 murine melanoma cells. The purpose of the present study was to determine if the immunomodulatory agent imiquimod might have an adjuvant effect in this immunization model. Imiquimod is a synthetic agent that has shown therapeutic efficacy in a variety of skin diseases including condyloma accuminata, basal cell carcinoma and stage 0 melanoma.

The authors found that topical application of imiquimod prior to immunization with the TRP-2 vaccine led to early death of the mice due to overwhelming *Listeria* infection. In subsequent experiments, immunized mice were challenged with B16 cells followed by application of imiquimod to the injection site. This resulted in a significant inhibition of tumor growth in these animals compared to controls.

The effect of imiquimod appeared to be systemic since protection was also afforded by application of the compound at a distant site. However, a powerful local effect was also demonstrated by the development of vitiligo at the site of application in 4 mice that were completely protected against tumor growth. Interestingly, addition of imiquimod to the vaccine protocol did not result in increased induction of antigen-specific cytotoxic T cells. Although the mechanisms underlying the effects seen in this animal tumor model have not been fully elucidated, it appears likely that they are related to one known activity of imiquimod as an agonist of TLR7, which plays an important role in innate immunity.

G. M. P. Galbraith, MD

Targeting the Local Tumor Microenvironment With Vaccinia Virus Expressing B7.1 for the Treatment of Melanoma
Kaufman HL, DeRaffele G, Mitcham J, et al (Columbia Univ, New York; Albert Einstein College of Medicine, New York; Therion Biologics Corp, Cambridge, Mass; et al)
J Clin Invest 115:1903-1912, 2005   17–62

Introduction.—Immunotherapy for the treatment of metastatic melanoma remains a major clinical challenge. The melanoma microenvironment may lead to local T cell tolerance in part through downregulation of costimulatory molecules, such as B7.1 (CD80). We report the results from the first clinical trial, to our knowledge, using a recombinant vaccinia virus expressing B7.1 (rV-B7.1) for monthly intralesional vaccination of accessible melanoma lesions. A standard 2-dose–escalation phase I clinical trial was conducted with 12 patients. The approach was well tolerated with only low-grade fever, myalgias, and fatigue reported and 2 patients experiencing vitiligo. An objective partial response was observed in 1 patient and disease stabilization in 2 patients, 1 of whom is alive without disease 59 months following vaccination. All patients demonstrated an increase in postvaccination antibody and T cell responses against vaccinia virus. Systemic immunity was tested in HLA-A*0201 patients who demonstrated an increased frequency of gp100 and T cells specific to melanoma antigen recognized by T cells 1 (MART-1), also known as Melan-A, by ELISPOT assay following local rV-B7.1 vaccination. Local immunity was evaluated by quantitative real-time RT-PCR, which suggested that tumor regression was associated with increased expression of CD8 and IFN-γ. The local delivery of vaccinia virus expressing B7.1 was well tolerated and represents an innovative strategy for altering the local tumor microenvironment in patients with melanoma.

▶ Although many previous studies have demonstrated tumor-specific T-lymphocyte induction in patients with melanoma, there is evidence to suggest that the function of such cells at the site of the tumor may be impaired. These authors report the results of a small clinical trial in which 12 patients with melanoma who did not respond to treatment with vaccination and IL-2 or chemotherapy abiologic modifiers such as interferon-γ were injected at the tumor site with a recombinant vaccinia virus that expressed the B7.1 molecule. B7.1 (CD80) is normally expressed by antigen-presenting cells and binds to the T-cell marker CD28 upon T-cell antigen recognition, imparting a potent costimulatory signal to the T cell. The investigators hypothesized that providing such a boost to the tumor-reactive lymphocytes within the melanoma microenvironment might overcome the supposed functional impairment of these cells. The results of B7.1 delivery in the 11 patients who completed the trial were modest, with clinical response in 3 individuals and stabilization of disease at the treated site in 2 additional patients in whom the disease progressed overall. Systemic T-cell responses were studied in 6 patients whose tumors expressed the gp100 and MART-1 melanoma antigens. A variable increase in T-cell reactivity to these antigens was observed in these subjects after B7.1 delivery to the tumor. However, a dramatic increase in reactivity was seen in the single patient who experienced stabilization of disease at the target site and complete remission of metastases. Further studies will be needed to validate this interesting immunotherapeutic approach to cancer treatment.

G. M. P. Galbraith, MD

18 Lymphoproliferative Disorders

Polymorphism of the CD30 Promoter Microsatellite Repressive Element Is Associated With Development of Primary Cutaneous Lymphoproliferative Disorders
Franchina M, Kadin ME, Abraham LJ (Univ of Western Australia, Perth; Harvard Med School, Boston)
Cancer Epidemiol Biomarkers Prev 14:1322-1325, 2005   18–1

Background.—Lymphomatoid papulosis is a preneoplastic cutaneous lymphoproliferative disorder. It is characterized by overexpression of CD30, a member of the tumor necrosis factor superfamily. CD30 signaling is known to have an effect on the growth and survival of lymphoid cells. The increased risk of neoplasia in patients with lymphomatoid papulosis suggests the presence of an underlying genetic defect associated with this disorder.

Previous studies have established that the CD30 gene may be regulated in an allele-specific manner. A microsatellite of the type $[(CCAT)_{2-12}CCACTTATGAT]_n$ has been identified between positions -1.2 kb and -336 bp of the gene at the transcriptional level. This study evaluated the efficacy of using the highly polymorphic microsatellite within the promoter region of the CD30 gene as a marker for prediction of susceptibility to the development of lymphomatoid papulosis and associated lymphoproliferative disorders and the likelihood or progression of lymphomatoid papulosis to lymphoma.

Methods.—The patient cohort included 32 unrelated patients with lymphomatoid papulosis with or without existing lymphoma and 8 unrelated patients with primary cutaneous anaplastic large cell lymphoma. A control group was composed of 57 healthy volunteers and patients with non-lymphoid malignances. The patients and control subjects were gender matched. A small sample of peripheral blood was obtained from all subjects, and genomic DNA was isolated from dried blood spots. CD30 microsatellite typing was performed.

Results.—Two allelic forms of the CD30 promoter microsatellite repressive element, designated 20M377 and 30M362, were found to be associated with the development of lymphomatoid papulosis and CD30+ lymphomas in lymphomatoid papulosis patients, respectively.

Conclusion.—Allele-specific differences in the control of CD30 transcription may determine the pathogenesis of the spectrum of CD30+ cutaneous lymphoproliferative disorders.

▶ CD30 is a membrane marker that is included in the tumor necrosis receptor superfamily and plays a role in lymphoid cell growth. Increased expression of this marker has been observed in T-lymphocyte proliferative conditions including lymphomatoid papulosis and lymphomas including anaplastic large cell lymphoma. Studies of the CD30 gene have revealed a highly polymorphic microsatellite region within the CD30 promoter that is involved in repression of gene activation.

Franchina and colleagues examined the possibility that the possession of certain alleles of this microsatellite might be associated with the development of lymphomatoid papulosis and its progression to lymphoma in certain patients. The distribution of 13 microsatellite alleles was determined in a population of 32 patients with either lymphomatoid papulosis alone (n = 21) or in association with Hodgkin's disease, mycosis fungoides, or anaplastic large cell lymphoma (n = 11). The control group of 57 subjects included healthy individuals and patients with nonlymphoid malignancies.

The results obtained showed that the frequency of 1 allele (named 30M377) was significantly increased in the total patient group as compared to the control group ($P = .037$). No association of any allele was found in patients with both lymphomatoid papulosis and lymphoma when compared to the control population. Studies of larger patient populations will be required to determine if this polymorphic system may be useful in the prediction of lymphoma development in patients with lymphomatoid papulosis.

G. M. P. Galbraith, MD

Human Herpesvirus 8 Infection in Patients With Cutaneous Lymphoproliferative Diseases

Trento E, Castilletti C, Ferraro C, et al (San Gallicano Dermatology Inst, Rome; Lab of Clinical Pathology and Gen Hosp "S Giovanni Calibita," Rome; Univ of Jena, Germany)
Arch Dermatol 141:1235-1242, 2005   18–2

Objective.—To investigate the prevalence of human herpesvirus 8 (HHV-8; Kaposi sarcoma–associated herpesvirus) infection in patients with lymphoproliferative skin diseases such as large-plaque parapsoriasis (LPP) and mycosis fungoides compared with inflammatory cutaneous conditions or healthy control subjects.

Design.—A survey study was undertaken in 123 subjects with various clinical conditions.

Setting.—All patients had been seen in the Dermatology Department of the San Gallicano Dermatology Institute, Rome, Italy, in the last 2 years.

Patients.—Forty-five patients with inflammatory or autoimmune cutaneous diseases, 50 healthy control subjects, 10 patients with LPP, 12 patients with mycosis fungoides, and 6 patients with classic Kaposi sarcoma were included in the study.

Main Outcome Measures.—The prevalence of HHV-8 infection was investigated with serologic studies using the gold standard assay based on body cavity–based B-cell lymphoma-1 cells latently infected with HHV-8. The presence of HHV-8 conserved sequence, corresponding to open reading frame 26, was also assessed in the peripheral blood and lesion tissue samples from patients with lymphoproliferative cutaneous diseases with nested polymerase chain reaction. The presence and distribution of cell types infected with HHV-8 in the lesion tissues was determined with immunohistochemical staining with the monoclonal antibody directed against the latent nuclear antigen-1 of HHV-8 encoded by open reading frame 73.

Results.—In healthy control subjects and patients with inflammatory skin diseases, 13.9% were found to have antibody against HHV-8, consistent with the seroprevalence population in Italy. A highly significant association of HHV-8 infection and LPP was found (100%) compared with mycosis fungoides (25%). The peripheral blood mononuclear cells in 8 of 10 patients with LPP were found to harbor viral sequences at nested polymerase chain reaction, whereas none of them had a detectable serum viral load. All LPP lesion tissue samples were positive for HHV-8–encoded open reading frame 26, and the presence of HHV-8–infected cells was confirmed by immunohistochemistry profiles performed on paraffin-embedded tissues from 4 of 10 patients. The positive cell types included endothelial cells and the infiltrating dermal lymphocytes, characteristic hallmarks of LPP. Analysis of T-cell receptor γ chain rearrangements in lesion tissue from our patients confirmed the lack of a significant association between T-cell clonality and LPP.

Conclusion.—These data suggest that HHV-8 may play a role in the onset of LPP, a disease whose cause and evolution are still undefined and which has often been considered the early stage of mycosis fungoides.

▶ Disorders previously associated with HHV-8 infection include Kaposi's sarcoma, body cavity–based B-cell lymphoma (or a primary effusion lymphoma), and the plasmacytic form of multicentric Castleman's disease in patients with AIDS. The proposed association with cutaneous lymphoproliferative disease, especially LPP, requires confirmation by additional studies.

B. H. Thiers, MD

Ultraviolet Radiation Exposure and Risk of Malignant Lymphomas
Smedby KE, Hjalgrim H, Melbye M, et al (Karolinska Institutet, Stockholm; Statens Serum Inst, Copenhagen; Odense Univ, Denmark; et al)
J Natl Cancer Inst 97:199-209, 2005   18–3

Background.—The incidence of malignant lymphomas has been increasing rapidly, but the causes of these malignancies remain poorly understood.

One hypothesis holds that exposure to ultraviolet (UV) radiation increases lymphoma risk. We tested this hypothesis in a population-based case-control study in Denmark and Sweden.

Methods.—A total of 3740 patients diagnosed between October 1, 1999, and August 30, 2002, with incident malignant lymphomas, including non-Hodgkin lymphoma, chronic lymphocytic leukemia, and Hodgkin lymphoma, and 3187 population controls provided detailed information on history of UV exposure and skin cancer and information on other possible risk factors for lymphomas. Odds ratios (ORs) with 95% confidence intervals (CIs) were calculated by logistic regression. Statistical tests were two-sided.

Results.—Multivariable-adjusted analyses revealed consistent, statistically significant negative associations between various measures of UV light exposure and risk of non-Hodgkin lymphoma. A high frequency of sun bathing and sunburns at age 20 years and 5-10 years before the interview and sun vacations abroad were associated with 30%-40% reduced risks of non-Hodgkin lymphoma (e.g., for sunbathing four times a week or more at age 20 versus never sunbathing, OR = 0.7, 95% CI = 0.6 to 0.9; for two or more sunburns a year at age 20 versus no sunburns, OR = 0.6, 95% CI = 0.5 to 0.8). These inverse associations increased in strength with increasing levels of exposure (all $P_{trend} \le .01$). Similar, albeit weaker, associations were observed for Hodgkin lymphoma. There were no clear differences among non-Hodgkin lymphoma subtypes, although associations were stronger for B-cell than for T-cell lymphomas. A history of skin cancer was associated with a doubling in risks of both non-Hodgkin and Hodgkin lymphoma.

Conclusions.—A history of high UV exposure was associated with reduced risk of non-Hodgkin lymphoma. The positive association between skin cancer and malignant lymphomas is, therefore, unlikely to be mediated by UV exposure.

▶ Smedby et al studied 3740 patients with lymphoma and a similar number of patients without the disease. They found that increased exposure to UV radiation through sunbathing and sunburns was associated with a reduced incidence of non-Hodgkin lymphoma. In an accompanying editorial, Egan et al suggest that the variable responsible for this protective effective may be vitamin D.[1]

The data presented here challenge the concept of UV radiation as being a factor in the previously reported association between skin cancer and malignant lymphoma. Similarly, the presumed protective role of vitamin D can also be challenged. As pointed out by Kalish in subsequent correspondence, in patients with skin cancer who had extensive sun exposure, lymphoma risk was actually increased, whereas it was decreased in patients with extensive sun exposure without skin cancer.[2] Because vitamin D levels should be elevated in both groups, the difference in lymphoma risk cannot be explained by vitamin D levels alone.

B. H. Thiers, MD

References

1. Egan KM, Sosman JA, Blot WJ: Sunlight and reduced risk of skin cancer: Is the real story vitamin D? *J Natl Cancer Inst* 97:161-163, 2005.
2. Kalish RS: Re: Sun exposure and mortality from melanoma (letter). *J Natl Cancer Inst* 97:1158, 2005.

Hair Dye Use and Risk of Lymphoid Neoplasms and Soft Tissues Sarcomas

Tavani A, Negri E, Franceschi S, et al (Istituto di Ricerche Farmacologiche "Mario Negri," Milan, Italy; Internatl Agency for Research on Cancer, Lyon, France; Centro di Riferimento Oncologico, Aviano, Italy; et al)
Int J Cancer 113:629-631, 2005   18–4

Introduction.—We analyzed the relation between hair dye use and the risk of Hodgkin's disease (HD), non-Hodgkin's lymphoma (NHL), multiple myeloma (MM) and soft tissue sarcomas (STS) in a hospital-based case-control study conducted between 1985 and 1997 in northern Italy. Cases included 158 patients with histologically confirmed incident HD, 446 with NHL, 141 with MM, 221 with STS and controls included 1,295 patients with acute nonneoplastic conditions. Compared to never use of any type of hair dyes, the odds ratio (OR) for ever use was 0.68 (95% confidence interval, CI, 0.40-1.18) for HD, 1.03 (95% CI 0.73-1.44) for NHL, 1.17 (95% CI 0.70-1.97) for MM and 0.73 (95% CI 0.45-1.17) for STS. The OR were close to unity for permanent and semipermanent dyes analyzed separately or when the analysis was restricted to women. Our study indicates that there is no appreciable association between ever use of any type of hair dyes and the risk of HD, NHL, MM or STS.

Personal Use of Hair Dyes and Risk of Cancer: A Meta-analysis

Takkouche B, Etminan M, Montes-Martínez A (Univ of Santiago de Compostela, Spain; Royal Victoria Hosp, Montreal; Vancouver Coastal Health Inst, BC, Canada)
JAMA 293:2516-2525, 2005   18–5

Context.—Use of hair dyes has been suggested recently as a risk factor for several types of cancer in epidemiologic studies. This alarming news and controversial declarations by scientific organizations and general media have made necessary a systematic evaluation of the epidemiologic evidence.

Objective.—To examine the association between personal use of hair dyes and relative risk of cancer.

Data Sources.—We retrieved studies published in any language by systematically searching the MEDLINE (1966-January 2005), EMBASE, LILACS, and ISI Proceedings computerized databases and by manually examining the references of the original articles, reviews, and monographs re-trieved.

Study Selection.—We included cohort and case-control studies reporting relative risk estimates and 95% confidence intervals (CIs) (or data to calcu-late them) of personal hair dye use and cancer. We excluded studies that dealt with occupational exposure. We carried out separate analyses for bladder, breast, and hematopoietic cancers and cancers of other sites. Seventy-nine studies were included of 210 articles identified in the search.

Data Extraction.—Data were extracted independently by 2 investigators. We used a standardized questionnaire to record information on study de-sign, sample size, type of controls, year of publication, adjustment factors, and relative risks of cancer among ever users of hair dyes. When possible, we extracted association measures on use of permanent dyes and extensive use (>200 lifetime episodes of dye use).

Data Synthesis.—Study-specific relative risks were weighted by the in-verse of their variance to obtain fixed- and random-effects pooled estimates. The pooled relative risk for ever users of hair dyes was 1.06 (95% CI, 0.95-1.18) for breast cancer (14 studies), 1.01 (95% CI, 0.89-1.14) for bladder cancer (10 studies), and 1.15 (95% CI, 1.05-1.27) for hematopoietic cancers (40 studies). Other cancers were examined by only 1 or 2 studies, of which the pooled or single relative risk was elevated for brain cancer, ovarian can-cer, and cancer of the salivary glands. No effect was observed for use of per-manent dyes or for extensive use.

Conclusions.—We did not find strong evidence of a marked increase in the risk of cancer among personal hair dye users. Some aspects related to he-matopoietic cancer and other cancers that have shown evidence of increased risk in 1 or 2 studies should be investigated further.

▶ Previous studies have suggested the possibility that certain hair dyes may be mutagenic in vitro and carcinogenic in some animals. Tavani et al (Abstract 18–4) analyzed data from a case-control study of various lymphoproliferative disorders and STS and could find no association with the use of hair dyes. Takkouche et al (Abstract 18–5) noted the relation of personal use of hair dyes and the risk of lymphoma to be inconclusive and proposed the need for addi-tional investigation.

B. H. Thiers, MD

Narrowband Ultraviolet B Phototherapy to Clear and Maintain Clearance in Patients With Mycosis Fungoides

Boztepe G, Sahin S, Ayhan M, et al (Hacettepe Univ, Ankara, Turkey)
J Am Acad Dermatol 53:242-246, 2005   18–6

Background and Purpose.—Narrowband ultraviolet B (UVB) photo-therapy for early-stage mycosis fungoides (MF) has been found to be benefi-cial in some reports. Although rapid recurrences after discontinuation of therapy appear to interfere with its efficacy, optimal maintenance schedules for prolonged relapse-free intervals are not discussed in the literature. The purpose of this study was to review our experience with narrowband UVB in patients with MF.

Patients and Methods.—All available data that belong to 14 patients (10 male, 4 female; age range, 28-74 years) with histologically proven MF, at disease stages IA-IB (n = 10) and IIΛ (n = 4) who received narrowband UVB were retrospectively evaluated.

Results.—Complete response (CR) was achieved in 11 of 14 cases (78%) after a mean of 25 treatments. Ten of 11 patients were followed up for a median of 22 months (range, 7-43 months) after CR; one patient was lost to follow-up immediately after CR. Eight patients completed the recommended maintenance narrowband UVB therapy protocol. The median duration of maintenance was 18 months (range, 12-30 months). No patient had relapse during maintenance. Mean relapse-free duration was 26.0 ± 9.9 months.

Limitations.—The number of patients in the study group was relatively few.

Conclusion.—This study provides evidence that narrowband UVB might be an efficient treatment option for MF patients at stages IA and IB, as well as at stage IIA. Results suggest that using maintenance phototherapy after CR is a logical approach, which may prolong the duration of remission in MF.

▶ I have found narrowband UVB therapy to be a viable alternative to psoralen plus UVA for patients with early stage MF.

B. H. Thiers, MD

Long-term Follow-up of Patients With Early-Stage Cutaneous T-Cell Lymphoma Who Achieved Complete Remission With Psoralen Plus UV-A Monotherapy

Querfeld C, Rosen ST, Kuzel TM, et al (Northwestern Univ, Chicago)
Arch Dermatol 141:305-311, 2005   18–7

Objectives.—To evaluate long-term outcomes, impact of maintenance therapy and potential curability of patients with mycosis fungoides (MF) treated with psoralen plus UV-A (PUVA) monotherapy.

Design.—Single-center retrospective cohort analysis.

Setting.—Academic referral center for cutaneous lymphoma.

Patients.—A total of 66 of 104 patients with clinical stages IA to IIA MF who achieved complete remission (CR) after PUVA monotherapy between 1979 and 1995.

Main Outcome Measures.—Kaplan-Meier actuarial survival and disease-free survival curves were compared between stage IA and IB/IIA cases. Patients were stratified into relapse and nonrelapse groups based on whether their MF relapsed during study follow-up. Baseline characteristics and treatment were compared between these groups.

Results.—Median follow-up time was 94 months (range, 5-242 months). Thirty-three patients maintained CR for 84 months (range, 5-238 months), and 33 patients experienced relapse with a median disease-free interval of 39 months (range, 2-127 months). There was no significant difference in baseline characteristics between patients in the nonrelapse and relapse groups. Those in the nonrelapse group received a higher cumulative dosage to CR ($P = .03$) and required longer treatment periods to achieve CR ($P = .03$). Disease-free survival rates at 5 and 10 years for all patients with stage IA were 56% and 30%, respectively, and for stage IB/IIA, 74% and 50%. Actuarial survival rates at 5, 10, and 15 years were 94%, 82%, and 82%, respectively, in patients with stage IA, and 80%, 69%, and 58% in patients with stage IB/IIA. The overall survival rate for the nonrelapse and relapse groups did not show any statistical difference. One third of the patients developed signs of chronic photodamage and secondary cutaneous malignancies.

Conclusions.—Psoralen UV-A is an effective treatment for MF, inducing long-term remissions and perhaps in some cases disease "cure." Thirty percent to 50% of patients remain disease free for 10 years, but late relapses occur. Long-term survival is not affected by relapse status, and the risk of photodamage needs to be measured against the possible benefit of greater disease elimination.

▶ The data confirm the efficacy of PUVA therapy for early stage cutaneous T-cell lymphoma. Interestingly, long-term survival does not appear to be influenced by relapse status. Although many patients remain disease free for years, to call them "cured" may not be totally accurate, as some experience late relapses. Whether narrow-band UVB treatment can yield the same benefits without the considerable risk of photodamage and cutaneous carcinogenesis, associated with PUVA therapy, remains to be determined.

B. H. Thiers, MD

Treatment of Patch and Plaque Stage Mycosis Fungoides With Imiquimod 5% Cream
Deeths MJ, Chapman JT, Dellavalle RP, et al (Univ of Colorado, Denver)
J Am Acad Dermatol 52:275-280, 2005   18–8

Background.—Systemic interferon is effective in the treatment of mycosis fungoides (MF). Imiquimod is effective in the treatment of some epidermal neoplasms and induces localized interferon production.

Objective.—To evaluate the safety and efficacy of topical imiquimod 5% cream for the treatment of patch and plaque stage MF.

Methods.—Six patients with stage IA to IIB MF were treated with topical imiquimod 5% cream 3 times per week for 12 weeks in this open label pilot study. Index lesions were biopsied pre- and post- treatment, and up to 4 additional treated lesions were monitored for 16 weeks.

Results.—Three of 6 patients had histologic clearance of disease in index lesions, and also demonstrated significant improvement in the clinical scores for all treated lesions. A fourth patient had 2 of 4 lesions respond clinically. Application site reactions were limited to those patients responding to treatment.

Conclusion.—In this preliminary open label study topical imiquimod 5% cream was well tolerated and associated with a histologic and clinical response rate of 50%.

▶ Older therapies for MF, such as topical mechlorethamine or phototherapy, are generally applied to or directed at the entire skin surface, the assumption being that this is a multifocal disease that requires total body treatment. Newer therapies such as topical bexarotene and, now, imiquimod are applied solely to the clinically affected skin. More needs to be known about the pathogenesis of this fascinating disease before we can conclude which is the most appropriate strategy.[1,2]

B. H. Thiers, MD

References

1. Girardi M, Heald PW, Wilson LD: The pathogenesis of mycosis fungoides. *N Engl J Med* 350:1978-1988, 2004.
2. Girardi M, Taraszka K: Treatment of cutaneous T cell lymphoma. 2003 YEAR BOOK OF DERMATOLOGY AND DERMATOLOGIC SURGERY, pp 1-26.

Bexarotene Treatment of Late-Stage Mycosis Fungoides and Sézary Syndrome: Development of Extracutaneous Lymphoma in 6 Patients
Bouwhuis SA, Davis MDP, el-Azhary RA, et al (Mayo Clinic, Rochester, Minn)
J Am Acad Dermatol 52:991-996, 2005   18–9

Background.—Bexarotene was approved by the Food and Drug Administration in 2000 for the treatment of cutaneous T-cell lymphoma (CTCL). Bexarotene is one of a subclass of retinoids called rexinoids that selectively bind to nuclear retinoic X receptors. This drug has been shown to be beneficial in the treatment of refractory early stage and late-stage CTCL. A recent study found that higher response rates were achieved with bexarotene in patients with advanced disease, without unacceptable side effects. However, it has been observed that in some patients receiving extracorporeal photopheresis (ECP), the initiation of bexarotene therapy was temporally associated with the progression of extracutaneous lymphoma. While this is not necessarily indicative of causation, its occurrence in 6 patients is important. The development of extracutaneous lymphoma after bexarotene therapy in these 6 patients was reported.

Methods.—Bexarotene was initiated as adjuvant therapy in various doses in 6 patients already receiving ECP. All but one of these patients continued to receive therapy with monthly ECP. The patients were examined every 4 weeks for subjective degree of pruritis, objective degree of skin erythema, presence and degree of lymph node enlargement, and clinical evidence of liver or spleen enlargement. Sézary cell counts were performed, and triglyceride, cholesterol, and thyroid hormone levels were measured. Total body CT scans, including the chest, abdomen, and pelvis, were obtained before the initiation of bexarotene therapy and every 6 months thereafter.

Results.—All the patients responded to bexarotene therapy, with improved symptoms and signs of cutaneous involvement of CTCL. However, lymphoma developed elsewhere in all the patients.

Conclusions.—It is possible that bexarotene contributed to the progression of internal disease in all of these patients despite improvement in their cutaneous signs and symptoms. Bexarotene therapy may alleviate the signs and symptoms of CTCL, but careful surveillance of lymph nodes and solid organs during treatment is advised.

▶ The authors correctly caution against assuming that bexarotene treatment was responsible for the extracutaneous manifestations noted in these patients. These patients all had progressive, late-stage, treatment-recalcitrant CTCL, in whom systemic manifestations might well have developed independent of treatment with bexarotene or any other agent. More unusual is the observation that in these patients, progression to systemic disease developed in a setting of improved skin signs.

B. H. Thiers, MD

Treatment of Primary Cutaneous B-cell Lymphoma With Rituximab
Fink-Puches R, Wolf IH, Zalaudek I, et al (Med Univ of Graz, Austria)
J Am Acad Dermatol 52:847-853, 2005   18–10

Background.—Rituximab is a genetically engineered antibody directed against the CD20 antigen. Intravenous administration of rituximab has been used for the treatment of patients with low-, intermediate-, and high-grade B-cell non-Hodgkin's lymphomas and is a registered treatment modality for this indication. Treatment of primary cutaneous B-cell lymphoma (CBCL) with intralesionally or systemically administered rituximab has been described only in a few cases.

Objective.—Our purpose was to assess the efficacy of rituximab in the treatment of CBCL.

Methods.—We performed a retrospective study on 9 patients with CBCL who were treated with intralesional or systemic administration of rituximab.

Results.—Two patients treated with systemic rituximab achieved complete remission. Complete remission could be observed in 6 of 7 patients after 1 to 8 cycles of intralesional treatment with rituximab. In one patient one of two lesions showed a partial remission after 4 cycles of treatment, whereas the second showed complete remission. A local recurrence was observed in one patient after 27 months of follow-up and in two patients recurrences developed at other body sites after 12 and 14 months of follow-up.

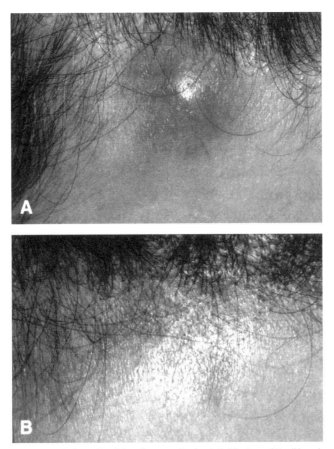

FIGURE 1.—**A**, Marginal zone B-cell lymphoma on forehead. **B**, No signs of B-cell lymphoma on forehead after intralesional treatment with rituximab (4 cycles). (Courtesy of Fink-Puches R, Wolf IH, Zalaudek I, et al: Treatment of primary cutaneous B-cell lymphoma with rituximab. *J Am Acad Dermatol* 52:847-853, 2005.)

No severe side effect occurred except for slight pain during intralesional injection.

Conclusion.—Rituximab therapy is a well-tolerated and effective treatment for primary CBCL. In comparison to intravenous administration, intralesional application of the drug allows the use of lower dosages. Intralesional therapy with rituximab deserves further investigation and comparison to systemic administration of the drug in controlled multicenter studies (Fig 1; see color plate XV).

▶ In this study, all patients had a predominant CD20+ population of lymphocytes. Although previous articles have suggested that a recurrence of skin lesions after rituximab therapy are characterized by a loss of CD20 expression, this was not the case in 2 of the patients described here, who were treated with intralesional rituximab and who had a cutaneous relapse with cells bearing the CD20 antigen.

B. H. Thiers, MD

19 Miscellaneous Topics in Dermatologic Surgery and Cutaneous Oncology

Brief Communication: Duration of Platelet Dysfunction After a 7-Day Course of Ibuprofen
Goldenberg NA, Jacobson L, Manco-Johnson MJ (Univ of Colorado, Aurora)
Ann Intern Med 142:506-509, 2005   19–1

Background.—Despite a paucity of evidence, clinicians routinely advise that patients discontinue using nonsteroidal anti-inflammatory drugs (NSAIDs), including ibuprofen, at least 1 week before most surgical procedures.

Objective.—To define the duration of ibuprofen-induced platelet dysfunction.

Design.—Prospective cohort study.

Setting.—Denver/Aurora, Colorado.

Participants.—11 healthy adult volunteers.

Measurements.—Individuals were tested at baseline and serially after completion of a 7-day course of ibuprofen (600 mg orally every 8 hours). The platelet function analyzer (PFA-100, Dade Behring, Newark, Delaware), a test that has replaced the bleeding time in many clinical settings, was used.

Results.—All participants exhibited normal platelet function before starting ibuprofen. Platelet dysfunction was apparent after completion of the ibuprofen course in 7 of the 11 participants and normalized by 24 hours after the last ibuprofen dose.

Limitations.—The sample size in this study was small, and no participants had a major illness. Correlation between PFA-100 results and clinical bleeding has not been established.

Conclusions.—Platelet function seems to normalize within 24 hours after cessation of regular ibuprofen use in healthy individuals. Further studies are warranted to provide a rational basis for timing of NSAID withdrawal in a range of patients undergoing surgery.

▶ Many surgeons recommend that patients discontinue using NSAIDS at least 1 week before an operative procedure. However, little experimental evidence supports such an assertion. Goldenberg et al present data to suggest that it may not be necessary to discontinue ibuprofen until 24 hours before surgery. One caution in interpreting these data is that the study evaluated platelet function in healthy adults using a platelet function analyzer and did not examine clinical bleeding.

B. H. Thiers, MD

Selective Serotonin Reuptake Inhibitors and Increased Bleeding Risk: Are We Missing Something?

Serebruany VL (Johns Hopkins Univ, Baltimore, Md)
Am J Med 119:113-116, 2006   19–2

Purpose.—Selective serotonin reuptake inhibitors (SSRIs) are first line agents to treat clinical depression. Although these medications exhibit a favorable safety profile, there are multiple case reports, registries, and uncontrolled studies suggesting that use of SSRIs might be associated in the increased risk of bleeding events. There is also emerging evidence that these side effects of SSRIs are due to blockade of serotonin reuptake in platelets and subsequent platelet dysfunction.

Methods.—The analysis of evidence linking SSRIs with bleeding episodes to define the prevalence, specific clinical characteristics, and estimated risk when SSRIs are used in combination with antiplatelet agents or/and anticoagulants.

Results.—There are over 120 MEDLINE-cited peer-reviewed research papers and more than 50 000 Web pages devoted to SSRI-related bleeding events.

Conclusion.—Independently of the brand, use of SSRIs is indeed associated with increased bleeding risk. Although such complications are rare, their frequency is growing, and physicians should be aware of SSRI-induced hemorrhages, especially in patients with hereditary platelet defects, and those treated with antiplatelet agents. Prospective studies are urgently needed to determine whether SSRIs will yield additional bleeding risks when used long term concomitantly with aspirin or clopidogrel.

▶ SSRIs have antiplatelet properties that may result in bleeding events. Most of the bleeding complications noted with the use of these drugs have been superficial and minor, although more severe internal bleeding events have been rarely encountered. The clinical relevance of SSRI intake for patients undergoing dermatologic surgery is uncertain, although this report drives home the necessity of taking a good drug history in all our patients. At the very least, concomitant administration of SSRIs with antiplatelet agents should be done with caution.

B. H. Thiers, MD

Decreased Efficacy of Topical Anesthetic Creams in Presence of Benzoyl Peroxide
Burkhart CG, Burkhart CN (Med Univ of Ohio at Toledo; Ohio Univ, Sylvania; Univ of North Carolina at Chapel Hill)
Dermatol Surg 31:1479-1480, 2005   19–3

Background.—Topical anesthetics are widely used to diminish the sensation of pain from various medical cutaneous procedures. Any topical agent that reduces the desired effect has clinical ramifications.

Materials and Methods.—Topical 6% benzocaine cream was applied to both inner forearms of five persons and covered with a bandage. One of the arms was additionally treated simultaneously with 5% benzoyl peroxide. The areas were tested with a pinprick examination every 10 minutes for the ensuing hour.

Results.—There was an estimated 75% increased perception of pain on the forearm to which benzoyl peroxide was applied in consort with the topical anesthetic at all examination times.

Conclusions.—Benzoyl peroxide chemically reacts with topical anesthetics such as tetracaine, procaine, pramoxine, prilocaine, and lidocaine, causing a significant reduction in their numbing effect. Clinically, make sure that the skin area to be topically anesthetized is devoid of any previous treatment with benzoyl peroxide or insist that the skin is thoroughly washed prior to application of the anesthetic.

▶ An interesting observation and one that the clinician needs to be aware of to ensure less-painful treatments.

J. Cook, MD

Digital Anesthesia With Epinephrine: An Old Myth Revisited
Krunic AL, Wang LC, Soltani K, et al (Univ of Texas, Dallas; Univ of Chicago)
J Am Acad Dermatol 51:755-759, 2004   19–4

Background.—The prohibition against the use epinephrine with local anesthetics for digital blocks or infiltrative anesthesia is an established dogma in dermatologic surgery. Major textbooks reinforce this teaching suggesting that there is substantial risk of digital gangrene caused by local anesthesia containing epinephrine.

Objective.—To provide a comprehensive literature review of the cases of digital necrosis associated with the use of local anesthesia containing epinephrine.

Methods.—A PubMed search of the National Library of Medicine database using the terms "lidocaine" and "epinephrine" and "finger" with no specified limits was performed.

Results.—A total of 16 papers were referenced and only 6 papers dealt with digital anesthesia. A total of 50 cases of digital gangrene were reported, mostly in the early part of the 20th century. In 21 cases digital gangrene was associated with anesthetic mixed with epinephrine. Actual concentration of epinephrine was known in only 4 cases. Careful analysis of all cases of necrosis did not support epinephrine itself as a cause. Other contributing factors including older compounds (cocaine, eukaine, and procaine), non-standardized inaccurate methods of mixing epinephrine with lidocaine, inappropriate use of a tourniquet, postoperative hot soaks, infection, or large anesthetic volume were also present. None of the reported cases were associated with the use of a commercial lidocaine-epinephrine mixture.

Conclusion.—A literature review failed to provide evidence to support the dogma that block or infiltrative anesthesia with lidocaine and epinephrine produces digital necrosis. Proper injection technique and adequate selection of patients (absence of thrombotic, vasospastic conditions, or uncontrolled hypertension) are mandatory to minimize complications. The addition of epinephrine, in fact, reduces the need for the use of tourniquets and large volumes of anesthetic and provides better and longer pain control during digital procedures.

▶ Many of us were taught in medical school or residency to avoid epinephrine-containing solutions when administering digital anesthesia. Like many propagated myths, this dictum may be erroneous. This report summarizes previously published studies documenting the safety of digital anesthesia with epinephrine-containing solutions.

The reduced hemorrhage certainly improves the ease of the surgical procedure. Nevertheless, the morbidity of distal necrosis of a finger or toe cannot be understated. Although prior studies have clearly documented the safety of epinephrine in digital anesthesia, the treating physician must be particularly careful in patients predisposed to concomitant microvascular injury (such as those with thromboangiitis obliterans and others).

J. Cook, MD

General Anesthesia for Pediatric Dermatologic Procedures: Risks and Complications
Cunningham BB, Gigler V, Wang K, et al (Univ of California, San Diego; Univ of California, Irvine; Northwestern Univ, Chicago; et al)
Arch Dermatol 141:573-576, 2005   19–5

Objective.—To assess the safety and adverse events associated with the use of general anesthesia in children undergoing elective dermatologic procedures.

Design.—A multicenter retrospective review.

Setting.—Children's Hospital and Health Center, San Diego, Calif, and Northwestern University School of Medicine, Chicago, Ill.

Patients.—The study population comprised 269 children and adolescents ranging in age from 2 months to 18 years (881 procedures performed by 6 pediatric dermatologic and laser surgeons).

Main Outcome Measures.—The risk of an adverse event occurring during general anesthesia for pediatric dermatologic procedures.

Results.—The risk of general anesthesia in elective pediatric dermatologic procedures was low: 90% of patients experienced no clinically relevant complications. The most common clinically relevant adverse effect of general anesthesia was perioperative nausea and emesis, which was noted in 4% of patients. There were no serious life-threatening events noted, and the mortality rate was 0%.

Conclusion.—The use of general anesthesia for dermatologic procedures in a children's hospital setting appears safe, with a low rate of complications.

▶ This study may serve as a point of reference for anxious parents of children undergoing anesthesia for dermatologic surgical procedures. The short duration of anesthesia for the low complexity procedures done by the dermatologic surgeon certainly increases the safety of the administration of anesthesia. I have done hundreds of pediatric dermatologic surgery procedures requiring general anesthesia and have found that parents are significantly more anxious over the anesthesia than the surgical procedure itself. This needs to be understood by the treating physician, and the data presented here bolster the safety of the technique.

J. Cook, MD

Primary Closure vs Second-Intention Treatment of Skin Punch Biopsy Sites: A Randomized Trial

Christenson LJ, Phillips PK, Weaver AL, et al (Mayo Clinic, Rochester, Minn)
Arch Dermatol 141:1093-1099, 2005   19–6

Objective.—To determine if healing of punch biopsy wounds by second intention is equivalent to healing with primary closure.

Design.—Prospective, randomized, method comparison equivalence study.

Setting.—Tertiary academic medical center.

Participants.—Study volunteers were recruited from the general population and enrolled between January 7, 2002, and August 20, 2002. Patients with immunodeficiency, peripheral vascular disease, or history of keloid formation and those receiving anticoagulation therapy or systemic corticosteroids were excluded.

Intervention.—Study volunteers had two 4-mm or two 8-mm punch biopsies performed on the upper outer arms, midlateral aspect of the thighs, or upper back. One biopsy site was closed with interrupted 4-0 nylon suture, and the contralateral biopsy site was allowed to heal by second intention.

Main Outcome Measures.—At 9 months, scar appearance was evaluated blindly and independently by 3 physicians using a visual analog scale (0 indicating poor and 100 indicating best).

Results.—Seventy-seven of 82 enrolled volunteers completed the study. Mean (SD) visual analog scale score was 57.1 (19.5) for biopsy sites allowed to heal by second intention and 58.9 (19.7) for biopsy sites that healed with primary closure. The median surface area of the biopsy scars at 9 months was 32 mm(2) for second intention and 33 mm^2 for primary closure. For the 8-mm biopsies, the volunteers preferred the appearance of the sites that healed with primary closure; however, for the 4-mm biopsies, volunteers had no significant preference for either biopsy method. Costs were lower for second intention, and complications were equivalent.

Conclusions.—Punch biopsy sites allowed to heal by second intention appear at least as good as biopsy sites closed primarily with suture. Although volunteers preferred suturing at larger biopsy sites, elimination of suturing of punch biopsy wounds would result in personnel efficiency and economic savings for both patients and medical institutions.

▶ This series shows largely equivalent outcomes in cosmesis with or without suturing punch biopsy sites. It is clear that patient's expectations and pros and cons of each technique need to be reviewed before deciding which is best for a given patient. It is my perception that scars resulting from larger biopsies such as the 8-mm punch biopsy performed in this series may at times be cosmetically unacceptable. Moreover, the physician is met almost uniformly with the comment from the patient that "the doctor didn't even stitch it up" if the scar from second intention healing is poor. For this reason, I suture larger biopsy sites regardless of the time and expense in an effort to achieve a better cosmetic outcome. It should be noted that I generally do not perform 8-mm punch biopsies because I feel better cosmetic results may be achieved using small elliptical excisions with layered closures.

J. Cook, MD

The Cutaneous Surgery Experience of Multiple Specialties in the Medicare Population
Shaffer CL, Feldman SR, Fleischer AB Jr, et al (Wake Forest Univ, Winston-Salem, NC; Tucson, Ariz)
J Am Acad Dermatol 52:1045-1048, 2005   19–7

Background.—There has been tremendous growth in the performance of ambulatory surgical procedures. Traditional forms of peer review, commonplace for hospital-based procedures, are not typically performed in the office-based setting. Hospital credentialing of physicians has been suggested to be a means of assuring patient safety. Credentialing committees may be unaware of the level of experience of typical office-based physicians who perform cutaneous surgery.

Purpose.—To compare the levels of cutaneous surgery experience of dermatologists and other surgical specialists.

Methods.—Medicare claims data on number of cutaneous surgery procedures performed by various medical disciplines, including dermatologists, plastic surgeons, general surgeons, and others, were obtained from the 1998-1999 Medicare Current Beneficiary Survey (MCBS) and analyzed. The number of physicians in each specialty was used to normalize the data to a per physician basis.

Results.—Dermatologists performed half (50%) of the complex repairs and most of the excisions (58%) and intermediate repairs (62%). Dermatologists performed more flaps (40% of all flaps) than any other specialty, while plastic surgeons performed more total grafts (38%) than any other specialty. Dermatologists and plastic surgeons performed similar numbers of full-thickness skin grafts, while plastic surgeons performed more split-thickness skin grafts.

Conclusion.—As dermatologists seek hospital credentials for performing cutaneous surgery procedures, these data should help surgical colleagues understand the typical level of experience of their dermatologist colleagues.

▶ The data presented here confirm what we all know: Dermatologists in this country are busy successfully and expertly performing cutaneous surgical procedures. The metamorphosis of our specialty into one embracing and pioneering reconstructive surgical techniques of the skin is welcome. Previously published studies clearly support the contention that dermatology represents the "standard of care" for treatment of skin cancer in the Medicare population.

J. Cook, MD

Adverse Event Reporting: Lessons Learned From 4 Years of Florida Office Data
Coldiron B, Fisher AH, Adelman E, et al (Skin Cancer Ctr, Cincinnati, Ohio; Wake Forest Univ, Winston-Salem, NC; Ohio State Univ, Columbus; et al)
Dermatol Surg 31:1079-1093, 2005   19–8

Background.—Patient safety regulations and medical error reporting systems have been at the forefront of current health care legislature. In 2000, Florida mandated that all physicians report, to a central collecting agency, all adverse events occurring in an office setting.

Purpose.—To analyze the scope and incidence of adverse events and deaths resulting from office surgical procedures in Florida from 2000 to 2004.

Methods.—We reviewed all reported adverse incidents (the death of a patient, serious injury, and subsequent hospital transfer) occurring in an office setting from March 1, 2000, through March 1, 2004, from the Florida Agency for Health Care Administration. We determined physician board certification status, hospital privileges, and office accreditation via telephone follow-up and Internet searches.

Results.—Of 286 reported office adverse events, 77 occurred in association with an office surgical procedure (19 deaths and 58 hospital transfers). There were seven complications and five deaths associated with the use of intravenous sedation or general anesthesia. There were no adverse events associated with the use of dilute local (tumescent) anesthesia. Liposuction and/or abdominoplasty under general anesthesia or intravenous sedation were the most common surgical procedures associated with a death or complication. Fifty-three percent of offices reporting an adverse incident were accredited by the Joint Commission on Accreditation of Healthcare Organizations, American Association for Accreditation of Ambulatory Surgical Facilities, or American Association for Ambulatory Health Care. Ninety-four percent of the involved physicians were board certified, and 97% had hospital privileges. Forty-two percent of the reported deaths were delayed by several hours to weeks after uneventful discharge or after hospital transfer.

Conclusions.—Requiring physician board certification, physician hospital privileges, or office accreditation is not likely to reduce office adverse events. Restrictions on dilute local (tumescent) anesthesia for liposuction would not reduce adverse events and could increase adverse events if patients are shifted to riskier approaches. State and/or national legislation establishing adverse event reporting systems should be supported and should require the reporting of delayed deaths.

▶ In the current era of evidence-based medicine, is it not ironic that those demanding everything from board recertification to office accreditation are not subjected to the same scrutiny? Where is the evidence that any of this would improve patient care or patient safety?

B. H. Thiers, MD

The Incidence of Major Complications From Mohs Micrographic Surgery Performed in Office-Based and Hospital-Based Settings
Kimyai-Asadi A, Goldberg LH, Peterson SR, et al (DermSurgery Associates, Houston; Methodist Hosp, Provo, Utah)
J Am Acad Dermatol 53:628-634, 2005   19–9

Background.—There has been significant interest in the safety of office-based surgery.

Objective.—Our purpose was to compare the safety of Mohs micrographic surgery and related surgical repairs performed in office- and hospital-based settings.

Methods.—The study included 3937 consecutive patients undergoing Mohs surgery. Surgery was performed at either an outpatient office or a hospital-based setting.

Results.—Mohs surgery was performed on 1540 patients in the hospital and 2397 patients underwent surgery in the office. The mean patient age was 66 years, and 61% were men. Ninety-three percent of lesions were basal cell or squamous cell carcinomas, and 86% were located on the head and neck.

The average tumor measured 1.1 × 1.0 cm, required 1.7 stages of Mohs surgery, and resulted in a defect measuring 2.4 × 1.8 cm. Linear closures, flaps, grafts, and second-intention healing were utilized in 69%, 14%, 6%, and 11% of defects, respectively. There were no differences in patient or tumor characteristics or the types of closures used at the two operating facilities. The only serious surgical complication was gastrointestinal hemorrhage due to naproxen prescribed postoperatively for auricular chondritis in one patient.

Conclusion.—Mohs micrographic surgery and repair of associated defects can be safely performed in either an office- or hospital-based setting.

▶ This study supports the findings of a previously published work demonstrating the safety of Mohs surgery in the office or hospital-based setting.[1]

J. Cook, MD

Reference

1. Cook JL, Perone JB: A prospective evaluation of the incidence of complications associated with Mohs micrographic surgery. *Arch Dermatol* 139:143-152, 2003.

Histopathological Differential Diagnosis of Keloid and Hypertrophic Scar
Lee JY-Y, Yang C-C, Chao S-C, et al (Natl Cheng Kung Univ, Tainan, Taiwan)
Am J Dermatopathol 26:379-384, 2004   19–10

Introduction.—Distinguishing hypertrophic scar (HS) from keloid histopathologically is sometimes difficult because thickened hyalinized collagen (keloidal collagen), the hallmark of keloid, is not always detectable and α-smooth muscle actin (α-SMA), a differentiating marker of HS, is variably expressed in both forms of scar. The aim of this study was to investigate additional distinguishing features to facilitate differentiation between keloid and HS. We compared various histologic features and the expression of α-SMA in 40 specimens of keloid and 10 specimens of HS. The features more commonly seen in keloids were: (a) no flattening of the overlying epidermis, (b) no scarring of the papillary dermis, (c) presence of keloidal collagen, (d) absence of prominent vertically oriented blood vessels, (e) presence of prominent disarray of fibrous fascicles/nodules, (f) presence of a tongue-like advancing edge underneath normal-appearing epidermis and papillary dermis, (g) horizontal cellular fibrous band in the upper reticular dermis, and (h) prominent fascia-like fibrous band. The last three features were found in keloid specimens only, including the ones lacking detectable keloidal collagen. Our study confirmed the diagnostic value of keloidal collagen, but it was only found in 55% of keloid specimens. α-SMA expression was found in both HS (70%) and keloid (45%), thus it would not be a differentiating marker. In scars with no detectable keloidal collagen, the presence of the following feature(s) favors the diagnosis of keloid: non-flattened epidermis, non-fibrotic papillary dermis, a tongue-like advancing edge, horizontal cellular fibrous band in the upper reticular dermis, and prominent fascia-like band.

▶ In most instances, the diagnosis of keloid is based on clinical criteria. In some cases, however, it may be necessary to obtain additional evidence before undertaking interventional therapy. This study sought to define histopathologic criteria for distinguishing HS from keloid. The gold standard was the clinical characteristics of the lesion.

The authors found that there were 4 histopathologic features in addition to nodules of thick, hyalinized collagen bundles that were helpful in distinguishing keloids from HSs. These features included a normal dermal papilla pattern, lack of fibrosis of the papillary dermis, and a tongue-like advancing edge to the area of fibroplasia. These features seem to indicate that keloids are histopathologically as well as clinically distinguishable from HSs. This information may be useful to clinicians and researchers alike in evaluating therapies for keloids.

J. C. Maize, MD

Intralesional 5-Fluorouracil in the Treatment of Keloids: An Open Clinical and Histopathological Study
Kontochristopoulos G, Stefanaki C, Panagiotopoulos A, et al (Andreas Sygros Skin Hosp, Athens; Agia Sofia Children's Hosp, Athens)
J Am Acad Dermatol 52:474-479, 2005   19–11

Background.—The treatment of keloids remains unsatisfactory. Intralesional 5-fluorouracil (FU) has not been much investigated as a monotherapy in the treatment of keloids.

Objective.—We sought to evaluate the use of intralesional injections of 5-FU in the treatment of keloids.

Methods.—A total of 20 patients (11 male and 9 female) were treated once weekly with intralesional injections of 5-FU (50 mg/mL). Patients received an average of 7 treatments. Average injection volumes were 0.2 to 0.4 mL/cm². All patients had full blood cell count, liver function tests, and renal function tests before and after treatment was commenced. A total of 10 patients had biopsy specimens taken before starting treatment as a baseline and after 6 sessions. Routine hematoxylin-eosin and immunohistochemical analysis detecting Ki-67 and transforming growth factor-β were performed on paraffin sections. All patients were followed up for 12 months, or until recurrence was noted.

Results.—Of 20 patients, 17 (85%) showed more than 50% improvement. Only one did not respond favorably. Small and previously untreated lesions improved the most. Pain (20 of 20), hyperpigmentation (20 of 20), and tissue sloughing (6 of 20) were the main adverse effects. Histopathologic and immunohistochemical evaluation were consistent with the clinical observations. Ki-67 proliferative index was significantly reduced ($P = .0001$) after treatment. Transforming growth factor-β was reduced less significantly. Recurrence was noted in 47% (9 of 19) of patients who responded to treatment within 1 year. A correlation was found ($P = .028$) between the duration of the lesions and recurrence.

Conclusion.—Our study demonstrates that intralesional 5-FU may be effective in the treatment of keloids, but recurrence is common and further investigation is required.

5-Fluorouracil Selectivity Inhibits Collagen Synthesis

Bulstrode NW, Mudera V, McGrouther DA, et al (RAFT Inst of Plastic Surgery, Middlesex, England; Univ College of London)
Plast Reconstr Surg 116:209-221, 2005   19–12

Background.—Fibroproliferative disorders, such as Dupuytren's contracture of the hand, are characterized by excessive production of collagen. 5-Fluorouracil has been used to treat fibroproliferative disorders of the eye and skin and is thought to inhibit thymidylate synthetase blocking DNA replication. 5-Fluorouracil has been shown to down-regulate fibroblast proliferation and differentiation in vitro.

Methods.—This study investigated the dose-dependent effect of 5-fluorouracil on fibroblast extracellular matrix production. Fibroblasts were derived from tendon and primary Dupuytren's disease of the hand, a fibroproliferative disorder of the palmar aponeurosis ($n = 4$ patients). Total collagen synthesis was determined by means of the incorporation of radiolabeled proline. Fibroblast secretion of the profibrotic factor transforming growth factor-$\beta 1$ (TGF-$\beta 1$) was measured by a sandwich enzyme-linked immunosorbent assay. Gene expression of collagen types I and III and TGF-$\beta 1$ were quantified by means of reverse-transcriptase polymerase chain reaction assays.

Results.—The authors found that 5-fluorouracil caused a dose-dependent, selective, and specific decrease in collagen production by Dupuytren's fibroblasts compared with noncollagenous protein synthesis. By contrast, procollagen types I and III mRNA were unaffected by 5-fluorouracil treatment. These changes did not appear to be mediated by alterations in the endogenous secretion of TGF-beta1 or its autocrine effect on collagen metabolism.

Conclusions.—The clinical implication is that 5-fluorouracil could possibly reduce extracellular matrix production and therefore reduce recurrence of Dupuytren's disease of the hand.

▶ Kontochristopoulos et al (Abstract 19–11) demonstrate significant efficacy using intralesional 5-FU for the treatment of keloids. I have found similar success after using 5-FU with or without triamcinolone for stubborn keloids and hypertrophic scars. I have encountered no significant complications using such therapy. Interestingly, Bulstrode et al (Abstract 19–12) found that 5-FU caused a dose-dependent decrease in collagen production. It appears that these changes are not mediated by alterations in the endogenous secretion of

TGF-β1. Intralesional 5-FU may be considered for patients with more resistant scars with or without adjuvant therapy.

J. Cook, MD

Postsurgical Use of Imiquimod 5% Cream in the Prevention of Earlobe Keloid Recurrences: Results of an Open-Label, Pilot Study

Martín-García RF, Busquets AC (Univ of Puerto Rico, San Juan)
Dermatol Surg 31:1394-1398, 2005   19–13

Background.—Traditional surgical modalities for the management of earlobe keloids are often associated with high recurrence rates. A recent report suggests that imiquimod 5% cream can be effective in the prevention of keloid recurrences after surgical excision.

Objectives.—To establish the safety and efficacy of imiquimod 5% cream in the prevention of recurrences of excised earlobe keloids.

Methods.—Patients who attended a dermatologic surgery clinic for the treatment of earlobe keloids were recruited into the study. Earlobe keloids underwent parallel shave excision. Imiquimod 5% cream was applied daily for 8 weeks followed by an observation period of 16 weeks. In patients who presented with bilateral earlobe keloids, paired comparisons of imiquimod versus intralesional steroid injections were performed.

Results.—Eight earlobes were treated with imiquimod 5% cream after parallel keloid removal. Twenty-four weeks after surgery, six (75%) remained recurrence free. Four patients underwent bilateral paired comparisons. At the end of the observation period, two patients (50%) remained recurrence free in the imiquimod-treated areas while experiencing recurrences in the intralesional steroid-treated areas. Local irritation secondary to imiquimod application required rest periods in three cases. In all cases, patients were able to resume therapy and completed the study without further complications.

Conclusion.—Although small and uncontrolled, the results of this open-label, pilot study suggest that imiquimod 5% cream may prove to be a reasonably effective adjuvant therapeutic alternative for the prevention of recurrences in excised earlobe keloids.

▶ This small and uncontrolled study suggests that imiquimod may have some role in the prevention of recurrences of surgically resected keloids. My experience is quite different in that I have not seen significant efficacy with application of imiquimod after keloid resection. Nevertheless, this small investigation suggests that larger, well-controlled prospective trials are warranted to assess its efficacy and safety for this indication.

J. Cook, MD

Double-blind, Randomized, Placebo-controlled, Prospective Study Evaluating the Tolerability and Effectiveness of Imiquimod Applied to Postsurgical Excisions on Scar Cosmesis

Berman B, Frankel S, Villa AM, et al (Univ of Miami, Fla)
Dermatol Surg 31:1399-1403, 2005   19–14

Background.—It has been reported that topical application of imiquimod 5% cream induces interferon-α, an antifibrotic cytokine.

Objective.—To determine the tolerability and effectiveness on the cosmetic outcome of the application of imiquimod to postsurgical excision sites.

Materials and Methods.—A prospective, double-blinded, randomized, vehicle-controlled trial was conducted among 20 patients with two skin lesions clinically diagnosed as melanocytic nevi. Imiquimod 5% cream was applied to one of the sutured surgical wounds starting the night of the excision nightly for a period of 4 weeks. The second sutured excision site was treated with vehicle cream. Scar cosmesis, erythema, pigmentary alterations, induration, tenderness, and pain were assessed using a visual analogue scale 2, 4, and 8 weeks after surgery.

Results.—Eighteen subjects completed the study, with a total of 36 excision sites; no wound site dehisced, and no signs of infection were noted. Surgical wounds treated with imiquimod had more erythema, pigmentary alterations, and lower cosmesis rated by the investigator compared with wounds treated with placebo, both becoming nonsignificant in further evaluations. For pigmentary alterations, induration, and cosmesis rated by the patients, no statistically significant difference between treatment groups was observed at week 8.

Conclusion.—Treatment of surgical excision-site wounds with imiquimod was well tolerated and without serious adverse events. Evaluations for cosmesis of placebo-treated surgical sites were better than imiquimod-treated sites at week 8, becoming nonsignificant later.

▶ In this study, scars treated with imiquimod showed, over the short term, a poor cosmetic outcome. Longer follow-up showed no statistically significant difference or improvement in scar cosmesis versus placebo. The search continues for adjuvant topical preparations that show demonstrable improvement in scar cosmesis in well-controlled clinical trials.

J. Cook, MD

Ultrapotent Topical Corticosteroid Treatment of Hemangiomas of Infancy

Garzon MC, Lucky AW, Hawrot A, et al (Columbia Univ, New York; Univ of Cincinnati, Ohio; Baylor College of Medicine, Houston; et al)

J Am Acad Dermatol 52:281-286, 2005   19–15

Background.—Superficial cutaneous hemangiomas of infancy represent a therapeutic challenge. Two small case series using ultrapotent topical corticosteroids for periocular hemangiomas were reported in the ophthalmologic literature. The use of this therapy for hemangiomas of infancy at other sites on the body has not been reported.

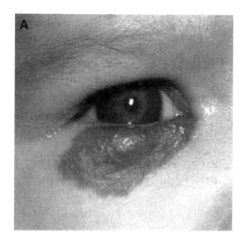

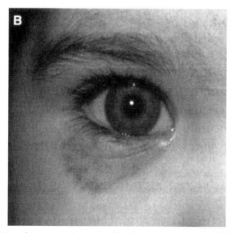

FIGURE 1.—Case 1 (good response): 2-month-old girl pretreatment (**A**) and following 8 weeks of treatment with clobetasol propionate 0.05% ointment (**B**; photo taken at 18 months of age). (Reprinted by permission of the publisher from Garzon MC, Lucky AW, Hawrot A, et al: Ultrapotent topical corticosteroid treatment of hemangiomas of infancy. *J Am Acad Dermatol* 52:281-286, 2005. Copyright 2005 by Elsevier.)

Objective.—We sought to assess the clinical effects of short-term application of ultrapotent topical corticosteroids for the treatment of hemangiomas of infancy.

Methods.—The records of 34 infants with proliferating hemangiomas of infancy that were treated with ultrapotent topical steroids were reviewed retrospectively. Treatment response was based on: (1) cessation of growth; (2) shrinkage or flattening of the lesion; and (3) lightening of the surface color. Lesions demonstrating responses of two of the three criteria were judged to have good response; one criterion, partial response; and no improvement, no response.

Results.—Of the patients, 35% demonstrated good response, 38% partial response, and 27% no response.

Conclusions.—Hemangiomas in 74% of the infants demonstrated either good or partial response to treatment with ultrapotent topical corticosteroids. Of the responders, the majority reported cessation of growth before what would have been expected for their age. Improvement varied, with thinner superficial hemangiomas demonstrating better cosmetic improvement than thicker lesions (Fig 1; see color plate XVI).

▶ The authors report a partial to good response in 74% of hemangiomas treated with ultrapotent topical corticosteroids for 2 to 21 weeks, the majority (71%) of which were superficial lesions. Temporary hypopigmentation around treated hemangiomas was the only side effect reported. Four periorbital lesions were treated; these patients were followed up by an ophthalmologist. Although the possibility of the development of glaucoma or cataracts would be a concern when treating eyelid lesions with ultrapotent corticosteroids, none of these conditions developed in the 4 patients whose eyelids were treated. A trial application of ultrapotent topical corticosteroids to hemangiomas in cosmetically sensitive areas or in locations where enlargement might impair function seems worthwhile because this method of treatment would be less painful and likely safer than intralesional corticosteroids. Close follow-up by an ophthalmologist would be recommended when treating eyelid lesions.

S. Raimer, MD

Response of Ulcerated Perineal Hemangiomas of Infancy to Becaplermin Gel, a Recombinant Human Platelet-Derived Growth Factor
Metz BJ, Rubenstein MC, Levy ML, et al (Baylor College of Medicine, Houston)
Arch Dermatol 140:867-870, 2004   19–16

Background.—Hemangiomas of infancy are the most common tumors of childhood, and ulceration is the most common complication. Many treatments have been used for hemangioma ulceration, although none are uniformly effective. A recent report described the successful use of 0.01% becaplermin gel, a recombinant human platelet-derived growth factor, for an ulcerated hemangioma refractory to standard care. We sought to further assess the responsiveness of hemangioma ulceration to 0.01% becaplermin gel and to compare its cost to that of conventional modalities.

Observations.—We report a case series of 8 infants treated with becaplermin gel for ulcerated perineal hemangiomas of infancy. All infants were seen between January and June 2003 in the pediatric dermatology clinic at Texas Children's Hospital. Six female and 2 male infants were included. All of the hemangiomas were large ($\geq$6 cm^2), and of superficial or mixed superficial and deep morphology. Rapid ulcer healing occurred in all patients within 3 to 21 days (average, 10.25 days).

Conclusions.—In this small series, 0.01% becaplermin gel was a safe and effective treatment for perineal hemangioma ulceration. The rapid healing achieved with 0.01% becaplermin gel allows a reduction in the risk of secondary infection, pain, and need for hospitalization, as well as in the costs that often accumulate from multiple follow-up visits and long-term therapy.

▶ In this report, children with painful ulcerated hemangiomas healed remarkably quickly with application of a gel preparation containing 0.01% becaplermin (Regranex), a recombinant human platelet-derived growth factor. The gel is quite expensive (the authors quote a price of $519 per 15 g); however, for large lesions that would otherwise require frequent office visits, hospitalization, or surgery, the gel would seem to be cost effective. Becaplermin gel also appears to work very rapidly; therefore, a trial of this medication is worthwhile for children with severe, painful ulcerated hemangiomas.

S. Raimer, MD

20 Miscellaneous Topics in Cosmetic and Laser Surgery

Influences on Decision-Making for Undergoing Plastic Surgery: A Mental Models and Quantitative Assessment
Darisi T, Thorne S, Iacobelli C (Univ of Guelph, Ontario, Canada; Decision Partners, LLC, Pittsburgh, Pa)
Plast Reconstr Surg 116:907-916, 2005   20–1

Background.—Research was conducted to gain insight into potential clients' decisions to undergo plastic surgery, their perception of benefits and risks, their judgment of outcomes, and their selection of a plastic surgeon.

Methods.—Semistructured, open-ended interviews were conducted with 60 people who expressed interest in plastic surgery. Qualitative analysis revealed their "mental models" regarding influences on their decision to undergo plastic surgery and their choice of a surgeon. Interview results were used to design a Web-based survey in which 644 individuals considering plastic surgery responded.

Results.—The desire for change was the most direct motivator to undergo plastic surgery. Improvements to physical well-being were related to emotional and social benefits. When prompted about risks, participants mentioned physical, emotional, and social risks. Surgeon selection was a critical influence on decisions to undergo plastic surgery. Participants gave considerable weight to personal consultation and believed that finding the "right" plastic surgeon would minimize potential risks. Findings from the Web-based survey were similar to the mental models interviews in terms of benefit ratings but differed in risk ratings and surgeon selection criteria.

Conclusions.—The mental models interviews revealed that interview participants were thoughtful about their decision to undergo plastic surgery and focused on finding the right plastic surgeon.

▶ This was a nonrandomized study of patients intent on having plastic surgery that was conducted by telephone polling and using a Web-based survey; thus, it cannot be considered unbiased. Nevertheless, it is clear that some patients may have unrealistic expectations about the outcomes of cosmetic proce-dures. Counseling regarding risks, benefits, and expectations is an essential component of the preoperative visit.

B. H. Thiers, MD

Long-term Effects of Hormone Therapy on Skin Rigidity and Wrinkles
Wolff EF, Narayan D, Taylor HS (Yale Univ, New Haven, Conn)
Fertil Steril 84:285-288, 2005   20–2

Objective.—To evaluate the effects of long-term hormone therapy (HT) on skin rigidity and wrinkling.

Design.—Single blinded cross-sectional analysis.

Setting.—Academic medical center.

Patient(s).—Sixty-five long-term HT users who underwent menopause at least 5 years before evaluation and who have either consistently used HT or have never used HT.

Intervention(s).—Visual assessment of severity of wrinkles at 11 facial lo-cations using the Lemperle scale by a plastic surgeon blinded to HT use. Measurement of skin rigidity at the cheek and forehead with a durometer.

Main Outcome Measure(s).—Lemperle wrinkle score and skin rigidity.

Result(s).—Twenty women met inclusion criteria. Eleven women who had not used HT were compared to nine long-term HT users. Demographics including age, race, sun exposure, sunscreen use, tobacco use, and skin type were similar. Rigidity was significantly decreased in HT users compared to nonusers at both the cheek (1.1 vs. 2.7) and forehead (20 vs. 29). Average wrinkle scores were lower in hormone users than in nonhormone users (1.5 vs. 2.2).

Conclusion(s).—Long-term postmenopausal HT users have more elastic skin and less severe wrinkling than women who never used HT, suggesting that hormone therapy may have cosmetic benefits.

▶ The authors demonstrate that long-term HT in postmenopausal women is associated with significantly fewer wrinkles and less skin rigidity. Neverthe-less, given the potential risks of HT, its use solely for that reason would prob-ably not be justified.

B. H. Thiers, MD

Prevention of the Ultraviolet B-Mediated Skin Photoaging by a Nuclear Factor κB Inhibitor, Parthenolide
Tanaka K, Hasegawa J, Asamitsu K, et al (Nagoya City Univ Graduate School of Med Sciences, Japan; Ichimaru Pharcos Co, Ltd, Motosu, Japan)
J Pharmacol Exp Ther 315:624-630, 2005   20–3

Introduction.—The skin photoaging is characterized by keratinocyte hy-perproliferation and degradation of collagen fibers, causing skin wrinkling and laxity and melanocyte proliferation that leads to pigmentation. UV is considered to be a major cause of such skin changes. It is well established that nuclear factor κB (NF-κB) is activated upon UV irradiation and induces various genes including interleukin-1 (IL-1), tumor necrosis factor α (TNFα), and matrix metalloprotease-1 (MMP-1). It is also known that basic fibroblast growth factor (bFGF) production is induced by UV and promotes the proliferation of skin keratinocytes and melanocytes. We found that

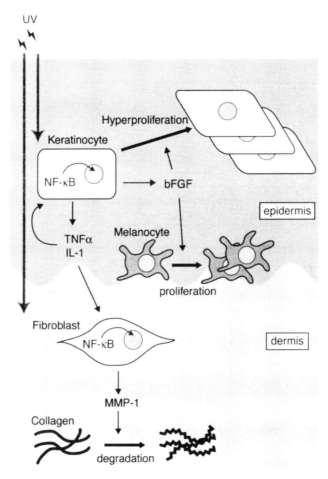

FIGURE 7.—Diagrammatic representation of the action of NF-κB in the process of UVB-mediated cutaneous alterations (photoaging). Environmental stimuli, such as UV irradiation and inflammatory signaling, induce the NF-κB activation that leads to the production of MMP-1 and bFGF in epidermal keratinocytes. The upregulation of bFGF promotes proliferation of keratinocytes and melanocytes as a protection mechanism to these environmental insults. In dermis, skin fibroblasts are stimulated by UV and proinflammatory cytokines, such as IL-1 and TNFα, produced by keratinocytes, and then NF-κB is activated, leading to the MMP-1 production. Thus, NF-κB inhibitors are considered to be effective in preventing the UVB-mediated cutaneous alterations and eventually the skin photoaging process. (Courtesy of Tanaka K, Hasegawa J, Asamitsu K, et al: Prevention of the ultraviolet B-mediated skin photoaging by a nuclear factor κB inhibitor, parthenolide. *J Pharmacol Exp Ther* 315:624-630, 2005.)

UVB, IL-1, and TNFα induced NF-κB activation and then produced MMP-1 and bFGF in HaCaT keratinocytes and skin fibroblasts. In this experiment, we examined if parthenolide, an NF-κB inhibitor, could block the UVB-mediated skin changes. We found that parthenolide could effectively inhibit the gene expression mediated by NF-κB and the production of bFGF and MMP-1 from cells overexpressing p65, a major subunit of NF-κB. We also found that parthenolide could inhibit the UVB-induced proliferation of keratinocytes and melanocytes in the mouse skin. These findings suggest that NF-κB inhibitors should be useful for the prevention of skin photoaging (Fig 7).

▶ The findings suggest that NF-κB plays both a direct and indirect role in UVB-mediated skin changes and that inhibition of NF-κB activation by intraperitoneal injection of parthenolide helps prevent or ameliorate UVB-mediated cutaneous alterations and photoaging in mice. NF-κB plays an important role in immunologic and inflammatory responses. Thus, a therapeutic role for NF-κB may be problematic as prolonged treatment might be associated with untoward side effects such as immunosuppression and decreased host defenses.

B. H. Thiers, MD

Patterns of Saphenous Reflux in Women With Primary Varicose Veins

Engelhorn CA, Engelhorn ALV, Cassou MF, et al (Pontifícia Universidade Católica do Paraná, Curitiba, Paraná, Brazil)
J Vasc Surg 41:45-51, 2005   20–4

Objective.—Varicose veins have been linked to great saphenous vein (GSV) reflux and in particular, with reflux at the saphenofemoral junction (SFJ). Early stages of disease, however, may be associated with limited, localized reflux in segments of the GSV and/or small saphenous vein (SSV). Ultrasound mapping of saphenous veins was performed to determine patterns of GSV and SSV reflux in women with simple, primary varicose veins.

Methods.—Ultrasound mapping was performed prospectively in 590 extremities of 326 women with varicose veins (CEAP C_2 class) but without edema, skin changes, or ulcers (C_3 to C_6). Average age was 42 ± 13 (SD) years (range, 8 to 87). Patterns of GSV and SSV reflux, obtained in the upright position, were classified as I: perijunctional, originating from the SFJ or saphenopopliteal junction (SPJ) tributaries into the GSV or SSV; II: proximal, from the SFJ or SPJ to a tributary or perforating vein above the level of the malleoli; III: distal, from a tributary or perforating vein to the paramalleolar GSV or SSV; IV: segmental, from a tributary or perforating vein to another tributary or perforating vein above the malleoli; V: multisegmental, if two or more distinct refluxing segments were detected; and VI: diffused, involving the entire GSV or SSV from the SFJ or SPJ to the malleoli.

Results.—Reflux was detected in 472 extremities (80%): 100 (17%) had reflux in both the GSV and SSV, 353 (60%) had GSV reflux only, and 19

TABLE 2.—Anatomy Involved in Great Saphenous Vein
Reflux in 590 Extremities in Women With
Primary Varicose Veins

Location	Number	Percentage
Saphenofemoral junction	72	12
Thigh segment	220	37
Knee segment	96	16
Calf segment	345	58

(Reprinted by permission of the publisher from Engelhorn CA, Engelhorn ALV, Cassou MF, et al: Patterns of saphenous reflux in women with primary varicose veins. *J Vasc Surg* 41:645-651, 2005. Copyright 2005 by Elsevier.)

(3%) had SSV reflux only, for a total prevalence of 77% at the GSV and 20% at the SSV. The most common pattern of GSV reflux was segmental (types IV and V) in 342 (58%) of 590; either one segment in 213 (36%) or more than one segment with competent SFJ in 99 (17%), or incompetent SFJ in 30 (5%), followed by distal GSV reflux (type III) in 65 (11%), proximal GSV reflux (type II) in 32 (5%), diffused throughout the entire GSV (type VI) in 10 (2%), and perijunctional (type I) in 4 (<1%). GSV refluxing segments were noted in the SFJ in 72 (12%) and in the thigh in 220 (37%), and leg (or both) in 345 (58%) (Table 2).

Conclusions.—The high prevalence of reflux justifies ultrasound mapping of the saphenous veins in women with primary varicose veins. Correction of SFJ reflux, however, may be needed in $\leq 12\%$ of the extremities, and only about one third CEAP C_2 limbs may require treatment of a refluxing GSV in the thigh.

▶ Management of GSV reflux is essential in the treatment of patients with varicose veins. Much emphasis has been placed on the association of varicosities with GSV reflux at the SFJ. In this study, which used duplex US scanning to map out the GSV, only 12% of women had reflux at the SFJ. The most common location of GSV reflux was the calf, with the second most common area being the thigh. Thus, the authors suggest that many women with varicosities will benefit from treatment directed at only the varicosities themselves.

P. G. Lang, Jr, MD

Stability of Foam in Sclerotherapy: Differences Between Sodium Tetradecyl Sulfate and Polidocanol and the Type of Connector Used in the Double-Syringe System Technique

Rao J, Goldman MP (Dermatology/Cosmetic Laser Associates of La Jolla, Inc, Calif)
Dermatol Surg 31:19-22, 2005   20–5

Background.—Foam sclerotherapy is an increasingly popular modality in the treatment of varicose veins. Worldwide, the most popular agents used are sodium tetradecyl sulfate (STS) and polidocanol (POL). The double-syringe system technique to make foam out of a sclerosing solution and air has received wide attention for its ease and reproducibility. This study examined the possibility that the relative silicone content of various disposable connectors may affect overall foam stability. We also evaluated the differences in the stability of foam between STS and POL.

Materials and Methods.—In the first part of the study, one nondisposable stainless steel connector and five disposable plastic connectors were used to create foam from STS 0.50% and air. The procedure was then repeated to produce foam from POL 0.50% and air from each of the six different connector types. As a measure of foam stability, once foam was created with each type of connector, the time required for half of the original volume of sclerosing solution to settle was recorded. In the second part of the study, foam was created with a nondisposable stainless steel connector only and various concentrations of STS and POL. Foam stability was then measured for these different concentrations of sclerosants.

Results.—The time for sclerosing solution to settle to half of its initial volume was found to vary according to the specific sclerosant and concentration used, with no statistically significant variation based on connector type.

Conclusions.—The type of connector used in the double-syringe system technique to produce foam for sclerotherapy is not a factor in foam stability. Sclerosing solutions differ in their foaming stability.

► In recent years, the foaming of sclerosants has been popularized as a means of improving efficacy and decreasing side effects such as skin necrosis. In this study, except for a 0.25% concentration, POL exhibited greater foam stability than STS. Whether this has any clinical significance remains to be demonstrated.

P. G. Lang, Jr, MD

Lymphangioma Circumscriptum: Treatment With Hypertonic Saline Sclerotherapy

Bikowski JB, Dumont AMG (Ohio State Univ, Columbus; Lake Erie College of Osteopathic Medicine, Pa)
J Am Acad Dermatol 53:442-444, 2005   20–6

Introduction.—A 38-year-old woman came for treatment of multiple clear vesicles and hemorrhagic papules on the posterior aspect of the right shoulder and the right axillary vault of 5 years' duration. These lesions would spontaneously manifest as clear or blood-filled vesicles (or both) and appear to be exacerbated by physical contact from certain articles of clothing. A biopsy was done and the results revealed lymphangioma circumscriptum. The purpose of this case study was to evaluate a new form of treatment of lymphangioma circumscriptum with the use of 23.4% hypertonic saline sclerotherapy. The patient's lymphangioma circumscriptum significantly resolved with minimal side effects, such as mild hyperpigmentation. Decreased sensitivity was noted and no further treatment was indicated.

This case showed that hypertonic saline 23.4% solution can be effective in treating the appearance of vesicles containing clear fluid or lymph and those containing red blood cells in superficial lymphangiomas and that this treatment can be considered for long-term management of lymphangioma circumscriptum.

▶ Lymphangioma circumscriptum is difficult to treat. Excisional surgery is often ineffective and may worsen the disease. In recent years, one of the more popular treatments has been the use of the CO_2 laser to ablate the superficial dilated lymphatics. However, affected patients often continue to develop new lesions and may experience scarring. Another approach that has been utilized to obliterate the abnormal lymphatics has been the use of a sclerosing agent, in this case hypertonic saline. Although the results in this patient appear impressive, there is a significant risk of skin necrosis and scarring. We need more data on this treatment modality to determine its safety and efficacy.

P. G. Lang, Jr, MD

Health-Related Quality of Life After Thoracoscopic Sympathectomy for Palmar Hyperhidrosis

Kumagai K, Kawase H, Kawanishi M (Fujita Health Univ, Nakagawa-ku Nagoya, Japan)
Ann Thorac Surg 80:461-466, 2005   20–7

Background.—Palmar hyperhidrosis is a benign functional disorder regarded as a psychological and social handicap. Improvement of the quality of life is a major goal of treatment. However, little attention has been given to quality of life after thoracoscopic sympathectomy, which is the first line of treatment for palmar hyperhidrosis. This study investigated the impact of thoracoscopic sympathectomy on subjective health-related quality of life (HRQoL) and psychological properties.

Methods.—Forty patients who underwent thoracoscopic sympathectomy were followed up for 6 months. The HRQoL measures were the Medical Outcomes Study Short Form 36 (SF-36), the Spielberger State Trait Anxiety Inventory (STAI), and the Zung Self-Rating Depression Scale (SDS). Patients were administered these questionnaires before procedure and then again at 1, 3, and 6 months after sympathectomy.

Results.—A comparison between the current sample and Japanese normative data for the SF-36 showed mild impairment of HRQoL before sympathectomy. However, it also showed significant improvement of the social functioning domain after sympathectomy. While there was worsening of the bodily pain and role physical domains 1 month after sympathectomy, both domains recovered in 3 months. The results of STAI showed significant improvement of both trait and state anxiety after sympathectomy. However, the results of SDS showed patients remained neurotic.

Conclusions.—This study is the first to show the pattern of impairment in health status and therapeutic impact in palmar hyperhidrosis patients. Hyperhidrosis is associated with impaired HRQoL. It was also demonstrated that thoracoscopic sympathectomy is safe, minimally invasive, and improves HRQoL, even if compensatory hyperhidrosis occurs.

▶ The important conclusion that can be drawn from the data presented is that palmar hyperhidrosis is associated with a significant impairment of HRQoL, and that thoracoscopic sympathectomy is a safe and minimally invasive procedure that improves HRQoL, despite compensatory hyperhidrosis.

B. H. Thiers, MD

Clinical Experience in 397 Consecutive Thoracoscopic Sympathectomies
Kwong KF, Cooper LB, Bennett LA, et al (Univ of Maryland, Baltimore)
Ann Thorac Surg 80:1063-1066, 2005   20–8

Background.—The purpose of this study is to evaluate the safety and efficacy of thoracoscopic sympathectomy for the treatment of hyperhidrosis, blushing, reflex sympathetic dystrophy, and digital ischemia.

Methods.—We conducted a retrospective review of 202 patients who underwent thoracoscopic sympathectomy at the University of Maryland from March 1992 to April 2003.

Results.—Three hundred ninety-seven procedures were performed on 202 patients (105 women, 97 men). Mean age was 29 years (range, 9 to 65). Indications for surgery included hyperhidrosis, facial blushing, digital ischemia, and reflex sympathetic dystrophy. Synchronous bilateral sympathectomies were performed in 194 patients; right side alone (n = 6); left side alone (n = 1); 1 patient had staged bilateral sympathectomies. Single incision with lung isolation technique was used. There was no mortality. Preoperative symptoms resolved completely or significantly improved in greater than 90% of patients. One patient with reflex sympathetic dystrophy recurred and 1 patient with hyperhidrosis complained of significant compensatory sweating. Compensatory sweating to a lesser degree occurred in approximately one third of patients. Complications included asymptomatic pleural effusion (n = 1), pneumothorax (n = 1), and reoperation for chylothorax that was identified early (n = 1). In 2 patients treated for facial blushing, Horner's syndrome developed postoperatively; 1 of them subsequently underwent blepharoplasty. In 3 patients, hyperesthesias developed at the incision.

Conclusions.—Thoracoscopic sympathectomy can be performed safely and with excellent results. Compensatory sweating is the main side effect, although significant complaints from this are rare. Horner's syndrome remains an extremely uncommon complication as a result of thoracoscopic sympathectomy at our institution.

▶ The authors reviewed the outcomes of more than 200 patients who underwent thoracoscopic sympathectomy for a variety of conditions over an 11-year period. Hyperhidrosis was the leading indication for the procedure in this series. The authors found compensatory sweating to be the main side effect, although most patients reported that this was well tolerated and a small price to pay for the significant alleviation or elimination of their preoperative symptoms.

B. H. Thiers, MD

The Treatment of Melasma With Fractional Photothermolysis: A Pilot Study

Rokhsar CK, Fitzpatrick RE (Albert Einstein College of Medicine, Bronx, NY; Dermatology Associates of San Diego County, Encinitas, Calif)
Dermatol Surg 31:1645-1650, 2005   20–9

Background.—Melasma is a common pigmentary disorder that remains resistant to available therapies. Facial resurfacing with the pulsed CO2 laser has been reported successful but requires significant downtime, and there is a risk of adverse sequelae.

Objective.—To determine if melasma will respond to a new treatment paradigm, fractional resurfacing.

Methods.—Ten female patients (Fitzpatrick skin types III-V) who were unresponsive to previous treatment were treated at 1- to 2-week intervals with the Fraxel laser (Reliant Technologies, Palo Alto, CA, USA). Wavelengths of 1,535 and 1,550 nm were both used, and 6 to 12 mJ per microthermal zone with 2,000 to 3,500 mtz/cm^2 were the treatment parameters. Four to six treatment sessions were performed. Responses were evaluated according to the percentage of lightening of original pigmentation. Two physicians evaluated the photographs, and each patient evaluated her own response.

Results.—The physician evaluation was that 60% of patients achieved 75 to 100% clearing and 30% had less than 25% improvement. The patients' evaluations agreed, except for one patient, who graded herself as 50 to 75% improved as opposed to the physician grading of over 75%. There was one patient with postinflammatory hyperpigmentation and no patient with hypopigmentation. No downtime was necessary for wound healing.

Conclusions.—Fractional resurfacing affords a new treatment algorithm for the treatment of melasma that combines decreased risk and downtime with significant efficacy. This treatment modality deserves further exploration to maximize benefits.

▶ Fractional resurfacing is one of the new exciting developments in dermatologic surgery. This study, albeit with very short follow-up, showed improvement of melasma with this technique. Larger prospective trials with longer follow-up will be necessary to assess the durability of improvement given the high incidence of repigmentation of melasma after what appeared to be successful therapy. Before such technology can be widely accepted and recommended, more critical scientific analysis is needed.

J. Cook, MD

Long-Pulsed Dye Laser Treatment for Facial Telangiectasias and Erythema: Evaluation of a Single Purpuric Pass Versus Multiple Subpurpuric Passes

Iyer S, Fitzpatrick RE (Univ of California, Los Angeles; La Jolla Cosmetic Surgery Centre, Calif)

Dermatol Surg 31:898-902, 2005   20–10

Background and Objective.—Subpurpuric treatments with the pulsed dye laser can be effective for treatment of vascular lesions, although less so than when purpuric fluences are used. Increased efficacy may be achieved by performing multiple passes at the time of treatment. We performed a split-face bilateral paired comparison of multiple low-fluence subpurpuric passes compared with a single high-fluence purpuric pass in the treatment of facial telangiectasias.

Materials and Methods.—Nine patients were included in the study. One cheek was chosen to be treated with four passes of a nonpurpuric fluence, and the contralateral cheek was treated with a single purpuric pass. Reductions in vessel density, diameter, arborization, and background erythema were evaluated 3 weeks after treatment.

Results.—We found a 43.4% reduction in surface area covered by telangiectasias on the cheek treated with a single purpuric pass compared with 35.9% on the cheek treated with four subpurpuric passes. The purpuric fluences produced greater reduction in vessel diameter and arborization, whereas the subpurpuric protocol was more effective in reducing background erythema. Purpuric fluences were also noted to produce more significant edema and transient hyperpigmentation in one patient.

Conclusion.—The multipass subpurpuric approach to treatment with the pulsed dye laser is both cosmetically acceptable and effective, although purpuric treatments may be required to effectively eliminate larger-caliber, more highly networked vessels.

▶ The induction of purpura with the pulsed-dye laser is a sign of successful vessel ablation; it is, nevertheless, a cosmetically concerning side-effect to many patients. In this study, multiple subpurpuric passes were efficacious, but not on larger caliber vessels. However, the multiplicity of treatments required using subpurpuric thresholds significantly adds to the time and expense of vessel treatment. In my experience, patients prefer a quicker, more efficacious, and cheaper treatment alternative, and thus purpuric passes are routinely utilized.

J. Cook, MD

Subject Index

Author Index